Donated to

Dr. K. Bh

Practical Gastrointestinal
Endoscopy

THIRD EDITION

Practical Gastrointestinal Endoscopy

Peter B. Cotton MD FRCP
Professor of Medicine,
Duke University Medical Centre,
Durham, North Carolina

Christopher B. Williams BM FRCP
Consultant Physician, Endoscopy Unit,
St Mark's and
St Bartholomew's Hospitals, London

FOREWORD BY
Marvin H. Sleisenger MD
Professor of Medicine,
University of California, San Francisco

OXFORD
BLACKWELL SCIENTIFIC PUBLICATIONS
LONDON   EDINBURGH   BOSTON
MELBOURNE   PARIS   BERLIN   VIENNA

© 1980, 1982, 1990 by
Blackwell Scientific Publications
Editorial Offices:
Osney Mead, Oxford OX2 0EL
25 John Street, London WC1N 2BL
23 Ainslie Place, Edinburgh EH3 6AJ
3 Cambridge Center, Cambridge,
    Massachusetts 02142, USA
54 University Street, Carlton,
    Victoria 3053, Australia

Other Editorial Offices:
Arnette SA
2, rue Casimir-Delavigne
75006 Paris
France

Blackwell Wissenschaft
Meinekestrasse 4
D-1000 Berlin 15
Germany

Blackwell MZV
Feldgasse 13
A-1238 Wien
Austria

First published 1980
Reprinted 1981
Second edition 1982
Reprinted 1984, 1985, 1987, 1988
Third edition 1990
Reprinted 1991

Italian editions 1980, 1986
German edition 1985
French edition 1986

Set by Oxprint Ltd, Oxford
Printed and bound in Great Britain at
the University Press, Cambridge

DISTRIBUTORS

Marston Book Services Ltd
PO Box 87
Oxford OX2 0DT
(*Orders*: Tel: 0865 791155
        Fax: 0865 791927
        Telex: 837515)

USA
    Mosby-Year Book, Inc.
    11830 Westline Industrial Drive
    St Louis, Missouri 63146
    (*Orders*: Tel: (800) 633-6699)

Canada
    Mosby-Year Book, Inc.
    5240 Finch Avenue East
    Scarborough, Ontario
    (*Orders*: Tel: (416) 298-1588)

Australia
    Blackwell Scientific Publications
    (Australia) Pty Ltd
    54 University Street
    Carlton, Victoria 3053
    (*Orders*: Tel: (03) 347-0300)

British Library
Cataloguing in Publication Data
Cotton, Peter B.
    Practical gastrointestinal endoscopy.
        —3rd ed.   1. Man. Digestive system.
        Diagnosis. Endoscopy   I. Title
        II. Williams, Christopher B.
    (Christopher Beverley), *1938*–
    616.307545

    ISBN 0-632-02706-1

Contents

Foreword to the First Edition

I look upon it as a sign of the close liaison between the UK and the USA in gastroenterology to have been asked by Drs Cotton and Williams to introduce this fine new volume, *Practical Gastro-intestinal Endoscopy*. Although not personally involved in endoscopy, I have maintained a close watch on developments, particularly in our own units in the University of California in San Francisco. I hope therefore that I can step back and take an objective view.

Flexible instruments have started a revolution in diagnostic gastroenterology, one which will continue to evolve as we assess their real indications and usefulness. The time is ripe for this most complete volume devoted mainly to technique. It encompasses every worthwhile detail with which endoscopists must become closely familiar, ranging from the type and choice of instrument to discussions of the more recent endoscopic–therapeutic procedures, e.g. removal of common bile duct stones. Being intelligent physicians, the authors also discuss indications and the significance of these procedures to both patient and referring physician.

The information on the diagnostic usefulness of upper intestinal endoscopy goes beyond technique; it includes important points of differential diagnosis and indications for biopsy. The discussion of upper alimentary bleeding correctly assumes that endoscopy is now usually the first diagnostic procedure. The authors introduce us to the most modern endoscopic techniques for dealing with bleeding lesions but are wisely circumspect about assigning degrees of definitiveness to them at present.

The chapters on ERCP and endoscopic sphincterotomy are compact and complete. The technique is particularly useful in the diagnosis and management of common duct stones; the authors wisely emphasize the potential dangers in attempting to remove the largest stones—and in the use of pancreatography in patients with pancreatic pseudocysts. I also admire their cautious stand on the role of sphincterotomy for patients with so-called 'stenosing papillitis'. Endoscopy of the colon has also developed rapidly and the reader is provided with full details of technique, indications and hazards. Of particular interest these days is the usefulness of the procedure in the diagnosis and management of colonic polyps. The authors assume that all polyps should be removed, including those less than 5 mm in diameter which have heretofore been considered to be 'hyperplastic'. Whilst the efficacy of prophylactic polypectomy in reducing the problems of colonic carcinoma remains to be proven, the practice of polypectomy is rapidly increasing. The guidelines for safe colonoscopy and polypectomy are explicit and detailed.

There are other fine features of this book, including discussions of the establishment and maintenance of a proper endoscopy suite, of the role of the endoscopy nurse/assistant, the repeated and appropriate emphasis on endoscopy as part of a group effort, and much useful information on good endoscopic housekeeping. Throughout the book, the illustrations are appropriate, clear and informative.

The ultimate indications and usefulness of endoscopic procedures will be defined, perhaps in the next decade. Long-term studies of this question launched by the American Gastroenterology Association and the American Society for Gastrointestinal Endoscopy may help resolve some of the important questions. In the meanwhile, enough evidence is at hand to warrant these procedures in a large number of circumstances, and we are indebted to Drs Cotton and Williams for their illuminating exposition. This book will be of great use to all those who are interested in gastrointestinal endoscopy.

Marvin H. Sleisenger

Preface to the Third Edition

Much has happened since the second edition. Therapeutic techniques have proliferated and matured, video-endoscopy has arrived, both authors have turned 50, and one has changed continents. The latter fact has introduced an American flavour (not 'flavor', since we have chosen to maintain English spelling).

It is difficult to keep track of all developments in such a large field. We have asked several friends to criticize certain sections in draft, and are enormously grateful for their suggestions—particularly from John Baillie (general review), Willie Webb (oesophagus), Joe Bowden (intra-operative endoscopy and gastrostomy), David Fleischer (GI bleeding, lasers and tumour therapy) and Marilyn Schaffner (GI nursing). For simplicity, not chauvinism, we refer to all patients and doctors as 'he', and nurses as 'she'. Why aren't there more female gastroenterologists?

We have attempted to maintain the practical 'cook-book' approach which has made earlier editions popular. Increasingly there are more comprehensive texts to which enthusiasts can refer, and we especially recommend the massive, multi-authored *Gastroenterologic Endoscopy*, edited meticulously by Michael Sivak. We also hope that you will find it worthwhile to scan the new *Annual of Gastrointestinal Endoscopy* (published by Current Science, London), which we edit with Guido Tytgat.

In concentrating on techniques, we do not wish to appear not to be interested in their clinical role (and have written extensively elsewhere on this topic). Objective evaluation of these powerful tools is a major responsibility of all endoscopists. Some references are given in the appropriate chapters.

Sincere thanks are due to our families, colleagues and friends on both sides of the Atlantic, and to our indefatigable secretaries, Rita Oden and Helen Lando.

March 1990

P.B. Cotton
C.B. Williams

Introduction 1

The human gut is long and tortuous. Diagnosis and localization of its afflictions has relied for many decades on barium radiology, which provides indirect data in black and white. Man is by nature inquisitive and direct inspection in colour is instinctively preferable and probably more accurate. Rigid open-ended instruments allow direct visual examination (and biopsy sampling) of only the proximal 40 cm and distal 25 cm of the gut. Semi-flexible lens gastroscopes were introduced in the 1930s and 1940s and used by a few experts; examinations were uncomfortable and incomplete, and biopsy facilities were poor.

The situation has changed dramatically since the late 1960s with the introduction of fully flexible and manoeuvrable endoscopes. Upper GI endoscopy is now a routine procedure which has superseded the barium meal as the primary diagnostic tool. Duodenoscopy allows direct cannulation of the papilla of Vater for cholangiography and pancreatography (ERCP). The whole colon can be examined, and methods are available for small intestinal endoscopy. Tissue specimens can be removed from all of these areas under direct vision, using biopsy forceps, cytology brushes and snare loops.

A further revolution occurred in the 1970s with the arrival of endoscopic therapy. Trans-endoscopic snare removal has revolutionized the management of polyps, and flexible endoscopes now allow removal of foreign bodies, sphincterotomy for gallstones, insertion of stents, dilatation of strictures, and direct attack on bleeding lesions and tumours.

GI endoscopy is a skill which requires motivation, determination and dexterity. Patients may suffer if examinations are not performed correctly, and endoscopic techniques themselves may fall into disrepute if results are sub-optimal or unnecessary complications occur. The speed of development and the consequent clinical demand for endoscopy initially outstripped the evolution of training facilities. Many of the present 'experts' (including the authors) were self-taught, but instruction and experience of endoscopy should now be an integral part of GI training programmes.

This volume attempts to provide a basic framework for this process, and includes some 'tricks of the trade' which we find helpful.

2 Basic Endoscopic Instrumentation

The flexible endoscope is a complex tool (Fig. 2.1). It consists basically of a control head with eyepiece and controls, and a flexible shaft which has a manoeuvrable tip. The head is connected to a light source via a connecting 'umbilical' cord, through which pass other tubes transmitting air, water and suction, etc. Accessories include flexible biopsy forceps for passage through the instrument, a side arm for assistant's viewing, and cameras (Fig. 2.1). The image is transmitted either by fibreoptics or electronically from a CCD video chip. The principles will be described briefly.

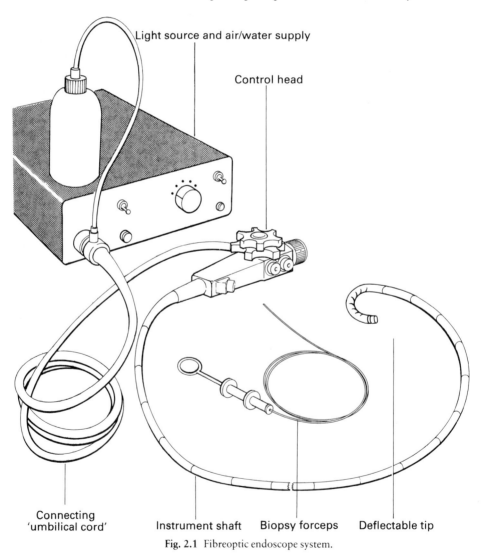

Light source and air/water supply

Control head

Connecting 'umbilical cord'

Instrument shaft   Biopsy forceps   Deflectable tip

Fig. 2.1 Fibreoptic endoscope system.

Fibreoptics

At the heart of any fibreoptic instrument are the viewing and light-carrying bundles, well described as 'highly flexible pieces of illuminated spaghetti'. The viewing bundle of a standard fibre-endoscope is 2–3 mm in diameter and contains 20–40 000 fine glass fibres, each close to 10 μm in diameter. Light focused onto the face of each fibre is transmitted by repeated internal reflections (Fig. 2.2). Faithful transmission of an image depends upon the spatial orientation of the individual fibres being the same at both ends of the bundle (a 'coherent' bundle). Each individual glass fibre is coated with glass of a lower optical density, to prevent leakage of light from within the fibre; since this coating does not transmit light, it and the space between the fibres causes a dark 'packing fraction', which is responsible for the fine mesh frequently apparent in the fibreoptic image (Fig. 2.3). For this reason, the image quality, though excellent, can never equal that of a rigid lens system. However, the fibreoptic image-carrying system is extremely flexible, and an image can be transmitted even when the bundle is tied in a knot.

In most modern instruments the distal lens which focuses the image onto the bundle is fixed, and a pin-hole aperture gives a depth of focus from 10–15 cm down to about 3 mm. The image reconstructed at the top of the bundle is transmitted to the eye via a focusing lens which provides correction for individual differences in refraction.

Video-endoscopes

First-generation video-endoscopes are mechanically identical to fibre-endoscopes, with a CCD 'chip' and supporting electronics mounted at the tip, to and fro wiring replacing the optical bundle and further electronics and switches occupying the site of the ocular lens on the upper part of the control head. The removal of any need to hold these instruments close to the endoscopist's face gives, as well as the hygienic advantages of avoidance of splash contamination, the opportunity for radical changes of instrument design and handling techniques in the future.

The subtleties of different CCD systems in design and performance are beyond the authors', and this book's, capability. In essence, however, a CCD is an array of 33–100 000 individual photo cells (known as picture elements or pixels) receiving photons reflected back from the mucosal surface and producing electrons in proportion to the light received. In common with all other television systems the individual receptors of the CCD respond only to degrees of light and dark and not to colour. 'Colour' CCDs have extra pixels to allow for an overlay of multiple primary-colour filter stripes, making the pixels under a particular stripe respond only to light of that particular colour. Black and white (more correctly, sequential-system) CCDs can be made smaller, or potentially of higher resolution, by the expedient of illuminating *all* the pixels with intermittent primary-colour strobe-effect lighting produced by rotating

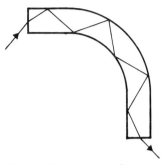

Fig. 2.2 'Total internal reflection' of light down a glass fibre.

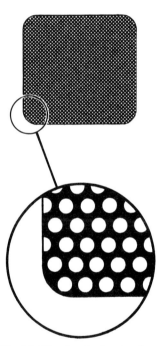

Fig. 2.3 Fibre bundle showing the 'packing fraction' or dead space between fibres.

a colour filter wheel within the light source. The sequential primary colour images (in the gut mostly red, some green and little blue) are stored transiently in banks of memory chips in the processor and fed out to the red/blue/green electron guns of the TV monitor every 30th of a second. The thousands of chips and sophisticated computer technology used to optimize the underlying single CCD output account for the excellence of the image produced by sequential CCD systems and the high price involved, as well as the relatively large processor. By contrast, a 'colour' CCD uses white light from a conventional light source and its electronics input directly into the monitor, requiring a cheaper and smaller processing unit.

From the user's point of view there are other advantages and disadvantages. The first-generation sequential system video-endoscopes give an extremely crisp colour view when the view is good, but bubbles and other rapid changes in the visual field (altering faster than the 1/30th second frame-store rate) produce an unpleasant strobe-effect on the screen. This is undesirable in gastro-enterology, although it may be of less importance during bronchoscopy or flexible cystoscopy, for which the smaller size of the sequential black and white CCD approach will continue to have advantages. All the CCDs, but especially the sequential variety, perform rather poorly in red light such as a blood-filled intestinal lumen, in which the view becomes fuzzy and fluorescent in quality. Video-scopes are therefore not well suited to bleeding emergency endoscopy where tried and true fibreoptic large-channel instruments, coupled with the remarkable range of light-sensitivity and image-processing capability provided by the human retina and optical cortex, give results so far unequalled by electronic systems.

Video-endoscope or fibre-endoscope?

Leaving aside the problems in bleeding patients, the screen-image quality of present video-endoscopes, in both colour and resolution, otherwise approximately equals that of present fibrescopes. Video-endoscopy scores greatly by the fact that everyone can view simultaneously with a clarity previously restricted to the endoscopist alone (teaching side-arms and add-on television cameras introduce optical interference and reduced quality). Whereas optical fibre technology is near its maximum theoretical performance (since below the 6–8 μm fibre diameter approached in modern bundles there is massive loss of light transmission), there is no reason why the 10 μm pixel size of present CCDs should not reduce to around 1 μm. This means that future CCDs can be smaller, but also that the greatly increased numbers of pixels will allow the use of high-definition TV monitors giving excellent resolution. The objection that video-endoscopes introduce 'artificial colour' values is untenable, since: (i) they can be shown in technical studies to give a remarkably faithful rendering of test charts; (ii) the visual assessment of pathology depends little on absolute colour values and anyway is backed by histopathology; and (iii) there is the inescapable fact that individual perception of colour varies significantly—the extreme example being colour-blindness. In terms of hard-copy imaging there is also a clear advantage in employing only the ocular lens system at the instrument tip without the degrading effects of transmission down an optical bundle and through a secondary lens system.

The mechanical transition to handling video-endoscopes whilst viewing the TV monitor is mastered in a few minutes. Thereafter most endoscopists tend instinctually to work this way even with fibre-endoscopes if a camera system is available. The ease of stance, brighter view and the natural visual field, combining a macular view of the image and peripheral view of the patient and others in the endoscopy room, makes video-endoscopes extremely relaxing to use, which is beneficial to good endoscopy and patient communication. Although in individual practice no user of fibre-endoscopes need feel disadvantaged, the bonus for larger institutions or teaching hospitals of the shared view, including the ability for the experienced endoscopist to see precisely the same image as obtained by an apprentice, scores highly in favour of using video-endoscopes. The mechanical manipulation of endoscope controls and subtle management of its shaft, including de-looping or rotatory movements, are significantly easier with video-endoscopes, since the manipulating left hand can move freely without relationship to the endoscopist's eye.

Overall it seems likely that video-endoscopes will rapidly take over a majority position in GI endoscopic units, although fibreoptic instruments will, by virtue of their simplicity and small diameter capability, retain a valuable role, for instance where portability is relevant, as well as in other special circumstances.

Illumination

No image is observed unless the area is illuminated by light transmitted from an external high intensity source through one or more light-carrying bundles. Since these light bundles do not transmit a spatial image, the fibres within them need not be 'coherent' and are randomly arranged. Because light intensity is reduced at any optical interface, light bundles run uninterruptedly from the tip of the instrument through its connecting 'umbilical' cord directly to the point of focus of the lamp.

Light sources

Illumination is provided either by a xenon arc (300 W), or a halogen-filled tungsten filament lamp (150 W), focused by a parabolic mirror onto the face of the bundle; the transmitted intensity is controlled by filters and/or a mechanical diaphragm. The light source contains a cooling fan and a pump for the air and water supply. The light sources made by different companies are not always interchangeable; adapters may be provided, but involve a further optical interface and some loss of light. Small sources are mobile and

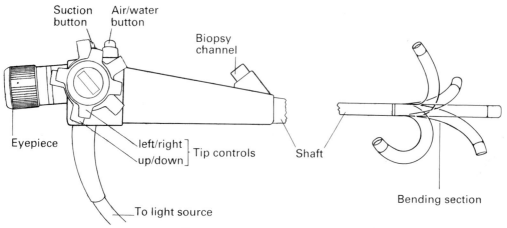

Fig. 2.4 Basic design—control head and bending section.

relatively cheap and provide sufficient illumination for simple observation and standard photography. However, they may be inadequate when the view is being shared through a teaching side arm, particularly when using smaller endoscopes. Large light sources are necessary for optimal photography and television applications when using fibrescopes or video-endoscopes. These utilize high temperature xenon arc lamps which give a bluish light and require the use of daylight type film for photography.

Control of the instrument tip

Tip movement depends upon pull wires attached at the tip just beneath its outer protective shaft, and passing back through the length of the instrument shaft to the angling controls in the control head (Fig. 2.4). The two angling wheels/knobs (for up/down and right/left movement) incorporate a friction braking system, so that the tip can be fixed temporarily in any desired position. The instrument shaft is relatively torque stable so that rotatory 'corkscrewing' movements applied to the head are transmitted to the tip —if the shaft is straight at the time.

Instrument channels

An 'operating' channel (usually 2–3 mm in diameter) allows the passage of fine flexible accessories (e.g. biopsy forceps, cytology brushes, sclerotherapy needles, diathermy snares) from a port on the endoscope control head (Fig. 2.4) through to the tip and out into the field of view (Fig. 2.5). In instruments with a lateral-viewing lens system the tip of the channel incorporates a small deflectable elevator or bridge, which permits some directional control of the forceps and other accessories independent of the instrument tip (Fig. 2.6); this elevator or bridge is controlled by a further thumb lever. In single-channel instruments, the operating channel is also

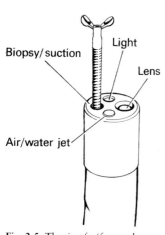

Fig. 2.5 The tip of a 'forward-viewer.'

used for aspiration; an external suction pump is connected to the 'umbilical' cord of the instrument near the light source and suction is diverted into the instrument channel by pressing the suction button.

In most instruments the accessories emerge from the suction port distally in the bottom right hand corner of the field, which is where fluid or polyp specimens should be best placed for suctioning.

The larger channel (≥ 3.7 mm) of 'operative' or 'therapeutic' endoscopes allows both better suction and passage of larger accessories. Twin-channel endoscopes exist for specialized applications.

An ancillary small channel transmits air to distend the organ being examined; the air is supplied from a pump in the light source and is controlled by another button (Fig. 2.4). The air system also pressurizes the water bottle so that a jet of water can be squirted across the distal lens to clean it. In colonoscopes there is a separate proximal opening for the water channel, to allow high-pressure flushing with a syringe.

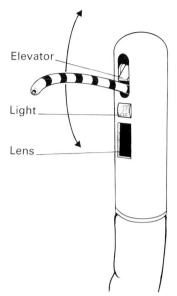

Fig. 2.6 A side-viewer with cannula protruding from the elevator.

Different instruments

The above basic design principles apply to most endoscopes but specific instruments differ in length, size, sophistication and distal lens orientation. Most gastrointestinal endoscopy is performed with instruments providing direct forward vision (Fig. 2.5), via a 90–130° wide angle lens (the angle being measured across the diagonal of square image endoscopes). However, there are circumstances in which it is preferable to view laterally (Fig. 2.6)—see Chapter 4 for details.

The overall diameter of an endoscope is a compromise between engineering ideals and patient tolerance. The shaft must contain and protect many bundles, wires, and tubes, all of which are stronger and more efficient when larger. A colonoscope can reasonably approach 15 mm in diameter to provide resilience and torque stability, but this size is acceptable in the upper gut only for specialized therapeutic instruments. Most routine upper GI endoscopes are between 8 and 11 mm in diameter. Smaller endoscopes are available; they are better tolerated by all patients and have specific application in children. However, smaller instruments inevitably involve some compromise in durability, image quality and the biopsy size. All modern endoscopes can be completely immersed for cleaning and disinfection; non-immersible instruments are obsolete.

Biopsy forceps, cytology brushes, etc.

The ability to take target tissue specimens is a crucial part of endoscopy. Forceps consist of a pair of sharpened cups (Fig. 2.7), a spiral metal cable, and a control handle (Fig. 2.8). The maximum diameter is limited by the size of the operating channel of the specific instrument and the length of the cups is limited by the radius of curvature through which they must pass in the instrument tip. In

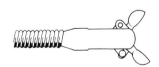

Fig. 2.7 Biopsy cups open.

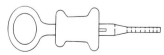

Fig. 2.8 Control handle for forceps.

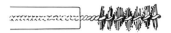

Fig. 2.9 Cytology brush with outer sleeve.

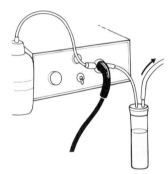

Fig. 2.10 A suction trap to collect fluid specimens.

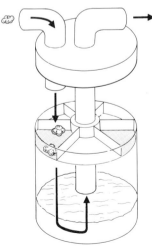

Fig. 2.11 A filtered suction trap is better for tissue specimens.

side-viewing instruments with a forceps elevator, this curvature is acute. When it is necessary to take biopsy specimens from a lesion which can only be approached tangentially (e.g. the wall of the oesophagus), forceps with a central spike may be helpful; however, these present a significant puncture hazard, and should probably not be used, to avoid accidental infectious inoculation. Cytology brushes have a covering plastic sleeve to protect the specimen during withdrawal (Fig. 2.9). A simple Teflon tube can be passed down the instrument channel to clear mucus or blood from areas of interest with a jet of water or to highlight mucosal detail by 'dye-spraying'. Other diagnostic and therapeutic devices will be described in the relevant sections.

Additional useful equipment

Suction traps

The device used for collecting samples of sputum during bronchial aspiration is equally useful for taking samples of intestinal secretions and bile. It is fitted temporarily into the suction line (Fig. 2.10) and allows collection of samples for microbiology, chemistry and 'salvage' cytology. Solid or snare-loop specimens can also be retrieved in an ingenious filtered suction trap available commercially (Fig. 2.11).

Flushing ancillaries

In addition to the jet of water passing across the lens to clear off secretions it is useful also to be able to direct a jet of fluid at a lesion such as an ulcer, particularly in the presence of food residue or acute bleeding. With a standard endoscope, this can be done by applying a syringe with a suitable nozzle through the biopsy port. Some therapeutic instruments have an in-built forward-facing flushing channel at the tip. It may be convenient to use a pump—either a manual bulb (Fig. 2.12) or an electrical pulsatile water Pik such as those marketed for cleaning teeth.

Overtubes (sleeves)

There are circumstances when it is useful to use an overtube. These are flexible hoses 24–45 cm long (depending on the indication) designed to slide over the shaft of an upper GI or colon endoscope. Sophisticated low friction PTFE versions are produced but suitable alternatives can be made from plastic hose; the internal diameter needs to be tailored to the size of the endoscope; the walls should be as thin as possible (to minimize patient discomfort) but should have sufficient strength not to kink, and to maintain shape when the endoscope is removed. The top end of the tube should have a flange which abuts against the mouthguard, or any device which can be gripped by the assistant (to prevent it from disappearing into the mouth or anus).

Overtubes are mainly used when repeated intubation is anticipated, e.g. for change of endoscopes, removal of multiple polyps, or use of muzzle-loaded forceps and biopsy capsules. The endoscope is passed in the usual way, with the overtube at the top of the shaft. Once the endoscope is in position, the overtube is lubricated and slid in over the shaft. It is then simple to remove and to replace the endoscope without significant patient discomfort.

Alternatively, the upper GI overtube can be passed first over a large flexible lavage tube or dilator (Fig. 2.13). Once in place, the lavage tube can be used to empty or lavage the oesophagus and stomach. When this is completed, the lavage tube is withdrawn, leaving the overtube in place; this protects the airway and allows the endoscope to be passed through it without additional patient discomfort.

Longer and large overtubes are used for removal of sharp foreign bodies from the stomach and, by some practitioners, windowed overtubes have been found useful during variceal injection sclerotherapy, especially during active bleeding. The use of colonic (split) overtubes is described in Chapter 9.

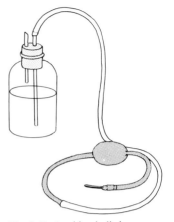

Fig. 2.12 A rubber bulb for flushing through the instrumentation channel.

Some basic practical principles

Details of instruments for specific purposes, and precise methods for cleaning and disinfection are outlined in separate chapters. This section serves to introduce the true beginner to some principles which are common to all endoscopes and procedures.

Handling, storage and security

Endoscopes are expensive and complex tools. They should be stored safely, hanging vertically and in cupboards through which air can circulate. Care must be taken whilst carrying instruments, the rigid optics at either end are easily damaged if left to dangle or knocked against a hard surface. The head, tip and umbilical should be held (Fig. 2.14); paradoxically, the flexible parts are least easily damaged, unless crushed.

Dress

There are no accepted standards for endoscopy dress. The procedures are not sterile and a complete change is unnecessary. Many endoscopists do routine procedures in their usual clinical clothes. We prefer to change into operating room 'scrubs', or at least the top part, when doing complex or messy procedures. Infection control considerations now dictate the need to wear an impervious gown and disposable gloves. Policies concerning masks and goggles vary in different units. Common sense dictates that extra protection should be used during procedures which carry a significant risk of splashing (e.g. variceal sclerotherapy) although video-endoscopes take the biopsy splash port further from the endoscopist. These aspects are further discussed in Chapter 12.

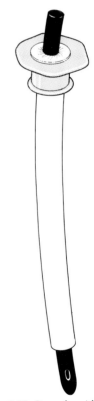

Fig. 2.13 Overtube with toothguard over rubber lavage tube.

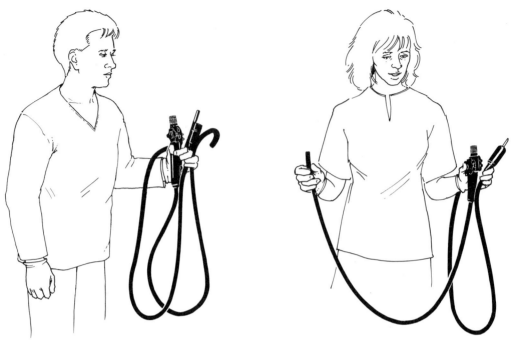

Fig. 2.14 Carry endoscopes carefully—to avoid knocks to the optics in the control head and tip.

Lead aprons (and exposure monitoring badges) should always be worn during procedures involving X-rays.

Instrument checks

The instrument will normally be set up with the water bottle and other accessories suitably cleaned and disinfected by the GI staff and all appropriate connections made. However, the endoscopist must check that everything has been done satisfactorily and that the equipment is ready and safe for use. He thus needs to understand the basic principles of cleaning and disinfection routine and the mechanisms, connections and plumbing of the endoscopes.

Before passing an instrument, the endoscopist should test that the controls are all functional (including tip deflection, air/water and suction) and that the image is clear.

Clearing blockages

One of the commonest endoscope problems is blockage of the air/water or suction systems. When failure occurs, the various systems and connections (instrument umbilical, water bottle cap or tube, etc.) must be checked, including the tightness and the presence of rubber O-rings where relevant. If a blockage is confirmed, it is usually possible to clear the different channels with a syringe and a suitable introducer such as an intracath, or plastic micropipette tip. Water can be injected down any channel and, since water is not compressed, more force can be applied than with air. Remember that a small syringe (1–5 cm^3) generates more pressure than a large one, whereas a large one (50 cm^3) generates more suction. The air or suction connections at the umbilical, or the water tube within the water bottle can be syringed until water emerges from the instrument tip. Another method for unclogging the suction channel is to remove the suction button, and apply the suction hose directly at the port. Care should be taken to cover or depress the relevant control buttons while syringing. Irreversible air-channel blockages are invariably due to coagulated residue inside or just above the small angled tube inserted at the instrument tip and held in place by a small grub screw covered with soft mastic. As a last resort this can be removed, with a very small screwdriver. The best way to avoid such blockages is to insist on scrupulous cleaning regimes including the use of enzyme detergents (see Chapter 12).

The grip

An endoscope, like a golf club or violin, has to be held correctly to produce good results. Its head should be placed in the palm of the left hand, and gripped between the fourth and fifth fingers and the base of the thumb, with the tip of the thumb resting on the up/down control (Fig. 2.15). This grip leaves the first finger (forefinger) free to activate the air/water and suction buttons. The second (middle) finger assists the thumb as a 'ratchet' during the major movements of the up/down control. With practice, the left/right control can also be managed with the left thumb (Fig. 2.16). The left thumb is also used to control the lever for the forceps elevator where present. The right hand thus remains free to push, pull and torque the instrument and also to control ancillaries such as biopsy forceps and cameras. The right hand may be used intermittently to manage the left/right tip control and the brakes, but for fluent 'single-handed' endoscopy this is avoided as much as possible.

The basic left-hand grip should be maintained throughout the examination. Acute rotation of the instrument should be effected

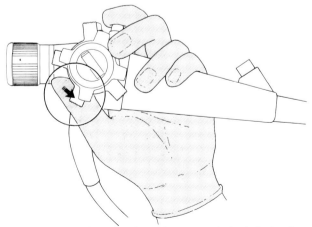

Fig. 2.15 The thumb rests on the up/down control wheel, the forefinger on the air/water button and the middle finger can also assist.

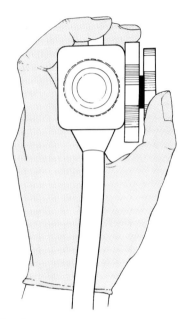

Fig. 2.16 The thumb can reach across to the left/right control.

by rotating the hand, not by rotating the instrument in the hand. Some endoscopists find it convenient to ask the nurse to push and pull the instrument, leaving both hands free to manage the controls. This method may be easier for beginners but is not generally recommended.

The stance

To stand up or sit down is a matter of personal preference and stamina. However, it is important to maintain the instrument shaft as straight as possible, because it is then under the minimum strain and is maximally responsive. Incompetent endoscopists can be identified from a distance as they perform contortions which cannot be transmitted to the instrument tip and stress the equipment as well as the patient (Fig. 2.17). Always maintain a balanced comfortable stance and a relatively straight instrument (Fig. 2.18)—and be gentle.

Orientation conventions

When referring to tip deflection, it is convenient to use 'up/down' and 'left/right' in relation to the neutral position of the instrument head (i.e. buttons up), rather than to the ceiling or floor. Thus, turning the up/down control anti-clockwise as seen from the right (pushing the bottom of the wheel away from the endoscopist with the thumb) always moves the tip 'up' (Fig. 2.19). This applies whatever the shaft rotation; if the hand and the scope are rotated so that the buttons face the floor, 'up' deflection of the tip now points it towards the floor (Fig. 2.20). Fibreoptic instruments have a small

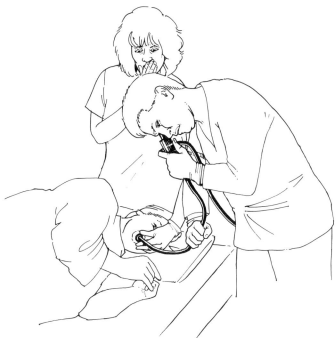

Fig. 2.17 Wrong: An obviously incompetent endoscopist with clumsy stance and handling.

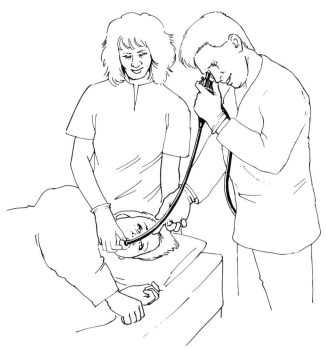

Fig. 2.18 Right: Confident and balanced stance with a straight instrument, gently handled.

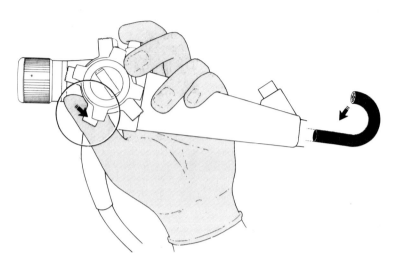

Fig. 2.19 The thumb pushes away from the endoscopist to angle the tip 'up'.

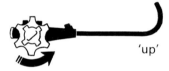

'up'

'up'

Fig. 2.20 Inversion of the endoscope and the 'up/down' convention.

mark at 12 o'clock in the field of view (Fig. 2.21) to facilitate orientation for photography and the endoscopist viewing down the teaching side arm, and 'up' deflection always deviates the tip towards that mark; video-endoscopes do not need this facility since the monitor does not rotate. Remember that tip movements cause the view to move in the opposite direction (Fig. 2.22). The lens in side viewing instruments always faces upwards towards the buttons and the same conventions apply.

12 o'clock marker

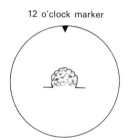

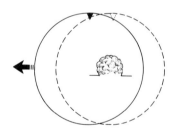

Fig. 2.21 Fibrescopes have a marker (for photography).

Fig. 2.22 Tip movements move the view in the opposite direction.

At the end of the procedure

Details of cleaning and disinfection schedules are given in Chapter 12. These must be initiated immediately after the instrument is removed from the patient and before proteinaceous secretions (and blood) can dry in the channels or become denatured during disinfection. A useful routine is for the endoscopist or assistant to place the tip of the instrument into water immediately after removing it from the patient, and then to press down on both buttons for 15–20 seconds. This flushes both the suction/biopsy and the air/ water channels. Where all-channel or other irrigating systems are supplied by the manufacturer, these should be employed.

Routine servicing?

Most car owners are persuaded of the need for routine servicing to reduce the likelihood of major expensive repairs. Preventive maintenance is equally logical for endoscopes, even though they do not have many parts which inevitably need changing. Most of this work is done in the unit by the GI staff especially regular 'leakage testing' of immersible endoscopes. However, a case can be made for returning instruments to the manufacturers or their servicing agents for detailed inspection and 'tightening up' from time to time. It is equally important to maintain complex accessories (particularly any diathermy equipment) in safe condition, properly calibrated and adjusted.

Further reading

Bat, L. and Williams, C. B. (1989) 'Usefulness of pediatric colonoscopes in adult colonoscopy'. *Gastrointestinal Endoscopy*, 35, 329–332.

Kawahara, I. and Ichikawa, H. (1987) 'Fiberoptic Instrument Technology', in *Gastroenterologic Endoscopy* (ed. Sivak, M. V. Jr.), pp. 20–41. W. B. Saunders, Philadelphia.

Sivak, M. V. (1988) 'Video endoscopy', in *Annual of Gastrointestinal Endoscopy* (ed. Cotton, P. B., Tytgat, G. N. J. and Williams, C. B.), pp. 115–127. Gower Academic Journals, London.

Williams, C. B. (1989) 'Endoscopic instrumentation', in *Annual of Gastrointestinal Endoscopy*, pp. 143–148. Current Science, London.

3 The Endoscopy Unit

A GI endoscopy service requires a range of instruments, competent operators and assistants, and a suitable environment. Many hospitals and clinics have developed highly sophisticated facilities. This section is designed to give some broad guidelines to those developing new units; details are best considered after visiting a number of active centres.

The facilities needed in an individual clinic or hospital depend upon the anticipated workload and spectrum of procedures. The workload can be expressed in total procedure numbers, or roughly translated into 'half-day sessions'. However, since endoscopy procedures vary enormously in complexity (which affects the time taken, equipment used and assistant staff requirements), they are better stratified in some way. This has been addressed in the USA by the 'relative value scale'. Sivak has suggested another scale in his excellent review of endoscopy unit organization in his book *Gastroenterologic Endoscopy*. We use a simplified scale, allocating points as follows.

1 point: diagnostic upper endoscopy, flexible sigmoidoscopy.
2 points: therapeutic uppers, diagnostic colons.
3 points: therapeutic colons, diagnostic ERCP.
6 points: therapeutic ERCP.

The point value is doubled for any procedure done outside normal working hours. Keeping track of the total points gives a better measure of workload than simple number of examinations, and can be useful when attempting to justify increases in staff and facilities.

GI endoscopy now requires dedicated space. The use of operating rooms is unnecessary and inappropriate (except for preoperative emergencies or perioperative examinations). However, when an institution has an efficient organization for day surgery (with recovery beds), sessional use of these facilities may initially appear attractive for GI endoscopy—sharing with several disciplines (e.g. bronchoscopy, cystoscopy). Such an arrangement has problems for storage of equipment and for emergency procedures; more important, clinical demands inevitably increase and more sessions are required. A purpose designed or adapted area dedicated to GI endoscopy is essential for efficient and safe procedures. Smaller centres may be able to lend space to colleagues for fibreoptic bronchoscopy.

Radiographic screening (fluoroscopy) is required for some diagnostic and therapeutic intubations. Units requiring X-ray screening (fluoroscopy) for only a few cases each week can share portable C-arm equipment. When screening is used on most days, it is more efficient to build in an X-ray unit which will be more reliable and involves less hazard from X-ray scatter. High-quality

Levels of activity/week				Reasonable facilities			
Case load	Sessions (half days)			Procedure rooms	Recovery beds	X-ray screening	ERCP
	Total	With X-ray screening	ERCP				
<50	<10	2	2	1–2	Share day case facility or own (and lend) 2–4	Book/ share fluoro	Travel to X-ray dept.
50–100	15	3	3	2–3	4–6	Own fluoro unit	
100–150	30	4+	4+	4–6	8–10	Own full X-ray unit	

Fig. 3.1 Endoscopy case load determines both the number of sessions and the facilities required.

X-ray apparatus (including a tipping table and fast processor) is required for procedures involving radiographs (such as ERCP). Many units do ERCP on only one or two days each week and must book appropriate times in the X-ray department. There will be difficulties with this arrangement, especially as demands increase, and it is inconvenient to transport all of the equipment. Units performing more than say 200 ERCP examinations each year are likely also to be doing many other sessions of endoscopy in which fluoroscopy is required; such units need full independent X-ray equipment (including instant processing). These different levels of activity can be tabulated by weekly numbers and 'half-day sessions' to give some idea of the required facilities (Fig. 3.1).

Design principles

Few people have the opportunity to design an ideal endoscopy unit for a new hospital or clinic. More often it is necessary to search for under-used space and to design a layout within its constraints. Certain principles should be kept in mind. The area must be accessible day and night and suitable for both out- and in-patients. If the institution has a day-care area or recovery area with spare capacity, it may be sensible to place the endoscopy unit nearby. It is convenient for doctors if the unit is close to other areas of work (wards, clinic, etc.), since it is then possible to supervise sessions without being completely tied to the procedure room. Extra toilets and facilities for giving enemas are required.

Whatever the ambitions of the unit, specific areas must be considered for specific functions: endoscopy procedures; instrument cleaning and storage; patient and relative reception; consultation and recovery; and office, teaching and social facilities. Their interrelationships should allow free and efficient flow, without cross-traffic.

Endoscopy examination rooms

Examination rooms should resemble modern kitchens, with a floor area of about 15 m² (150 ft²)—larger in teaching institutions—and contain large sinks, adequate work surfaces, cupboards and power points. Small rooms are not necessarily a disadvantage if well designed, but new developments and equipment can upset the best plans. The floor should be washable and smooth; anaesthetic considerations may dictate the need for antistatic flooring. Windows should have blackout curtains and roller blinds. General room light should be dimmable, with spotlights over the worktops. It is convenient for the endoscopist and nurses to be able to turn the main room light on and off without moving from their working positions (e.g. with a ceiling pull-switch) and to have easy access to intercom and telephone. Door openings should be wide, since it may occasionally be necessary to move beds or large pieces of equipment.

It is not necessary to have a formal examination table; trolleys (stretchers) are convenient for examination and recovery (Fig. 3.2). Adjustable height is an advantage. One trolley (stretcher) should have a radiolucent top if a portable X-ray fluoroscopy unit is to be used.

It is essential to have oxygen available and two suction points in each room, one for the instrument, and one for the patient. An alarm call system and resuscitation equipment must be available, including ECG monitor, defibrillator, incubation equipment and emergency drugs.

Since endoscopies may be performed outside the unit (e.g. ERCP

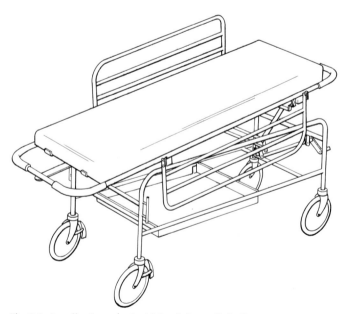

Fig. 3.2 A trolley (stretcher) with head-down tilt facility.

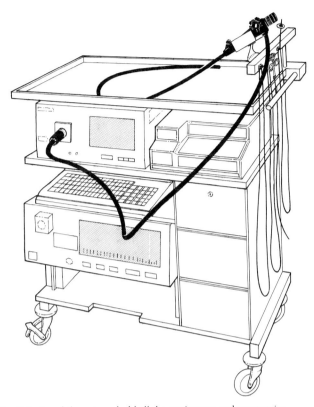

Fig. 3.3 A mobile cart can hold all the equipment and accessories.

in the radiology department, and emergencies in the intensive care unit), it is convenient to keep the light source and/or video-processor and much of the ancillary equipment on a mobile trolley (cart) (Fig. 3.3). This can be stored beneath or in front of a worktop, and also used during routine sessions.

Many different drugs, including narcotics, are used during endoscopy procedures. Special provision must be made for their efficient storage and for the safe disposal of syringes and needles.

Functional planning of the endoscopy room with the avoidance of cross-traffic is crucial to efficient work. Geographical spheres of activity should be defined for the doctor(s), nurses and trainees, with all their relevant equipment in that sector (Fig. 3.4). Direct access for in-patients and emergency cases should ideally be separated from that for well out-patients.

Patients often enter the examination room without sedation; the hardware may look rather frightening and can be hidden from view by appropriate planning or a railed curtain. The ambience should be cheerful rather than clinical, and the room should not resemble an operating room. Piped music may be appreciated. There must be adequate arrangements for maintaining reasonable temperature and for extracting odours, both clinical and chemical (disinfectants and anaesthetics).

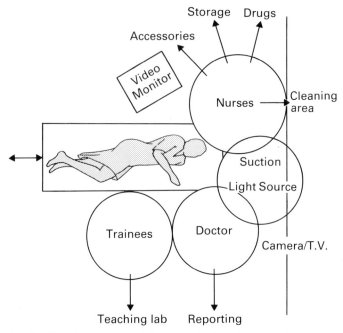

Fig. 3.4 Functional planning is important in the endoscopy unit.

Cleaning and storage of equipment

Delicate instruments require good arrangements for cleaning, disinfection and storage (Chapter 12). Instruments are best hung vertically in thin cupboards, which should be strong and lockable, well ventilated and not subject to extremes of temperature.

Doctors always underestimate the requirements for storage. There must be clean utility areas for instrument disinfection, linen, pre-packaged sterile supplies, and space for all the other equipment which accumulates. It is necessary to have areas designated for disposal of waste materials and for temporary storage of contaminated linen and equipment.

Porters (messengers), cleaners and other staff may also require storage facilities.

Patient reception, consultation and recovery

Although procedure rooms are the heart of a unit, patients undergoing endoscopy (and their relatives) spend more time elsewhere—in preparation and subsequent recovery. The design of the unit depends on the need for a recovery area (if there is no day-care area nearby), and whether patients are handled by a 'production-line' or 'personal' system.

In the personal system (Fig. 3.5), the patient is allocated an individual room (or bay) on arrival in the unit; it contains a stretcher (trolley), two chairs, a locker, a small hand basin and

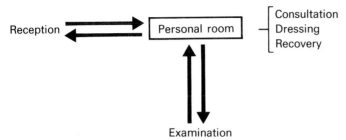

Fig. 3.5 'Personal' system of patient management for endoscopy.

mirror, suction and oxygen outlets and an emergency call system. Television surveillance may be appropriate. This room is used for the initial consultation and reassurance and for changing; clothes and valuables are placed in the locker. The patient gets on to the trolley and any medication is given. He is wheeled into the endoscopy area, examined and then returned on the trolley to the same room. The recovery phase is completed in a chair in the presence of a relative or friend. The patient leaves from the same room after recovery and discussion about the endoscopy findings with the doctor and/or nurse.

In the production-line system, patients have no personal base (Fig. 3.6). They are received into an interview room for discussion and reassurance and then change in a dressing area. Clothes and valuables are put in a fixed locker or carried in a basket which can then be stored underneath the examination stretcher. The patient walks into a medication area or directly into the endoscopy room and gets on to the stretcher. After examination he is wheeled on that stretcher into a recovery bay. When able to stand, he gets dressed and sits in a chair in a second stage recovery area, with a relative or friend who has been waiting outside. Prior to discharge he is again seen in the interview area by the doctor or nurse.

The personal system is preferable if staff and space permit. The rooms or bays need to be larger (and relatively sound-proof) and are more difficult for nurses to monitor than a series of small recovery bays separated only by curtains. Whichever system is used, suction and resuscitation equipment must be readily available to all patients.

Efficient endoscopy requires access to at least two recovery bays

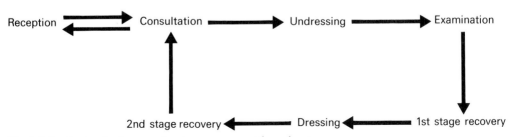

Fig. 3.6 'Production-line' system of patient management for endoscopy.

per procedure room. However, the precise number depends upon the type and volume of work, and also upon the medication regime used. Centres which use little or no sedation need fewer recovery facilities.

Office, teaching and social functions

Endoscopy reports should be dictated onto tape or entered onto a computerized database immediately after examination. An office area is needed for scheduling and maintenance of permanent records. Methods of documentation are discussed in Chapter 13, which also gives more detail about teaching. Training centres need to have a separate but adjacent teaching room, where trainees and visitors can withdraw at sensitive moments and study between sessions. Any service depends upon good communications and co-operation between its own staff and those of other departments. It is essential to have a small area where staff can relax, make coffee and keep their postcards and plants. Refreshments for patients can also be supplied from the same kitchen.

If the endoscopy unit is part of or close to the main gastro-enterology department, their office, teaching and social functions can usually be combined.

Endoscopy nurse/assistants

A purpose-designed endoscopy unit full of expensive equipment is of no avail without good assistants, who also require appropriate space in which to function. The vital contribution made by specifically trained endoscopy nurses is not always realized by those ignorant of modern techniques. The nurses' primary role is to care for the patient before, during and after procedures (Chapter 11). In most units the nurses also share reception and documentation duties with a secretary, and have an important technical role in the care and maintenance of delicate instruments. Larger units may be able to separate these functions, but none can survive unless they are provided for.

Further reading

Endoscopy Review (May 1990) Report of a conference on 'Endoscopy Unit Design and Organization'.
Sivak, M. V. (1987) 'The endoscopy unit', in *Gastroenterologic Endoscopy* (ed. Sivak, M. V.), pp. 42–66. W. B. Saunders, Philadelphia.

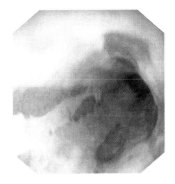

Plate 1 Ulcerative oesophagitis.

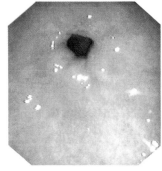

Plate 2 Normal pylorus.

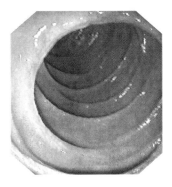

Plate 3 Normal descending duodenum.

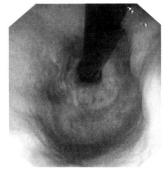

Plate 4 Normal retroversion in fundus of stomach.

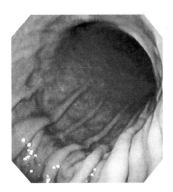

Plate 5 Normal gastric body.

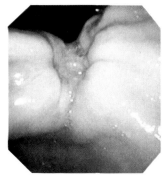

Plate 6 Gastric ulcer on angulus.

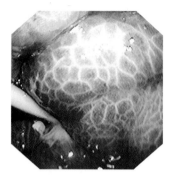

Plate 7 Endoscopic tube drainage of a pancreatic pseudocyst through the oedematous gastric wall.

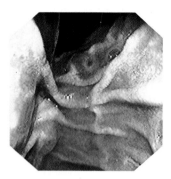

Plate 8 Main papilla (bottom left) with the accessory papilla in characteristic position above and to the right.

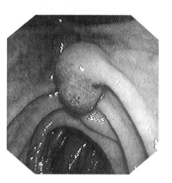

Plate 9 Swollen papilla due to impacted stone — direct needle-knife puncture over the stone may be needed.

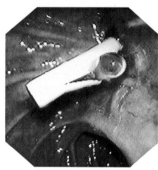

Plate 10 Stent draining bile — note short intraduodenal portion with flap well positioned.

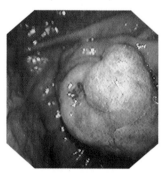

Plate 11 Benign tumour of the papilla; finding the axis to the duct(s) without causing bleeding is the problem.

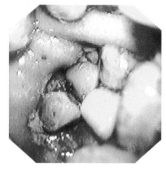

Plate 12 Multiple stones in the duodenum after sphincterotomy.

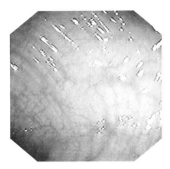

Plate 13 Normal colon showing vessel pattern and the highlights, and muscle rings indicating lumen direction (bottom left).

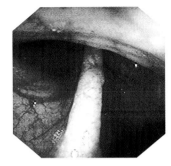

Plate 14 A prominent longitudinal taenia coli in a capacious colon indicates lumen direction (top).

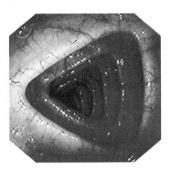

Plate 15 Triangular colon outline — often seen in the transverse, but sometimes elsewhere.

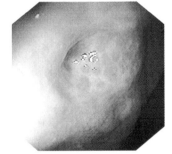

Plate 16 Appendix orifice — usually a crescentic slit but sometimes a whorl of folds.

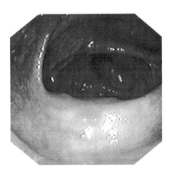

Plate 17 Bulge of the ileo-caecal valve, on the first circular fold back from the caecal pole.

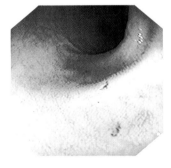

Plate 18 Terminal ileum — the villi look granular in air but stand up under water.

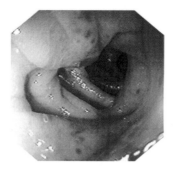

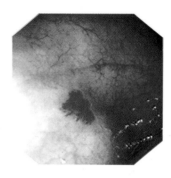

Plate 19 Traumatized redundant folds in diverticular disease, with petechiae and some inflammatory change.

Plate 20 A 3-mm angiodysplasia — not common but curable by coagulation.

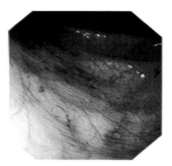

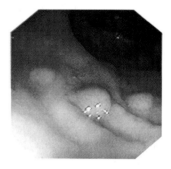

Plate 21 Dye-spray (dilute ink) shows fine mucosal detail (1-mm micro-adenomas in this adenomatous polyposis child).

Plate 22 Even 2–3-mm polyps in the colon are usually adenomas, but histology is needed.

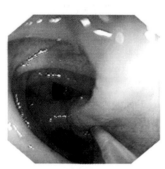

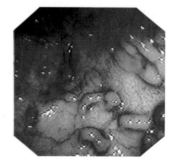

Plate 23 Adrenaline-sclerosant injection of a large polyp stalk before polypectomy.

Plate 24 Post-inflammatory polyps. They occur after severe colitis of any kind and have no cancer potential.

Diagnostic Upper Endoscopy

4

Patient preparation

Explanation

Many patients fear GI endoscopy. Natural anxiety may be aggravated by horror stories from 'friends' or inappropriate remarks by endoscopy staff. Good technique is essential and some medication is usually given, but the acceptability of endoscopy is also crucially dependent upon careful, sympathetic explanation and a reassuring friendly atmosphere at the time of reception as well as during the examination. Endoscopy can become such a routine to the doctors and nurses concerned that patients' natural anxieties may be ignored and thereby increased.

Patient education starts when the need for endoscopy is established. This is simple if the indication arises during consultation with the gastroenterologist who will himself perform the examination. However, patients are often referred to endoscopy units from other clinics or in-patient areas. Doctors with a long training in gastroenterology often wish to see the patient personally in consultation before agreeing to perform endoscopy; others are prepared to offer an open service. The first alternative is not always practical and some compromise must be reached which will be expressed in the design of any request/assessment form (Chapter 13). If the patient is sent from another clinic direct to the unit for endoscopy, the referring clinician must give the patient some idea of what is involved. References to swallowing a telescope or a camera may be helpful, but only if it is emphasized that these are miniaturized! It is perhaps better to speak of '*swallowing a small flexible tube through which we can see the lining of the stomach*' adding, where appropriate, '*you will be given a sedative injection and remember very little about it*'. The instruction document given or sent to the patient with the appointment should also include a reassuring explanation of the proposed procedure, which will contribute to the process of obtaining 'informed consent'.

Patients who are already in hospital should be seen by a member of the unit staff, to assess the indications for the procedure and its urgency, and to provide some explanation. Part of this role can be undertaken by unit nursing staff.

Wherever the patient comes from, and whatever discussion has gone before, there should always be an opportunity for the patient to discuss the procedure immediately beforehand with the doctor and nurse involved.

Safety evaluation

It is the responsibility of the doctor performing the endoscopy to satisfy himself that the examination is indicated, that there are no major contraindications, and the patient understands and consents. The extent to which the endoscopist should *personally* review the patient's fitness depends upon the circumstances, and some of this responsibility can be delegated to trained nurse assistants. They should be provided with a check-list of essential questions including the patient's arrangements for collection and future appointments, and maintain a record of the relevant answers. Most of these questions refer to safety aspects (see for example Chapter 13) and concern general medical problems (especially cardiac, respiratory and renal insufficiency), drug sensitivities, and current medications. The recommendations for antibiotic prophylaxis (especially in prevention of endocarditis) are given in Chapter 12. The patient's case record and any radiographs should always be available at the time of examination. The responsibility for safety lies ultimately with the endoscopist, who must be prepared to refuse examination or to delay it pending further discussion or preparation.

Informed consent

Good practice and simple prudence indicate that formal written informed consent should be obtained for all endoscopic procedures. The amount of explanation given and the type of form used will vary according to the custom of the institution and the laws of the country. The patient (before being relieved of his spectacles) should be asked to sign a form stating that he understands the nature and purpose of the examination. The doctor should countersign that he has given the patient the necessary information on which to make a judgement. For out-patients the form can include a phrase such as 'I understand that I should not drive a car or take charge of any machinery within 12 hours after this examination'.

Specific preparation and medication

Patients are instructed not to eat or drink for 4–6 hours before endoscopy (although small sips of water are permissible for comfort). It is thus kinder to perform examinations during the morning so that most patients can be fasted overnight. Patients with oesophageal or gastric outlet obstruction should be fasted for longer periods; aspiration of the oesophagus or formal gastric lavage may be necessary in these circumstances.

After initial discussion with the doctor and nurse, the patient should partly undress and put on a gown, or protective bib. Dentures and spectacles (including contact lenses) should normally be removed and stored safely.

Opinions and practices concerning analgesia and sedation vary widely between different centres and cultures. Most units use medication, but some experts rely solely on good technique, rapport and speed. Endoscopy without medication is better tolerated by older patients than by younger ones, and with small endoscopes (and lateral-viewing instruments which have a rounded tip); it is safer in patients with pulmonary problems. Endoscopy is also easier to organize when sedation is avoided; there is no need for formal recovery, and fit patients can drive or return immediately to work or play.

Pharyngeal anaesthesia

Local pharyngeal anaesthesia (by spray or lozenge) is particularly helpful when using little or no sedation, but is unnecessary when using heavy sedation, and may increase the risk of pulmonary aspiration. Spray application is preferred since it can be directed to the posterior pharyngeal wall to suppress the gag reflex. Do not ask the patient to say '*aaah*', since this may expose the larynx.

Benzodiazepines

The most popular sedative world wide is diazepam (Valium), but thrombophlebitis is a problem. This is avoided if it is presented in lipid emulsion (Diazemuls; KabiVitrum). Diazepam is given by slow intravenous injection (over 1–2 minutes) until the patient becomes dysarthric or develops ptosis. The appropriate dose must be judged by continuous observation and conversation with the patient. Less than 5 mg may induce coma in elderly patients (70 plus) and those with pulmonary or hepatic insufficiency, in whom half-dosage should be the norm. Conversely, 20 mg may have no effect in patients routinely taking similar tranquillizers or excess alcohol; there is little benefit and some hazard in giving much larger doses. It is a sensible rule to use 10 mg ampoules and 2 ml syringes, drawing up only 5 mg in each syringe so that the doctor has to make a conscious effort (by changing syringes) to give more than 5 mg. The usual dose of diazepam produces useful amnesia for the event. With larger doses, amnesia may be prolonged beyond the point where the patient appears to be awake and intelligent; consultations even 2 hours after the procedure may be forgotten. Blood levels of diazepam may show a secondary rise after some hours, and motor and cerebral function may be disturbed into a second day.

Midazolam (Versed) is a water-soluble alternative to diazepam with negligible risk of producing thrombophlebitis. Weight for weight it is more potent than diazepam and smaller doses must be given. Amnesia is more pronounced (which can be a problem as well as a virtue). Serious hypoxia has occurred when too much midazolam has been given too quickly, especially in the elderly.

When intravenous access is a problem, benzodiazepines can be given rectally resulting in full sedation in 5–10 minutes. Benzo-diazepine antagonists (e.g. adnexate) are available and are highly effective in an emergency.

Opiates

The prolonged effects of benzodiazepines and their occasional ineffectiveness have resulted in a search for other regimes. Intra-venous pethidine (Demerol) (50 mg) followed by a smaller dose of diazepam (2–10 mg) is a combination favoured by the authors, especially for younger patients (under 35) and alcohol abusers. Pethidine (Demerol) is particularly effective in suppressing the gag reflex. It also produces useful euphoria in the very anxious without the loss of control which can result from increasing the benzo-diazepine dose. The recovery time can be shortened by reversing the action of pethidine (Demerol) after the examination with naloxone (Narcan). Intravenous administration of 0.2–0.4 mg has a rapid but short-lived effect, and it is usually wise also to give the same dose intramuscularly. Both pethidine (Demerol) and diazepam indivi-dually can depress respiration. They should be used sparingly, if at all, in the elderly and in patients with respiratory problems.

Some units also use atropine (by muscular or intravenous injec-tion) to dry up secretions and to 'protect the heart'; there is no good evidence of benefit. Duodenoscopy usually requires suppression of duodenal motor activity, conveniently induced by an intravenous injection of Buscopan (hyoscine butylbromide, 20–40 mg). Since the effect lasts only 2–10 minutes, Buscopan is best given after the endoscope enters the duodenum if prolonged examination is in-tended. Glucagon (0.1–0.5 mg, i.v.) is an effective but expensive alternative where Buscopan is not available, or when the long-lasting effects of anticholinergics are undesirable (as in glaucoma, prostatism and unsedated drivers).

General anaesthesia

General anaesthesia may be required in special circumstances, such as complex and therapeutic procedures in young children, or un-controllable patients in whom normal sedative regimes are ineffec-tive (alcoholics, drug addicts, etc). General anaesthesia is safer than excessive doses of intravenous medication.

A standard medication regime

There is no agreed ideal medication regime, and each team will evolve a system with which it is familiar and content. A compromise practice can be briefly summarized. Unless the patient prefers no sedation we routinely use local pharyngeal anaesthesia and low-dose sedation. The patient lies down on the left side. Injections are given intravenously. There should be an established line into the *right* arm, since venous flow in the left arm may be reduced in the left lateral position; injections into the left arm may result in delayed effects, and an increased risk of thrombophlebitis. In younger patients we give pethidine (Demerol) by slow intravenous injection (usually 25–50 mg), followed immediately by diazepam (2–10 mg) whilst conversing with the patient and observing the effects. Pethidine is usually omitted in confident middle-aged patients and over the age of 70. Buscopan (20–40 mg), or glucagon (0.25–0.5 mg) is added intravenously when a duodenal lesion is suspected.

Routine upper GI examinations are usually complete within 10 minutes by which time the effects of sedation are wearing off. Some patients who have been given pethidine (Demerol) are also given naloxone (Narcan) at the end of the procedure (0.2 mg, i.v. and i.m.).

Recovery and discharge

The nature and duration of the recovery phase depend on the sedation given (if any) and whether naloxone has been used. With the regime outlined above, most patients rest for about 15–30 minutes on a trolley (stretcher) in view of the nursing staff. The accompanying relative or friend can sit with the patient if space permits. After 30 minutes most patients are able to sit in a chair. Drinking must be delayed for 20 minutes from the start of the procedure if pharyngeal anaesthesia has been used. Many patients are fit to leave by 30 minutes, and nearly all are discharged from our units into the care of a relative or friend within 1 hour of the examination. They are again instructed to go home, and not to drive or take any responsible action on the same day. These instructions should be given in writing. Patients who arrive in the unit unaccompanied (despite instructions) may need to be examined without sedation, or be re-scheduled.

Every patient should leave the unit with some idea of what has been discovered and what will happen next. Consultation should take place in the presence of any accompanying relative because of the somewhat unpredictable length of amnesia after sedation. Staff must ensure that the patient has further clinic appointments where appropriate.

Choice of instruments for upper endoscopy

A full range of endoscopes is now produced by several companies, and price differences are not currently a major consideration. However, since light sources and other accessories produced by different companies are not always interchangeable, most endoscopy units concentrate for convenience on equipment from only one manufacturer. Endoscopes are delicate and some breakages are inevitable. Only close communication, repair and back-up arrangements with an efficient company and its agents can maintain an endoscopy service. The quality of this contact is a crucial factor in choosing equipment and varies with different companies and countries.

Routine examinations are done with a long forward-viewing instrument (panendoscope). With the modern degree of tip deflection and wide-angle lens, it is usually possible to perform a complete survey of the stomach and duodenum. Some areas are slightly more difficult to see (Fig. 4.1) especially face on as is necessary for optimal tissue sampling (e.g. high lesser curve gastric ulcer), although a

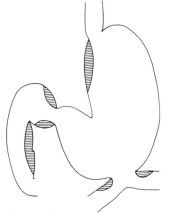

Fig. 4.1 Some areas are more difficult to see with a forward-viewing endoscope.

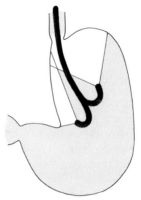
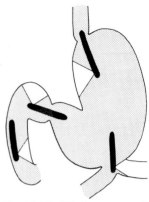
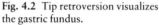

Fig. 4.2 Tip retroversion visualizes the gastric fundus.

Fig. 4.3 The blind areas are well seen with a side-viewer.

skilled endoscopist can usually achieve this by suitable manoeuvres, including tip retroversion (Fig. 4.2). The same areas are well seen with side-viewing instruments (Fig. 4.3), which are essential for examination (and cannulation) of the papilla of Vater. Rarely it may be necessary to withdraw the forward-viewing instrument, and replace it with a side-viewing endoscope. There is a trend towards smaller 'paediatric' endoscopes. These are essential for small children, and useful in patients with strictures. Surprisingly, very small experimental endoscopes (5–6 mm diameter) can be more difficult to pass than standard instruments, as the bending section is more floppy; it is easy to get lost in the pharynx unless insertion is under direct vision.

The proliferation of therapeutic techniques has lead to popularization of larger channel 'therapeutic' endoscopes. Their channel size is ≥ 3.5 mm, against the standard 2.8 mm. These channels allow passage of larger and more robust probes, and even more effective suction (e.g. blood).

Thus, a unit or clinic offering a comprehensive service for upper endoscopy should have a variety of instruments available, with back-up endoscopes for breakages, and more rapid turnover of patients without compromising disinfection procedures. For one procedure room, it is best to have available four endoscopes (two standard, one paediatric and one therapeutic). Busy units will alternate three endoscopes in one session of upper GI endoscopy. The more specialized instruments can be shared when there are several procedure rooms in use. Back-up instruments are necessary to cover breakages. Each room must have appropriate light sources and sufficient accessories (water bottles, biopsy forceps, etc.) to ensure that sterile replacements are always available.

If video-endoscopes (or CC TV systems) are selected, it is important to site the working monitor in a place convenient for the endoscopist and assistants, which means across from the patient in easy view of the endoscopist (Fig. 3.4). Patients and assistants appreciate a second monitor in a site convenient for them. If TV systems are not in use, a side-arm 'teaching attachment' must be available.

The examination

Some examiners like to start with the patients sitting up, or lying flat on their back; however, most have their patients in the left lateral position, with the head on a small pillow, covered with a disposable towel. The patient's head and neck should be in a straight longitudinal axis and not sagging, the head should be flexed forward slightly and the mouth if anything tilted downwards to facilitate dribbling or pooling of regurgitated secretions or saliva safely into the dependent parts of the mouth. Adjusting the pillow under the patient's head and having another one behind the back helps to achieve and maintain this good position. For paediatric gastroscopy ensure also that the whole of the upper body and arms are tightly swaddled in a binding sheet or blanket, so as to keep control once the procedure starts—rather than letting confusion reign, with risk to the instrument and the success of the procedure, for lack of small prior precautions. The nurse stands at the patient's head, to ensure an adequate airway (using suction as necessary), to hold or move the endoscope when instructed and to keep the mouthguard in position; this is important since bites to fingers and instruments are painful and expensive. The mouthguard should be held in such a way as not to threaten the patient's nasal airway. Some mouthguards have retaining straps. The nurse's hand should rest on the patient's head to prevent it retreating during intubation; she can also place her right arm across the patient's upper arm and chest to make it more difficult for the patient to reach up to the mouth (Fig. 4.4). Some endoscopists cover their patient's eyes; we do not.

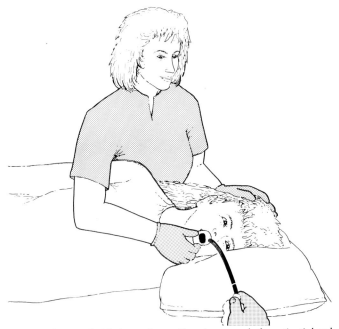

Fig. 4.4 The nurse holds the toothguard but also controls the patient's head and arms.

Passing the instrument

Pre-check the endoscope for proper functioning and lubricate the first 20–30 cm of the tip and shaft with jelly. Avoid waving the instrument around in front of a nervous patient; a little subtlety, sleight of hand, and smooth talking are appropriate at this moment.

It may sometimes be best to employ a toothguard even in edentulous patients, since this ensures the airway and also helps to keep the endoscope running in the mid-line axis during insertion. Just before insertion of the endoscope into the mouth or through the toothguard, pre-rehearse up/down movements of the controls to ensure that the tip moves in the correct longitudinal axis to follow the pharynx (Fig. 4.5). If necessary adjust the lateral knob or twist the shaft appropriately so that it does so, and tracks automatically down the mid-line, rather than impacting laterally into a piriform fossa.

There are three basic methods of passing an endoscope.

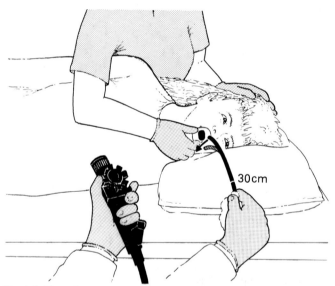

Fig. 4.5 The endoscopist pre-rehearses tip angulation in the correct axis before insertion.

Method 1 Steering down under direct vision

This is the safest, most exact, and (with a little practice) the quickest method of inserting a forward-viewing instrument. With the mouthguard in position hold the endoscope shaft at the 30-cm mark (so that changes of hand position are not needed during insertion), pre-rehearse up-angling to check the axis and then pass

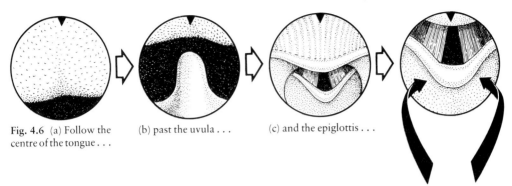

Fig. 4.6 (a) Follow the centre of the tongue . . .   (b) past the uvula . . .   (c) and the epiglottis . . .

(d) to pass below the crico-arytenoid on either side.

the tip just into the mouthguard. Look through the eyepiece or on the TV monitor for a rough, pale surface of the tongue horizontally in the upper (anterior) part of the view (Fig. 4.6a) and keep the interface between it and the red surface of the palate in the centre of view by angling up appropriately, whilst advancing inwards over the curve of the tongue. Simultaneously take care to stay in the mid-line by watching for the linear 'median raphae' of the tongue or the convexity of its mid-part, correcting if necessary by twisting the shaft; if the view is lost or the teeth are seen withdraw and start again. The uvula is often transiently seen in the lower part of the view (Fig. 4.6b). Then, as the tip advances, the epiglottis, and finally the crico-arytenoid cartilage with the vocal cords above it are visible (Fig. 4.6c). In a few patients with forcefully bulging tongues the view may be poor; in others gagging movements can be reduced by asking for deep breathing—which automatically reduces retching. The normal tonic contraction of the cricopharyngeal sphincter means that the entrance to the first, or pharyngeal, part of the oesophagus is poorly seen except transiently during swallowing. To reach it angle down (posteriorly) so that the tip passes inferior to the curve of the crico-arytenoid cartilage, preferably passing to one or other side of the mid-line since the mid-line bulge of the cartilage against the cervical spine makes central passage difficult (Fig. 4.6d). At this point there will often be a 'red-out' as the tip impacts into the crico-pharyngeal sphincter; insufflate air, keep up *gentle* inward pressure and the instrument should slip into the oesophagus within a few seconds. If necessary ask the patient to swallow, and push in quickly as the sphincter opens. Keep watching carefully to ensure smooth mucosal 'slide-by' as the instrument passes semi-blind into the upper oesophagus, for it is here that there is the occasional danger of entering a diverticulum.

Having been inserted to the cricopharyngeal region under direct vision the instrument can be guaranteed to be in the mid-line, with no possibility of impaction into one of the piriform fossae. The endoscopist can therefore have complete confidence that the instrument must pass correctly, safely and rapidly into the oesoph-agus, even when a less than perfect view is obtained. The adequate views of the region normally obtained, including the vocal chords, are a bonus denied to those using the old-fashioned 'blind' insertion technique.

Method 2 Blind tip manipulation

Standing facing the patient, the operator holds the instrument control head and tip close to each other. The nurse places the mouthguard, and holds the patient's head slightly flexed (Fig. 4.5). With the right hand, the endoscopist passes the instrument tip through the mouthguard and over the tongue to the back of the mouth; using the left thumb on the control knob, the tip is then actively deflected upwards so that it curls in the mid-line over the back of the tongue and into the mid-line of the pharynx. The tip is advanced slightly and the thumb is removed from the tip control. While slight forward pressure is maintained, the patient is asked to swallow to relax the cricopharyngeal sphincter, which lies at 15–18 cm from the incisor teeth. Most instruments have a mark at 20 cm from the tip, so the swallow is needed when that mark is just visible outside the mouthguard. As in the direct insertion method, constant reassurance and encouragement should accompany this phase (*'swallow please, this is the worst part, you've nearly done it, swallow please, well done, almost finished'*, etc.).

Passage of the tip through the cricopharyngeus is easily felt by the right hand as resistance is lost. If the tip does not pass after two or three good swallows, it is probably not in the mid-line. This can be checked by view or finger (see Method 3) but it is often better to remove the instrument, and to re-insert it after re-orientation and further reassurance to the patient.

Method 3 Finger guidance (back-up method not routinely recommended)

An assistant holds the control head of the instrument (avoiding contact with the control knobs), or the control head can be draped over the endoscopist's shoulder. The mouthguard is fitted over the shaft. The endoscopist puts the second and third fingers of his left hand over the back of the tongue. With the right hand he then passes the tip of the instrument over the tongue and uses the inserted fingers of the left hand to guide it into the mid-line of the pharynx (Fig. 4.7). The patient is asked to swallow after the fingers are withdrawn and the mouthguard is slid into place. If swallowing is not effective, the tip of the instrument has probably fallen into the left pyriform fossa; it may be necessary to re-insert a finger to lift the tip back into the mid-line.

Method 3 is probably easier for beginners or occasional endoscopists but it has hazards. The possibility of mutual infection is reduced by wearing gloves, but bites to the fingers and the instruments (unprotected by a guard at the crucial moment) can be painful and expensive. We strongly recommend Method 1—passing down under direct vision. Method 2 is applicable with lateral-viewing endoscopes, which have a smooth rounded tip. Passage of an endoscope is a co-operative venture between patient and endoscopist; rapport and safety should never be compromised by persisting when

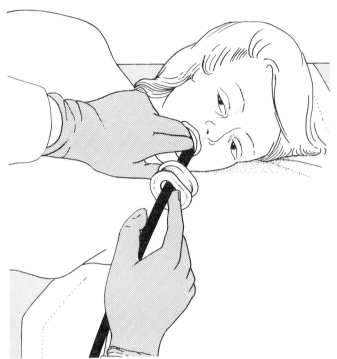

Fig. 4.7 Sometimes 'blind' insertion is helped by guiding the instrument between two fingers.

the patient is distressed. If in doubt remove the instrument and only try again when the patient is ready.

When endoscopy is performed under general anaesthesia and a laryngeal tube is in place it may be necessary to use a laryngoscope to elevate the larynx, so as to leave room to place the instrument tip in the upper oesophagus behind it. Under direct vision the endoscope follows the laryngeal tube down and then aims below it. Deflating the balloon of the endotracheal tube allows easier passage, especially of large instruments.

The routine survey

Whatever the precise indication, it is usually wise during every examination to examine the entire oesophagus, stomach and proximal duodenum where this is possible. A complete survey may sometimes be prevented by stricturing from disease or previous surgery or can be curtailed for other reasons. It is important to develop a systematic routine to reduce the possibility of missing any area.

Some endoscopists prefer to advance as quickly as possible to the duodenum, with only partial inflation of the stomach in the insertion phase so as to avoid difficulty in passing the greater curve; others complete the gastric survey before examining

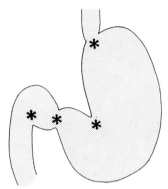

Fig. 4.8 Gastroscopy landmarks—cardia, angulus, pylorus and superior duodenal angle.

the duodenum. During examination the instrument is advanced under direct vision, using air insufflation and suction as required and delaying occasionally during active peristalsis. Mucosal views are often better during instrument withdrawal, when the organs are fully distended with air, but inspection during insertion is also important since minor trauma by the instrument tip (or excessive suction) may produce small mucosal lesions with consequent diagnostic confusion. Lesions noted during insertion are best examined in detail (and sampled for histology or cytology) following a complete routine survey of other areas.

After the cricopharyngeal sphincter, other landmarks seen during oesophagoscopy may include the indentation from the left main bronchus and pulsation of the left atrium and aorta. The most important landmarks thereafter are the: cardia, angulus of the stomach (incisura), pylorus and superior duodenal angle (Fig. 4.8). The oesophago-gastric mucosal junction is clearly seen (at 38–40 cm from the incisor teeth in adults) where pale pink squamous oesophageal mucosa abuts darker red gastric mucosa; this junction is often irregular and therefore called the 'Z-line'. The diaphragm normally clasps at or just below the oesophago-gastric junction. The position of the diaphragmatic hiatus can be highlighted by asking the patient to sniff or take deep breaths and recorded as distance (usually 38–40 cm) from the incisors. In any patient, the precise relationship of the Z-line to the diaphragmatic hiatus varies during an endoscopy (depending on the patient position, respiration, gastric distension, etc.). In normal patients, gastric mucosa is often seen at least 1 cm above the diaphragm; it is only justifiable to diagnose hiatus herniation if the Z-line remains > 2 cm above the hiatus. From the clinical point of view, however, the presence or degree of herniation is of less relevance than the presence or absence of oesophagitis.

Endoscopes are easy to pass through the cardia unless there is stenosis; the tip is simply advanced gently under direct vision. The distal oesophagus usually angles to the patient's left as it passes through the diaphragm, so it may be necessary to turn the instrument tip 'down' slightly to remain in the correct axis. Unless the cardia is unduly lax, the mucosal view is lost momentarily as the tip passes through, passage being felt by the advancing hand as a slight 'give'. If the tip is further advanced in the same plane, it will abut on the posterior wall of the lesser curvature of the stomach so that pushing in blindly risks retroflexing towards the cardia. Thus, as soon as the tip has passed through the cardia, the instrument should be rotated somewhat to the 'left' (counter-clockwise), further air inflated, and the tip withdrawn slightly to disimpact from the wall of the fundus on its posterior-greater curvature side (Fig. 4.9).

There are two golden rules of all endoscopic examinations:
1 Do not advance without vision.
2 If in doubt, withdraw.

With the patient in the left lateral position and the instrument held correctly (buttons up), the endoscopic view is predictable (Figs 4.10 and 4.11). The smooth lesser curvature is on the endoscopist's right

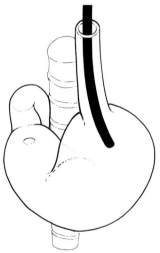

Fig. 4.9 The distal oesophagus angles the scope into the posterior wall of the lesser curve.

with the angulus distally, the longitudinal folds of the greater curve to the left and its posterior aspect below. The pool of gastric juice should be aspirated to avoid reflux or aspiration during the procedure and the stomach then inflated sufficiently to obtain a reasonable view during insertion. When the mucosal view is obscured by mucus or bubbles, it is helpful to inject a solution containing simethicone down the biopsy channel. The four walls of the stomach are examined sequentially by a combination of tip deflection, instrument rotation and advance/withdrawal. The field of view during advance of a four-way angling endoscope can be represented as a cylinder angulated over the vertebral bodies; the distended stomach takes up an exaggerated J-shape with the axis of the advancing instrument corkscrewing clockwise up and over the spine, following the greater curvature. Thus, the endoscopist, after first turning the tip to his left and somewhat down on entering the stomach, must increasingly angle it up, and rotate the shaft clockwise, following the longitudinal folds as the instrument is advanced down over the vertebral column and into the antrum (Fig. 4.12).

This clockwise corkscrew rotation through approximately 90° during insertion brings the angulus and antrum into end-on view (Fig. 4.13); downward deflection of the tip brings it into the axis of the antrum (Fig. 4.14). The antrum and pylorus should first be examined from a distance, waiting as necessary for peristaltic waves to pass.

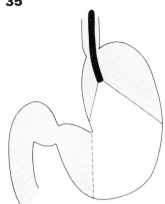

Fig. 4.10 With the gastroscope high on the lesser curve . . .

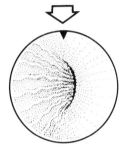

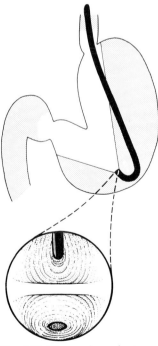

Fig. 4.11 . . . the view is of the angulus in the distance, with greater curve longitudinal folds on the left.

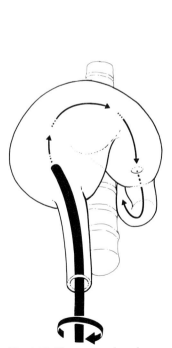

Fig. 4.12 The route to the pylorus and down the duodenum is a clockwise spiral around the vertebral column.

Fig. 4.13 The angulus and antrum come into view . . .

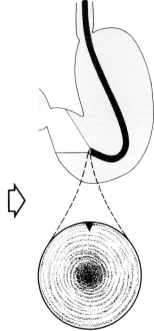

Fig. 4.14 . . . then angle down to see the pylorus in the axis of the antrum.

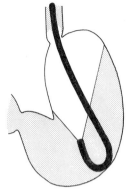

Fig. 4.15 180° angulation retroflexes the tip to see the lesser curve...

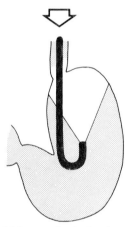

Fig. 4.16 ...and swinging the retroflexed tip around gives a view of the fundus and cardia.

Retroversion in the stomach

Complete 180° upward angulation with simultaneous inward pressure (when the tip is in the antrum and the stomach distended) retroflexes the tip and should demonstrate the angulus and the entire lesser curvature as the instrument is withdrawn (Fig. 4.15). This complete retroversion (sometimes called the J-manoeuvre) is probably best performed after examining the duodenum so as to avoid over-inflation on the way in. Some patients (particularly those with a lax cardia) find it difficult to hold enough air to permit an adequate view. This may be easier if the stomach is given more room to expand by rotating the patient slightly onto the back (but maintaining the patient's head on the side). Keeping the tip retroflexed, having examined the lesser curvature from below, the instrument shaft is rotated through 180° in either direction to swing the tip around and provide views of the greater curvature and fundus (Fig. 4.16). Close-up cardia views are obtained by withdrawing further still, again rotating the retroverted instrument as necessary.

During all these manoeuvres, try to keep the shaft of the instrument relatively straight from the patient's teeth to your hands (see Fig. 2.18). This reduces strains on the endoscope, aids orientation and ensures that rotatory movements are precisely transmitted to the tip as intended.

Having examined the proximal stomach and cardia, the instrument tip is straightened back to the neutral position. It is then again advanced past the angulus into the antrum (Fig. 4.17). The motor activity of the antrum, pyloric canal and pyloric ring should be carefully observed. Any asymmetry during a peristaltic wave is a useful indicator of present or previous disease.

Passing the pylorus

The pyloric ring is approached directly for passage into the duodenum. During this manoeuvre it is particularly convenient to use only the left hand to maintain the instrument tip in the correct axis. The left thumb controls up/down movement, and the small left/right

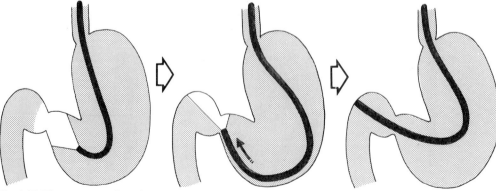

Fig. 4.17 The scope passes from the antrum...

Fig. 4.18 ...to the pylorus and duodenal cap...

Fig. 4.19 ...and tends to impact in the duodenum.

deflections are made by rotating (corkscrewing) the whole instrument, leaving the right hand free to advance and withdraw. When the pyloric ring fills the field of view, the tip is advanced and is seen or felt to pass into the duodenum cap (Figs 4.18 and 4.19), recognized by its more granular and paler surface.

As the instrument tip passes the pyloric resistance, the loop which has inevitably developed to follow the greater curvature of the stomach straightens out and accelerates the tip to the distal bulb (Fig. 4.19). This makes it necessary to withdraw the shaft considerably to disimpact the tip (insufflating some air) before a view is obtained (Fig. 4.20). Like the stomach, the bulb is scanned by circumferential manipulation of the tip during advance and withdrawal. The area immediately beyond the pyloric ring, especially the inferior part of the bulb, may be missed by the inexperienced, who fail to withdraw sufficiently for fear of falling back into the stomach. Buscopan (or glucagon) should be given if visualization is impaired by duodenal motility—but avoid excessive air insufflation, which will leave the patient uncomfortably distended.

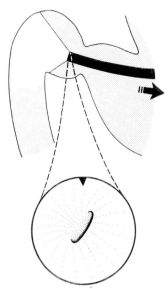

Fig. 4.20 Withdraw the scope to disimpact the tip and see the superior duodenal angle—an important landmark.

Entering the second part

Passing an instrument around the acute angle into the second part of the duodenum must be effected with care. The superior duodenal angle is the important landmark (Fig. 4.20). The instrument is advanced into the angle, so that the tip lies at the junction of the first and second parts of the duodenum. The shaft is rotated about 90° to the right, and the tip is then angled to the right and acutely up to corkscrew round the bend (Fig. 4.21), and provide a tunnel view of the descending duodenum (second part) and beyond. Paradoxically, the tip is often best advanced beyond the flexure by *withdrawing* the shaft since straightening the loop in the stomach presses the tip forwards, and the straightening shaft also corkscrews more efficiently round the superior duodenal angle (Figs 4.22 and 4.23).

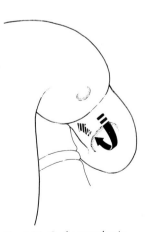

Fig. 4.21 Corkscrew the tip clockwise around the superior duodenal angle, using twist, right- and up-angulation simultaneously.

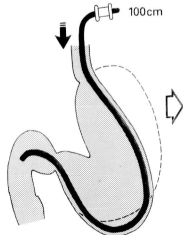

Fig. 4.22 Because of the loop in the greater curve . . .

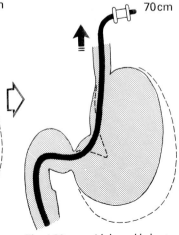

Fig. 4.23 . . . withdrawal helps to advance the scope into the second part of the duodenum.

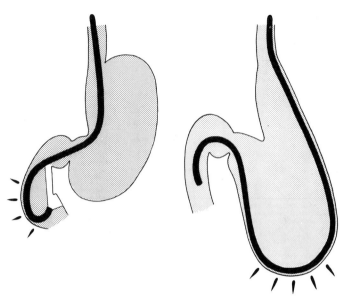

Fig. 4.24 Forceful partial retroflexion may give a view of the papilla, but take care.

Fig. 4.25 Trying to reach the third part by force simply forms a loop in the stomach.

A forward-viewing instrument gives tangential and often restricted views of the convex medial wall of the descending duodenum and the papilla of Vater. With small acute-angling instruments, it is sometimes possible to view this area more directly in a partly retroflexed manner (Fig. 4.24), but care should be taken.

Be gentle when trying to pass standard instruments further into the third part of the duodenum. Attempts at pushing simply form a loop in the stomach (Fig. 4.25). Further pressure may advance the tip but often at the cost of considerable discomfort to the patient; pulling back, deflating or even external hand pressure on the patient's upper abdomen may be more effective than just pushing.

The duodenum, stomach and oesophagus should be surveyed carefully once again during withdrawal. Under the different motility conditions and organ shapes produced by distension and instrument position, areas previously seen only tangentially on insertion may be brought into direct view on the way out.

Using a lateral-viewing endoscope

Lateral-viewing instruments are easy to swallow because they have rounded tips, but passing through the upper oesophagus is virtually blind. Nowadays few patients have a barium study before endoscopy, and the tip may be in a pharyngeal pouch or oesophageal diverticulum, or against an organic stenosis. The instrument must therefore not be pushed in forcibly when there is resistance; gentle pressure during swallowing should be sufficient. On the rare occasions when it is ineffective, the side-viewing instrument should

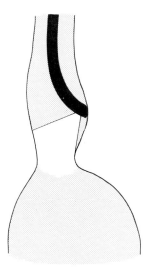

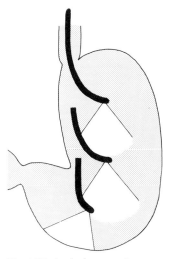

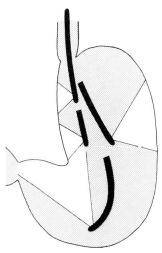

Fig. 4.26 Examination of the oesophagus is possible with a side-viewer by angling down, but take care.

Fig. 4.27 Angle down to give a forward view before advancing the side-viewer.

Fig. 4.28 Rotating the side-viewer gives face-on views of the whole stomach.

be withdrawn and the situation reviewed; the patient may need radiology or initial examination with a forward-viewing instrument.

Although a tunnel view is not obtained, most of the distal oesophagus can be seen with lateral-viewing instruments if air is insufflated and the tip angled slightly 'down' whilst pushing in or pulling out (Fig. 4.26). Excessive angulation may be hazardous and force should not be used.

Slight resistance is normally felt at the cardia (38–40 cm from the teeth), followed by the characteristic 'give' as the tip is advanced through it using gentle pressure. The instrument tip is then angled 'down' in the proximal stomach to view forwards; air is insufflated to obtain a view and any gastric juice aspirated. Advancing the endoscope through the body of the stomach with the tip angled down provides axial views (Fig. 4.27) similar to those given by a forward-viewing instrument with its tip straight. When rotated in the straight position, lateral-viewing instruments provide excellent face-on views of all four walls of the proximal stomach (Fig. 4.28). The cardia is seen if the endoscope is passed to the greater curvature and angled up (Fig. 4.29).

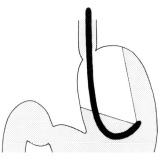

Fig. 4.29 Rotate to the greater curve and angle up to see the cardia with a side-viewer.

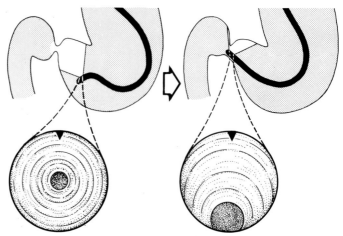

Fig. 4.30 Angle down to see the pylorus . . .

Fig. 4.31 . . . then angle up to let the tip enter the pyloric canal with a 'setting sun' view.

Passage of a lateral-viewing endoscope through the pylorus is partially a blind manoeuvre but provides no difficulty with experience. The tip is advanced through the antrum with a slight 'down' tip deflection to keep the pylorus in view (Fig. 4.30, top), whilst sliding the shaft in and around the greater curvature of the stomach. When close to the pyloric ring, the tip is angled 'up' into the neutral position (or slightly beyond it) and advanced (Fig. 4.31, top). The ideal view of the pylorus during this manoeuvre is described as the 'setting-sun' (Fig. 4.31, bottom). In a capacious stomach, the pylorus may 'set' out of the field of view, and some spatial judgement is needed to move the tip over the pylorus, then angling forcibly downwards so as to enter it blindly. This procedure may be even more difficult with some first-generation side-viewing videoscopes which have a longer tip beyond the viewing lens.

Passage through the pyloric ring is felt rather than seen; success depends upon having the instrument in the central axis of the antrum. If in difficulty, withdraw and check this orientation by angling the tip up. The angulus should be seen square on, not obliquely, so that further upward angulation would show the instrument shaft passing down the mid-line of the greater curvature of the gastric body (Fig. 4.32). The lateral angling controls or shaft twist should be used to achieve the correct mid-line position.

When the instrument passes the pylorus, the springiness of the redundant loop in the stomach propels the tip to the distal bulb (as with forward-viewing endoscopes (Fig. 4.19) resulting in a 'red-out'. Views are obtained only after withdrawing the instrument slightly, angling the tip sharply down (lens away from the mucosa) and insufflating some air; the tip is then virtually hooked in the pyloric ring, and the view is similar to that obtained with a forward-viewing endoscope (Fig. 4.33). The roof of the bulb is seen face-on, and lateral tip deflection and rotation provide views of the anterior and posterior walls. The inferior part or floor of the bulb is more

Pylorus   Endoscope

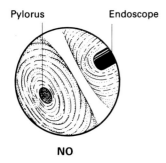

NO

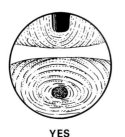

YES

Fig. 4.32 Use twist or the lateral control to square up the angulus before passing into the pylorus.

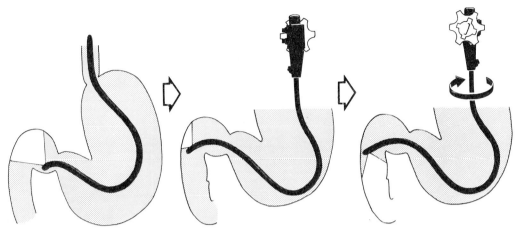

Fig. 4.33 Angle the tip down and withdraw into a hooked position to see the duodenum and cap . . .

Fig. 4.34 . . . then angle up again to advance over the superior duodenal angle . . .

Fig. 4.35 . . . and rotate 90° clockwise, whilst angling right and up, to view the descending duodenum.

difficult to survey; there is a tendency to fall back into the antrum during the necessary acute clockwise rotation.

Passing a lateral-viewing endoscope around the superior duodenal angle into the descending duodenum requires a corkscrew manoeuvre as used with forward-viewing instruments and also described and illustrated in detail in the context of ERCP (Chapter 6). From the bulb viewing position (Fig. 4.33), the tip is angled up to the neutral position and advanced until it is over the superior duodenal angle to the entry of the descending duodenum (Fig. 4.34). The tip is then angled acutely *right* and *up* at the same time as the instrument is rotated about 90° clockwise; this corkscrew rotation produces a tunnel view of the descending duodenum with its medial wall and ampulla in the upper part of the view (Fig. 4.35). Further tip advance can sometimes be achieved by simple pushing, but again (paradoxically) this is *much better done by pulling back*, which shortens the loop in the greater curve of the stomach—as in forward-viewing endoscopy (Fig. 4.23) and with the same resulting passage down the duodenum. When the shaft has been straightened (< 70 cm inside the patient), the tip lies beyond the papilla of Vater. The descending duodenum is surveyed on withdrawal, using tip manipulation and rotation.

Problems during endoscopy

Patient distress

Endoscopy should be quickly terminated if any patient shows distress, the cause of which is not immediately obvious and remediable. Many patients have an understandable anxiety about choking. The airway should be checked and any residual oral sections aspirated. If reassurance does not calm the patient, remove the instrument. If the cause is anxiety, extra pethidine (Demerol) is more effective than additional benzodiazepine (diazepam, midazolam), and will usually allow the procedure to be attempted again. Inadvertent bronchoscopy is not rare and is usually obvious from the unusual view and impressive coughing. Severe pain during endoscopy is very rare and indicates a complication such as perforation or a cardiac incident. Discomfort may arise from inappropriate pressure during intubation or excessive air insufflation. Elderly patients and those who abuse alcohol may become agitated through confusion. Discomfort after the procedure may be reduced if most of the insufflated air is sucked out of the stomach before withdrawal.

Getting lost

The endoscopist may become disorientated, and the instrument looped, in patients with congenital malrotations, major pathology (achalasia, large diverticula and hernias, cup and spill deformities) and after complex surgery. Careful study of any available radiographs should help. The commonest reason for disorientation in patients with normal anatomy is inadequate air insufflation due to a defect in the instrument or air pump (which should have been detected before starting the examination). Excessive air insufflation is uncomfortable and potentially dangerous. Most sedated patients are able to belch; but if performing endoscopy under general anaesthesia, it is wise to keep the abdomen exposed so that over-inflation can be detected. Inexperienced endoscopists often get lost in the fundus, especially when the stomach is angled acutely over the vertebral column. Having passed through the cardia into the stomach, the tip should be deflected to the endoscopist's left and slightly downwards (Fig. 4.36) into the main axis. A wrong turn to the right here brings the tip back up into the fundus. When in doubt, withdraw, insufflate, and turn *left* before rotating clockwise and

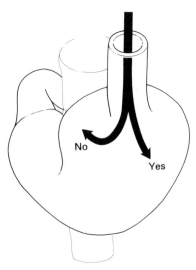

Fig. 4.36 Angling right (rather than left) on entering the fundus can cause retroflexion and result in getting lost.

inwards around the vertebral column, following the longitudinal folds down the stomach.

A curious endoscopic view may indicate perforation (which is not always immediately painful). If in any doubt, abandon the examination and obtain radiological studies.

No consistent mucosal view

Lack of a clear view means that the lens is lying against the mucosa or is obscured by fluid or food debris. Withdraw slightly and insufflate air; check that the air pump is working and that all connections are firm (which again should have been done before starting). Try washing the lens with the normal finger-controlled water jet. This may not be effective if the instrument lens is covered by debris (or mucosa) which has been sucked onto the orifice of the biopsy channel. Pressure can be released by brief removal of the rubber cap of the biopsy port, but it may be necessary to flush with water or air using a syringe.

Food residue

Small quantities of food or mucus obscuring an area of interest can be washed away with a jet of water. Foaming can be suppressed by adding a few drops of simethicone. Since most patients obey instructions to fast beforehand, the presence of excessive residue is an important sign of outlet obstruction. Standard endoscope channels are too small for aspiration of food; prolonged attempts simply result in blocked channels. The instrument can usually be guided along the lesser curvature over the top of the food to allow a search for a distal obstructing lesion. The greater curvature can also be examined if necessary by rotating the patient into the right lateral position. However, any examination in the presence of excess fluid or food carries a significant risk of regurgitation and pulmonary aspiration. The endoscopist should only persist if the immediate benefits are thought to justify the risk. It is usually wiser to stop and to repeat the examination only after proper lavage.

Remember to take the brakes off

The tip deflection controls include a braking system so that the tip can be fixed in any desired position. This facility is particularly useful when the hands are needed elsewhere, e.g. for biopsy sampling and photography. However, it is easy to forget to release the breaks before withdrawing the instrument, with potential hazard to the oesophagus.

Recognition of lesions

This book is concerned with the techniques rather than lesions. We recommend that beginners should study several of the excellent atlases which are now available. Certain points may be worth emphasis here.

Oesophagus

Oesophagitis normally follows acid reflux and is most apparent distally close to the mucosal junction. There is no clear macroscopic dividing line from normality; the earliest changes consist of mucosa congestion and oedema, which obscure the normal fine vascular pattern. At a more advanced stage, the mucosa becomes friable and bleeds easily on touching; there are patches of exudate and areas of reddening or ulceration, usually in the long axis of the oesophagus. The process culminates in a symmetrical stricture above which the mucosa (now protected from reflux) may appear almost normal.

Stricturing from primary oesophageal *carcinoma* is usually asymmetrical; there are areas of exuberant abnormal mucosa and raised edges to any ulcer. However, carcinoma of the gastric fundus may infiltrate upwards submucosally. The correct diagnosis is then easily made if the endoscope can be passed through the stricture to allow retroverted views of the cardia. Biopsies are taken to determine squamous or adenocarcinoma type.

Monilial oesophagitis (thrush) is characterized by white spots or plaques which do not readily wash off with a jet of water whereas milk residues do; moniliasis may occur in any part of the oesophagus.

Diverticula in the mid- or distal oesophagus are easily recognized, but the instrument may enter a pulsion diverticulum or pouch in the upper oesophagus without the true lumen being seen at all. Lack of view and resistance to inward movement are, as always during endoscopy, an indication to pull back and reassess. *Webs or rings*, such as the Schatski ring at or just proximal to the oesophago-gastric junction, may not be obvious to the endoscopist due to a combination of 'flat' bright illumination and the wide-angled lens view. If in doubt, skilled radiology (with video-taping) should be used to define the situation before therapeutic endoscopy.

Varices are usually obvious; they lie in the long axis of the oesophagus as tortuous bluish mounds covered with relatively normal mucosa and resemble varicose veins elsewhere in the body.

A *Mallory–Weiss tear* is a 5–20 mm mucosal split in the longitudinal axis of the oesophagus, lying either side of or across the oesophago-gastric mucosal junction. In the acute phase the tear is covered with exudate or clot and may sometimes be best seen in a retroverted view. When healing there is unimpressive linear ulceration.

Motility disturbances of the oesophagus should be diagnosed by radiology and manometry, but their consequences such as dilatation, pseudodiverticula, food retention and oesophagitis are well seen at endoscopy which is virtually always needed to rule out obstructing pathology. Hypermotility is probable when recurrent oesophageal contractions are seen in spite of antispasmodics and sedation.

The endoscope passes easily through the cardia of *achalasia*, in contrast to the fixed narrowing of some strictures whether from reflux oesophagitis or malignancy.

Stomach

The appearance of even normal gastric mucosa varies considerably.

Reddening (hyperaemia) may be generalized (particularly with bile reflux into the operated stomach), or localized, and sometimes occurs in long streaks along the ridges of mucosal folds. Localized (traumatic) reddening with or without petechiae or oedematous changes occurs in the posterior part of the upper lesser curve from patients who habitually retch from dysfunction or alcohol abuse. Macroscopic congestion does not correlate well with underlying histological gastritis, and care should be taken when considering clinical relevance. Biopsy samples should be taken from any odd-looking mucosa.

Gastric folds vary in size but the endoscopic assessment also depends upon the degree of gastric distension. Very prominent fleshy folds remain in spite of distension in Ménétrièr's disease, best diagnosed by a snare-loop biopsy. Patients with aggressive duodenal ulceration may have fleshy and oedematous gastric folds with spotty areas of congestion within the areae gastricae, and excess quantities of clear resting juice. With gastric atrophy, there are no mucosal folds when the stomach is distended and blood vessels are easily seen through the pale atrophic mucosa. Atrophy is often associated with intestinal metaplasia which appears as small grey–white plaques.

Erosions and *ulcers* are the commonest localized gastric lesions. A lesion is usually called an erosion at endoscopy if it is one of many, small (< 5 mm diameter) and shallow with no sign of scarring. Acute ulcers and erosions are most commonly seen in the antrum and are often capped with, and partially obscured by, clot. Oedematous erosions appear as small, smooth umbilicated raised areas often in chains along the folds of the gastric body. When these are multiple (and probably chronic) the condition has been called 'chronic erosive gastritis'. However, gastritis is a term best reserved for histological use.

The classical chronic benign *gastric ulcer* is usually single and is most frequently seen on the lesser curvature at, or above, the angulus. It is typically symmetrical with smooth margins and a clean base (unless eroding adjacent structures). Multiple, or very large but superficial, ulcers occur in patients on NSAID therapy. Features favouring *malignancy* include raised irregular margins (or different heights around the circumference), an irregular lumpy haemorrhagic base, and mucosal abnormality surrounding the ulcer. Mucosal folds around a benign ulcer usually radiate towards it and reach the margin. Inexperienced endoscopists cannot hope to separate benign from malignant ulcers on macroscopic appearance alone, and tissue specimens must be taken.

Outside Japan, gastric cancer is usually diagnosed at an advanced stage and is all too obvious at endoscopy, although diffusely infiltrating carcinomas (linitis plastica) may be missed unless motility is carefully studied. True early gastric cancer may mimic a small benign ulcer, chronic erosion or flat polyp, and its significance is usually missed unless biopsies are routinely taken of any possible abnormality seen. *Polypoid lesions* of < 1 cm in diameter in the stomach are usually inflammatory in origin, but the macroscopic distinction between adenoma and early carcinoma is impossible. Since all malignant lesions start small and are curable if detected at an early stage, odd mucosal lumps and bumps should not be ignored. Suitable specimens must be taken and follow-up arranged. *Submucosal tumours* are characterized by normal overlying mucosa and bridging folds; leiomyomas and plaques of aberrant pancreatic tissue usually have a central dimple or crater.

Duodenum

Persistent deformity of the pyloric ring indicates present or previous ulceration. *Duodenal ulcers* occur most commonly on the anterior and posterior walls of the bulb and are frequently multiple (kissing ulcers). When active they are surrounded by oedema and acute congestion. Scarring often results in a characteristic shelf-like deformity which partially divides the bulb and may produce a pseudodiverticulum; a small linear ulcer or scar is seen running along the apex of this fold. Between small ulcers and normality lie a number of mucosal changes of dubious clinical significance. Small areas of mucosal congestion with spotty white exudate ('pepper and salt ulceration') merge into even less definite macroscopic appearances labelled as 'duodenitis'. Minor mucosal changes should be described but not overemphasized. Primary duodenal tumours are rare and papillary lesions will be described elsewhere. Small mucosal lumps in the proximal duodenum usually reflect underlying Brunner's gland hyperplasia or ectopic islands of gastric mucosa (gastric metaplasia).

Dye-spraying techniques

Inconspicuous lesions may be recognized more easily if a dye is sprayed over the mucosal surface; the dye fills the interstices, highlighting irregularities in architecture. Methylene blue has been used most frequently, but simple pen ink (1:5 dilution of washable blue) is adequate. Best coating is achieved by spraying with a tube and fine nozzle, applied close to the mucosa.

An alternative approach to lesion enhancement is the use of intra-vital staining. Dyes placed onto the mucosa or injected intravenously may be taken up preferentially in diseased mucosa (such as intestinal metaplasia) and be recognizable directly or under special conditions such as ultraviolet illumination.

Taking tissue specimens

Using the correct endoscopes and techniques, tissue specimens can be taken for histological or cytological examination from any lesion seen in the oesophagus, stomach or duodenum. The relative value of forceps biopsy and brush cytology varies between different institutions and specialists. When working closely with an interested cytopathologist, it may be correct to use cytology as well as biopsy on every lesion. However, most centres rely mainly on biopsy, reserving cytology for lesions from which good biopsy specimens are difficult to obtain, such as tight oesophageal strictures.

Cytology specimens are taken under direct vision with a sleeved brush (Fig. 2.9) which is passed through the instrument channel. The head of the brush is advanced out of its sleeve, and rubbed and rolled repeatedly across the surface of the lesion; a circumferential sweep of the margin and base of an ulcer is desirable. The brush is then pulled back into the sleeve, both withdrawn together and left until the end of the procedure, as the sleeve protects the brush specimens from drying out. When convenient the brush is protruded, wiped over two to three glass slides and then rapidly fixed before drying damages the cells. The precise method of preparation (in the GI Unit or Cytology Laboratory) is determined by the preferences of the local cytologist. Most brushes are disposable, and should not be re-used. Those designed for re-use must be carefully washed and soaked in detergent to lyse any residual cells. Inadequate washing followed by glutaraldehyde or alcohol disinfection risks fixing whole cells in the bristles and causing serious errors of interpretation.

Biopsy specimens are taken with cupped forceps (Fig. 2.7). Those with a central spike make it easier to take specimens from lesions which have to be approached tangentially (as is often the case in the oesophagus), but carry an increased risk of accidental skin puncture and are best avoided. It is always preferable to approach a lesion face-on, so that firm and direct pressure can be applied to it with the widely opened cups; the forceps are then gently closed by an assistant and withdrawn. At least six good specimens should be taken from any lesion—perfectionists would ask for many more. Ulcer biopsies should include samples from the base and from the ulcer rim in all four quadrants; basal specimens are sometimes diagnostic, but usually yield only slough. When sampling proliferative tumours, it is wise to take several specimens from the same place to penetrate the outer necrotic layer. A larger final tumour biopsy may be obtained by grabbing a protuberant area but deliberately *not* pulling the forceps into the instrumentation channel but withdrawing the instrument with the specimen still at the tip. The methods for handling and fixing specimens should be established in each centre after discussion with the relevant pathologist; some prefer samples to be gently flattened on paper or other surfaces such as cellulose acetate filter (Millipore, etc.) or sliced cucumber. The cellulose filter method of biopsy mounting has considerable advantages for the management of multiple small endoscopic biopsies. They adhere well to the filter and are rarely lost, are mounted in sequence so that errors of location are impossible, and

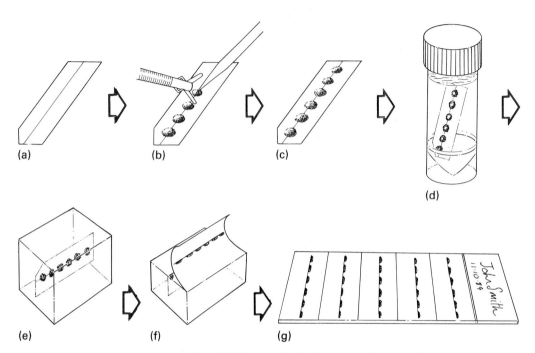

(a)   (b)   (c)   (d)

(e)   (f)   (g)

Fig. 4.37 Stages in placing biopsies on filter, then fixing, sectioning and mounting.

allow the histopathologist to view serial sections of six to eight biopsies at a time in a row across a single microscope slide. A 15-mm strip of cellulose filter (just less than the width of a glass slide) has a pencil-ruled or printed central line, and a notch or mark made at one end (Fig. 4.37a). Each biopsy as it is taken is eased out of the forceps cup with a micropipette tip (Fig. 4.37b) to avoid needle stick injuries, exactly onto the line, and patted flat (Fig. 4.37c). The strip with its line of biopsies is placed into fixative (Fig. 4.37d), then wax-mounted in correct orientation in the laboratory (Fig. 4.37e), sectioned (Fig. 4.37f), positioned on the microscope slide (Fig. 4.37g), and stained and examined without handling the biopsies individually at any stage.

A dissecting microscope or hand lens can be used to orientate mucosal specimens before fixation if information is required about mucosal architecture (e.g. duodenal biopsies in malabsorption). All specimens should reach the laboratory with precise details of their site of origin and the specific clinical question requiring an answer. A pathologist who routinely receives a copy of the endoscopy findings, and timely follow-up, is more likely to give relevant reports.

Biopsy and cytology sites often bleed trivially, but sometimes sufficiently to obscure the lesion before adequate samples have been taken; if so, the area should be washed with a jet of water or dilute adrenaline. Bleeding of clinical significance is exceptionally rare.

Standard biopsy forceps rarely traverse the muscularis mucosa, so that histology is usually normal in patients with submucosal lesions, such as benign tumours and lymphomas. Larger and deeper specimens can be taken with a diathermy snare loop; the technique is described with polypectomy in Chapter 10. Larger specimens can also be taken with experimental large jawed forceps, which have to be 'muzzled-loaded', i.e. the forceps are threaded backwards up the biopsy channel, before the instrument is passed into the patient—with an overtube (Fig. 2.13)—to protect the pharynx and oesophagus during intubation. An alternative method for obtaining deeper tissue is to use a needle to obtain aspiration samples for cytology.

A trap (Fig. 2.10) can be used to collect cytology specimens. It has been shown that suction through the channel after a biopsy procedure also produces useful cellular material ('salvage cytology').

Diagnostic endoscopy under special circumstances

Operated patients

It is often difficult to interpret barium radiographs taken in patients who have previously undergone surgery to the oesophagus, stomach and duodenum. Unless prevented by postoperative stenosis, endoscopy allows an excellent mucosal survey and is the best method for diagnosis and exclusion of recurrent ulcers and tumours. The endoscopist can document the size and arrangement of any outlet or anastomosis, but standard radiology and other techniques give more information about motility and disorders of emptying. Experience is needed to appreciate the wide range of 'normal' endoscopic appearance in the operated patient.

Partial gastrectomy, gastroenterostomy and pyloroplasty result in reflux of bile and intestinal juice; resultant foaming in the stomach may obscure the endoscopic view and should be suppressed by flushing with a solution containing simethicone. Gastric distension is difficult to maintain in patients with a large gastric outlet; avoid pumping in more air and distending the intestine. Most patients who have undergone partial gastrectomy or gastro-enterostomy have impressively hyperaemic mucosae. Initially this is most marked close to the stoma, but atrophic gastritis is progressive and plaques of grey–white intestinal metaplasia may be seen. There is an increased risk of cancer in the gastric remnant, particularly close to the stoma. Many cancers in this site have not been recognized endoscopically; during endoscopy of an operated stomach the opportunity should be taken to obtain multiple biopsy and cytology specimens from within 3 cm of the stoma—in every case, whatever the level of suspicion.

Ulcers following partial gastrectomy or gastroenterostomy usually occur at, or just beyond, the anastomosis. Endoscopic diagnosis is usually simple, but the area just beneath the stoma may sometimes be difficult to survey completely using a forward-viewing instrument. A lateral-viewing endoscope may also sometimes allow a more complete survey in a scarred and tortuous pyloro-plasty. Many surgeons use non-absorbable sutures when performing intestinal anastomosis. These can ulcerate through the mucosa and appear as black and green threads and loops. Their clinical significance remains controversial; when sutures are associated with ulcers, it is justifiable to attempt their removal with biopsy forceps or with a diathermy snare loop. Endoscopy is occasionally performed (for bleeding or stomal obstruction) within a few days of upper GI tract surgery; air insufflation should be kept to a minimum.

Acute upper GI bleeding

Endoscopy is more accurate than barium radiology in the diagnosis of patients admitted after haematemesis and melaena. Examinations should be performed by an experienced endoscopist within 24 hours, or earlier as an emergency (i.e. as soon as intravenous lines have been established and initial volume replacement achieved) in certain circumstances. Indications for more urgent endoscopy are as follows:
1 When there is evidence of continued active bleeding requiring immediate intervention.
2 When varices are suspected.
3 When the patient has had an aortic graft.
4 To check the upper tract before severe rectal bleeding is attributed to a colonic source.

Blood in the stomach and duodenum may obscure the view, but routine lavage is often not effective. We use a large channel 'thera-peutic' endoscope which does allow some flushing and suction of liquid blood. When views are totally inadequate (< 5% of cases), we remove the instrument, perform lavage immediately with a large bore tube and repeat the endoscopy. An alternative approach is to start the endoscopy with an overtube in place (Fig. 2.13). If excessive blood is encountered, lavage can be performed through the overtube and the endoscope replaced without difficulty. Changes of position can help (viz. right lateral or head up). When an urgent diagnosis is required but the endoscopic view is persistently obscured by blood (or the examination is poorly tolerated), the procedure should be repeated under general anaesthesia—preferably in the operating room with the surgeon in attendance and ready to proceed if necessary. A cuffed endotracheal tube abolishes the risk of regurgi-tation and aspiration, and allows generous gastric lavage where necessary. It is difficult to provide an endoscopic diagnosis when the patient is bleeding massively, but it should be possible at least to give the surgeon information about the oesophagus. Angiography also has a role in this context, where immediately available.

The lesions which cause acute bleeding are well known, but endoscopy has highlighted the importance of certain lesions which were rarely visualized by radiology, e.g. oesophagitis (especially in elderly recumbent patients) and Mallory–Weiss tears. About 20% of all bleeding patients are found to have two or more mucosal lesions (e.g. duodenal ulcer and acute gastric erosions). Thus a complete examination of the oesophagus, stomach and duodenum should be performed in every bleeding patient, no matter what is seen *en route*. A lesion should only be incriminated as the bleeding source if it is actually bleeding at the time of the examination, or is covered with clot which cannot be washed off with a jet of water. An ulcer whose base is haemorrhagic or contains a visible vessel (i.e. stigmas of recent haemorrhage), can be assumed to have bled recently. If the patient has presented with haematemesis, and endoscopy shows only a single lesion (even without any of these features), it is likely to be the bleeding source. This is not necessarily so if the presentation has been with melaena or if the examination takes place more than 48 hours after bleeding, since acute lesions such as Mallory–Weiss tears and erosions may already have healed.

Biopsy and cytology samples are usually not taken acutely from bleeding lesions. Endoscopy should be repeated for this purpose and general reassessment after the acute phase, if the patient has not been submitted to surgery.

Endoscopy is sometimes poorly tolerated by young drinkers, in whom diazepam sedation is often ineffective, indeed sometimes counterproductive; pethidine (Demerol) may be helpful. If the patient is well motivated, the examination can be performed without sedation. Since most young drinkers have acute lesions with a low risk of re-bleeding, attempts at endoscopy should not be prolonged.

The main problem of emergency endoscopy is organizing and maintaining an efficient expert service. Examinations should not be delegated to those early in training. Although it is essential to have an emergency rota, many cases can be fitted into normal working hours. In hospitals receiving many bleeding patients, an emergency endoscope trolley (cart) should be set up each evening equipped with appropriate endoscopes, light source and all accessories, which can be taken to the operating room or intensive care unit when necessary. It is also essential to have specially trained GI nurses on emergency call. These emergency examinations are amongst the most hazardous for patients and instruments as well as the most demanding for the endoscopist if a diagnosis is to be made or excluded with confidence or therapeutic procedures attempted. Fast, efficient assistance can make the difference between success and failure, especially in therapeutic interventions. Details of endoscopic haemostatic techniques are given in Chapter 5.

Endoscopy in children

Paediatric endoscopy is simple with appropriate instruments and preparation; examination techniques are similar to those used in adults, but a paediatrician equipped with the necessary paediatric resuscitation experience and equipment should always be present. The smaller (9–10 mm diameter) adult forward- and lateral-viewing instruments can be used down to the age of about 2 years. Smaller 'paediatric' instruments can be used even in neonates, but a bronchoscope may be needed to pass the pylorus or examine a premature baby.

Endoscopy can be performed with little or no sedation in the first year of life. Fasted babies usually swallow the instrument avidly. Some endoscopists prefer to use general anaesthesia beyond this age and into the mid-teens, but many are satisfied with heavy sedation alone—benzodiazepine and pethidine (Demerol). Even an apparently calm or well-sedated child may suddenly become briefly uncontrollable during insertion and it is essential to swaddle the upper body and arms completely within a blanket before beginning, and to have an experienced nurse in charge of the mouthguard (and sucker). There is a risk of excessive insufflation when using heavy sedation or anaesthesia; it is wise to keep the abdomen exposed during examination and to palpate it regularly. Careful monitoring of oxygenation and pulse is essential; impending shock in a neonate is indicated by the baby suddenly becoming still and floppy and this is an indication to abort the procedure rapidly.

Complications and precautions

Upper GI endoscopy should be a safe procedure, but there are many potential hazards. Operative endoscopy and diathermy procedures have specific risks. Large surveys suggest that simple diagnostic endoscopy carries a risk of significant complications in about one in 1000 procedures, and of death in about one in 10 000. Problems are more likely to be encountered in the elderly and acutely ill, and during emergency procedures. The most important factors are inexperience, incompetence and over-sedation.

Patient monitoring

The trained GI nurse/endoscopy assistant is the guardian of the patient's safety during the examination, whilst the doctor may be preoccupied with the technical aspects. The nurse must ensure that the airway and respiration are maintained, and keep a check on the pulse. Many centres recommend the use of a pulse oximeter during all endoscopies in which sedation is used. Oxygen, resuscitation equipment, and antidotes to sedatives (naloxone, adnexate) must be immediately available.

Medication reactions

Reactions may arise from idiosyncrasy or overdosage. Allergy to local anaesthetics is not unusual, and should always be checked prior to examination. Small doses of sedatives may produce coma in patients with respiratory or hepatic insufficiency. Medication problems may occur after patients leave the unit. Prolonged effects of various sedatives may affect co-ordination and judgement, and patients must not drive or operate machinery the same day. Anti-cholinergics will not affect treated glaucoma, but may precipitate an acute painful attack in occult chronic glaucoma, which is a good thing since it leads to diagnosis and appropriate treatment. There is therefore no ocular contraindication to the use of anticholinergics. Superficial thrombosis occasionally occurs at injection sites; the glycol carrier medium used for diazepam is particularly irritating and should not be given into small veins. Diazepam in lipid emulsion form (Diazemuls) or water-soluble midazolam (Versed) do not carry this risk.

Pulmonary problems

Mild hypoxia has been shown to be a common event with standard medication regimes, but hypoxia can be severe. The risk is best prevented by oximeter monitoring, and appropriate action (stimulation, oxygen, injection of antidotes) when it occurs. Aspiration pneumonia can also occur, especially in patients with oesophago-gastric retention (e.g. achalasia, pyloric stenosis) or in those with active bleeding. Aspiration is more likely to occur in elderly patients, and when the gag reflex has been suppressed by pharyngeal anaesthesia and excessive sedation.

Perforation

All levels in the upper gut have been perforated. Such accidents are more common in the pharynx and cervical oesophagus where the endoscope is passed blindly, but can also occur at the cardia and superior duodenal angle, especially when these areas are distorted or diseased. Perforation is more likely to occur during therapeutic dilatation, either when passing a stiff guidewire blindly or during the dilatation itself. Incompetence and imprudent force are usually responsible, but excessive air insufflation alone may occasionally result in perforation of an existing lesion. Perforation in the neck and mediastinum is immediately painful, but more distal perforation may not be immediately apparent. Perforation may be obvious (from a bizarre view), or later by subsequent development of subcutaneous emphysema, and by the characteristic appearances on abdominal radiographs. The management of evident or suspected perforation is discussed in Chapter 5 (oesophageal dilation).

Instrumental impaction

The tip of a highly flexible endoscope can impact in a hiatus hernia or the distal oesophagus during the retroversion manoeuvre. Blind and forceful withdrawal should not be attempted if impaction has occurred. Disimpaction is best achieved by *advancing* the instrument if necessary under fluoroscopic guidance. Rarely, a mechanical failure in a diagnostic device (cytology brush, biopsy forceps, or snare loop) may prevent its withdrawal through the instrument tip; the instrument and device must be carefully withdrawn together.

Bleeding

Endoscopic forceps biopsy carries a small risk of immediate or delayed bleeding in patients with impaired coagulation and in those with portal hypertension; biopsies should be undertaken only after due consideration. Aggravation of bleeding during urgent endoscopy is difficult to detect or disprove. Bleeding is more common after therapeutic procedures.

Cardiac dysrhythmias

Like other instrumental procedures, endoscopy can sometimes induce cardiac dysrhythmias (especially during periods of hypoxia), which are a potent source of the rare endoscopic fatalities. ECG monitoring (and oximetry) is advisable when endoscopy is performed in patients with cardiac problems. Full resuscitation equipment must always be available.

Transmission of infection

These problems are discussed in Chapter 12.

Selection of patients

A full assessment of the clinical role of upper GI endoscopy is outside the scope of this book. It varies with local circumstances, and the available radiological and endoscopic expertise.

Initially, endoscopy was mainly used to examine patients who had undergone barium studies which had not completely answered the clinical question, or had raised other questions. The endoscopic task was then straightforward, for the precise target and question were defined. However, even in such patients, a complete endoscopic survey should be performed in case other lesions are present. Nowadays, endoscopy has taken over the primary role in most situations, which makes the task more difficult and the endoscopist's responsibility greater, to achieve both accuracy and a high level of safety and patient acceptability. The examiner must be capable of doing a complete and reliable survey of the oesophagus, stomach and proximal duodenum. It is relatively easy to see, describe and sample a lesion, but much more experience and skill is needed to say that no lesion is present.

Endoscopy takes particular precedence over barium studies in bleeding and operated patients. The experienced examiner knows that endoscopy can also provide important information in many other patients whether radiographic reports are positive, negative or equivocal. Why not short-cut the whole process, eliminate the barium meal and endoscope everybody? This is a difficult question which each gastroenterologist and endoscopy unit must answer. Radiology is easier for the patient and has few direct complications. However, an incorrect diagnosis can also be hazardous, and endoscopy has greater diagnostic potential.

Much depends on local circumstances. Hospital based endoscopy units in some countries (including Britain) can have difficulty in coping even with selective referrals. The situation is different in private practice. The gastroenterologist with endoscopic skills may see little purpose in submitting patients to radiology when he has the ability to provide a precise diagnosis backed up by histology and cytology. In these circumstances, he will use barium studies only for the investigation of motility and outlet problems, and to provide a road map to show strictures or gross morphology prior to complex surgery.

Although endoscopes appear to be an expensive example of Western 'high-tech' medicine, they are cost effective and have become popular in developing countries, largely because X-ray facilities are far more expensive and good radiologists are rare.

The need for intermittent endoscopic surveillance in patients with pre-malignant conditions of the oesophagus and stomach (e.g. Barrett's oesophagus, pernicious anaemia, gastric polyps and the operated stomach) remains controversial. However, extra vigilance should be employed during any endoscopy on such patients, and it should be realized that significant lesions may be detected on biopsy even when visual appearances are not suggestive.

Further reading

Axon, A. T. R. (1989) 'Endoscopy of the the small bowel and duodenum', in *Annual of Gastrointestinal Endoscopy*. Current Science, London.

Cotton, P. B. (1973) 'Fibre optic endoscopy and the barium meal—results and implications'. *British Medical Journal*, **2**, 161.

Gilbert, D. A. and Silverstein F. E. (1987) 'Endoscopy in gastrointestinal bleeding', in *Gastroenterologic Endoscopy* (ed. Sivak, M. V.). W. B. Saunders, Philadelphia.

Habr-Gama, A. and Waye, J. D. (1989) 'Complications and hazards of gastrointestinal endoscopy'. *World Journal of Surgery*, **13**, 193–201.

Kleinman, R. E. (1989) 'Pediatric endoscopy', in *Annual of Gastrointestinal Endoscopy*. Current Science, London.

Misiewicz, J. J. *et al.* (1987) *Atlas of Clinical Gastroenterology*. Gower Medical Publishing, London.

Schuman, B. M. (1988) 'Endoscopy of the small bowel and duodenum', in *Annual of Gastrointestinal Endoscopy*. Gower Scientific Publications, London.

Schuman, B. M. (1989) 'Endoscopy of the stomach', in *Annual of Gastrointestinal Endoscopy*. Current Science, London.

Silverstein, F. E. (1988) 'Endoscopy of the stomach', in *Annual of Gastrointestinal Endoscopy*. Gower Scientific Publications, London.

Silverstein, F. E. and Tytgat, G. N. J. (1987) *Atlas of Gastrointestinal Endoscopy*. W. B. Saunders, Philadelphia.

Sivak, M. V. (1987) 'Techniques of upper gastrointestinal endoscopy', in *Gastroenterologic Endoscopy* (ed. Sivak, M. V.). W. B. Saunders, Philadelphia.

Swain, C. P. (1989) 'Endoscopy of upper gastrointestinal bleeding', in *Annual of Gastrointestinal Endoscopy*. Current Science, London.

Tytgat, G. N. J. (1988) 'Endoscopy of the esophagus', in *Annual of Gastrointestinal Endoscopy*. Gower Scientific Publications, London.

Tytgat, G. N. J. (1989) 'Endoscopy of the esophagus', in *Annual of Gastrointestinal Endoscopy*. Current Science, London.

Whitehead, R. (1973) *Mucosal Biopsy of the Gastrointestinal Tract*. W. B. Saunders, Philadelphia.

5 Therapeutic Upper Endoscopy

Gastroenterologists have taken over many of the therapeutic procedures which used to be performed by surgeons using rigid instruments and open operations. This applies particularly to the management of benign and malignant oesophageal strictures, and the management of foreign bodies and polyps. Therapeutic endoscopy is making an increasing impact in the management of patients with acute upper gastrointestinal bleeding.

Management of oesophageal strictures

The apparent simplicity of modern methods of dilatation should not blind the endoscopist to the potential risks, or to the need to ensure comprehensive and continuing management—which may mean surgical intervention in some cases.

Oesophageal dilatation is one of the endoscopic procedures which often produces bacteraemia; antibiotic prophylaxis against endocarditis should be given to patients with certain significant cardiac lesions (Chapter 12).

Benign oesophageal strictures

Relatively mild strictures can be dilated simply with mercury weighted bougies (such as Maloney's), but endoscopic and/or fluoroscopic control is required to ensure correct placement when the stenosis is tight or tortuous.

The variety of techniques and equipment can be bewildering for the beginner. Both balloon and bougie methods are effective, but their relative merits are still debated. It has been suggested that the radial force applied by distending a balloon within a stricture is likely to be more effective and safer than the tangential sheering force of pushing a bougie, but these claims have not been proven. Bougie techniques give a better 'feel' of the stricture.

Evaluation of the stricture

It is clearly necessary to evaluate the nature, site and extent of a stricture before considering the need for dilatation and the best technique. Evaluation methods include barium radiology, endoscopy with biopsy and cytology, and manometry (supplemented where necessary with other studies, such as pH monitoring). Many endoscopists rely almost exclusively on endoscopy (with tissue samples) but radiology is mandatory with tight and tortuous strictures, to provide a road map. The cause of the stricture may alter the therapeutic approach. Dilatation is used only as part of an overall treatment plan, with due attention to standard advice

56

about diet, medication, and the possible need for surgical intervention should medical management fail.

Scope-guided dilatation

It is possible to pass dilators (especially balloons) *alongside* an endoscope, and perform dilatation under visual control. The development of 'through the scope' (TTS) balloons has made things simpler for the endoscopist (and patient). The balloons are 3–8 cm in length, and of various diameters. We use 10, 15, and 18-mm diameter balloons, and usually prefer the 5-cm length. These are easier to pass than longer balloons, but less likely to 'pop out' of the stricture than shorter ones. They are passed through the biopsy channel of a standard endoscope (Fig. 5.1). Passage is easier if the balloons are well maintained and 'furled' in the same direction on each occasion. Lubrication should be applied, either directly to the balloon with a silicone spray, or by injecting 1–2 ml of silicone oil down the endoscope channel followed by 10 ml of air. Suction should be maintained on the balloon whilst it is passed through the channel. The stricture is examined endoscopically and the soft tip of an appropriate sized balloon is passed gently through the stricture under direct vision. The balloons are fairly translucent, so that it is usually possible to observe the 'waist' of the balloon endoscopically during the procedure, and to note the extent of dilatation. Manufacturers recommend inflation to a fixed pressure (35–50 p.s.i.) to avoid bursting smaller balloons, but, in the oesophagus, many experts dilate by feel. It is helpful to use a smaller syringe (15–20 ml) for easy inflation, changing to a larger one (50 ml) for more rapid evacuation. For tight strictures or maximal dilatation, the efficiency of balloon inflation is improved by using water (or contrast medium) rather than air, since fluids cannot be compressed. To do this, the balloon must be fluid-filled and all air extracted before insertion down the endoscope.

TTS balloon dilatation has become popular for obvious reasons. It can be performed immediately during initial endoscopy (with biopsy and cytology) and does not normally require fluoroscopic monitoring. The results of dilatation should be obvious immediately, and the endoscope can be passed through the stricture, if this was not previously possible, to complete the endoscopic examination (with emphasis on a retroverted view of the cardia in low lesions). Balloons have disadvantages: they are relatively expensive, and fragile if not handled with care, and it is often difficult to be sure that dilatation has reached the maximum diameter.

Similar balloon techniques can be applied to strictures beyond the oesophagus—including surgical stomas, the pylorus and

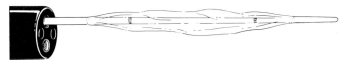

Fig. 5.1 'Through the scope' (TTS) balloon dilator—deflated.

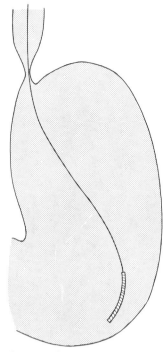

Fig. 5.2 Dilator guidewire positioned in the gastric antrum.

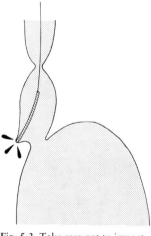

Fig. 5.3 Take care not to impact the guidewire.

duodenum. Results are good, at least in the short term. It is unwise to attempt dilatation in the presence of acute peptic ulceration.

Dilatation using endoscopically-placed guidewires

A standard (or 'paediatric') endoscope is used to examine the stricture and take any necessary tissue samples. A long guidewire, usually of solid metal with a flexible tip, is passed through the instrument channel and advanced gently through the stricture. The tip of the guidewire should be placed in the antrum of the stomach (Fig. 5.2) either under direct vision if the endoscope will pass through the stricture, or with fluoroscopic control; passing too much wire introduces the risk of forming a knot. It is essential to use fluoroscopy in tight and tortuous strictures, since the tip of the wire can impact within a stricture or hiatus hernia (Fig. 5.3). The endoscope is removed once the wire is in good position. Maintenance of this position is central to the safety of subsequent dilatation. The ideal is *always* to have fluoroscopic control. However, it is possible to control the position of the guidewire tip by keeping constant the amount of wire outside the patient's mouth. This can be done either by measurement, or with marked guidewires, or by fixing the external end of the wire against a piece of (fixed) furniture. The external tip is sharp, and can damage the eyes of assistants or patient; it should be capped when not in active use. Guidewires kink if care is not taken. Kinked wires should be discarded since the dilators no longer slide smoothly over them, which may result in the endoscopist using excessive (and dangerous) force.

Once the guidewire is in place, there is a wide choice of bougies to slide over them.

Types of bougies

In the USA, the *Savary–Guilliard (Wilson–Cook)* and *American Endoscopy (Bard)* bougies have become most poplar. These are simple soft plastic wands with a long taper (Fig. 5.4). They differ only in the length of the taper and the method used for making them radio-opaque. The Savary bougies have a radio-opaque band at the top and bottom of the taper, whereas the American Endoscopy variety are impregnated and radio-opaque throughout. Diameters range from 5 to 20 mm.

In Europe, the *Eder–Puestow* bougies were initially more popular. These are a series of olives which are attached to a shaft and leader (Fig. 5.5). They give good 'feel', but the dilatation is

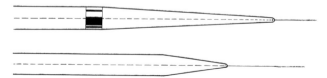

Fig. 5.4 Tips of Savary–Guilliard (above) and American Endoscopy (below) dilators for use over a guidewire.

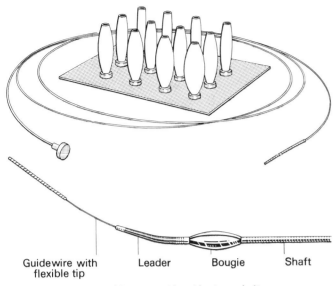

Guidewire with   Leader   Bougie   Shaft
flexible tip

Fig. 5.5 Eder–Puestow dilator set with guidewire and olives.

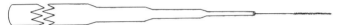

Fig. 5.6 Celestin stepped dilator and guidewire.

relatively abrupt. *Celestin* dilators have a series of short steps
(Fig. 5.6) but, with these (unless full insertion is possible), it can be
difficult to judge which step has been reached. There is a long
length of bougie within the stomach when the highest steps of a
Celestin dilator are reached, which makes their use potentially
hazardous in patients who have had gastric resection.

The major advantage of wire-guided bougies is the security of
knowing that the dilator is passing correctly through the stricture
into the main lumen (and not into a diverticulum or necrotic
tumour, or through the wall of a hiatus hernia). However, this
security really exists only if fluoroscopy is being used concurrently—
which is a problem since many endoscopists do not have immediate
X-ray access.

Balloons can be used over a guidewire under radiological control
with or without any endoscopic assistance. Indeed, in some institutions, many oesophageal dilatations are performed by radiologists.

The choice of endoscopic dilatation methods

It is clear that there are many techniques, and endoscopists vary in
their preference. It may be sensible and safer to use a familiar
technique rather than always to attempt to keep up with the
market.

Most endoscopists will have available Maloney mercury bougies,
TTS balloons, and one guidewire method. Maloney dilators can be

used for mild symmetrical strictures and for follow-up after other dilatations; TTS balloons are preferred where the lumen is asymmetrical (but obvious), and when an endoscope can be passed through it. For tight or tortuous strictures, it is wise to use guidewire methods under fluoroscopic control. The Savary system has probably become the most popular world wide.

The dilatation procedure

Choose a bougie which will pass relatively easily through the stricture and slide it over the guidewire down close to the mouth. Lubricate the tip of the bougie. Now choose a left- or right-hand action. Probably the most popular approach is to hold the bougie shaft in the right hand, and to use the left index finger to deflect the tip downwards over the back of the tongue. The GI assistant holds the end of the wire and applies counter-traction as the bougie is advanced. Some prefer to hold the bougie in the left hand and to apply counter-traction themselves with the right hand (checking the wire position by fluoroscopy where necessary). Whichever method is used it is wise to have the endoscopist's 'active' elbow extended (Fig. 5.7) so that the dilator cannot travel too far when resistance 'gives' (with the potential for distal perforation or a punch in the face for the patient).

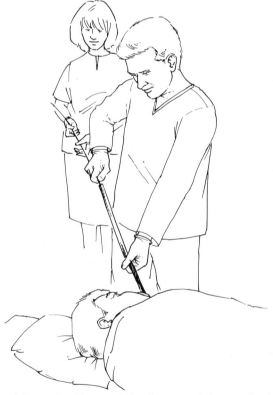

Fig. 5.7 Advance the dilator with the elbow extended to avoid sudden over-insertion.

After initial bouginage, increase the size stepwise, using (during a single session) *not more than three sizes above that at which significant resistance is felt*. Repeatedly check that the guidewire is in an appropriate position. At the end of the dilatation it is usually wise to check its effect by repeating the endoscopy; biopsy and cytology can also be taken.

Dilatation can be repeated within a few days in severe cases, and then sequentially every few weeks until swallowing has been restored fully.

Recovery and instructions

After a dilatation procedure patients should be kept under observation for longer than after a simple endoscopy—certainly for 1 hour, and for at least 3–4 hours if the stricture is complex and the dilatation has been difficult. Patients are kept 'nil by mouth' during this first period and observed in the recovery area for any sign of perforation (pain, distress or subcutaneous emphysema). The patient should always be reviewed by the endoscopist concerned (or his designated deputy) who should personally give the patient a trial drink of water if progress has been satisfactory. The patient is then discharged with instructions to keep to a soft diet overnight, with instructions about all medical measures, and a follow-up plan (to include possible further dilatations).

Complications

Oesophageal dilatation should be a relatively safe technique using these methods. However, perforations occur, especially with complex strictures approached by inexperienced or over-confident endoscopists. The main message is to take the dilatation step by step. Strictures form over months or years, and may take weeks or months (sometimes years) to relieve completely. Never try to dilate to the largest balloon or bougies simply because they are available.

Perforation should occur in < 1% of dilatations, even of complex strictures. The presence of a complication is usually obvious; the patient is distressed, anxious and in pain. Early suspicion and recognition of perforation is the key to successful management, and no complaint should be ignored. Clinical signs of subcutaneous emphysema may not develop for several hours. ECG, chest X-ray and water-soluble X-ray contrast swallow examinations should be performed. Surgical consultation is mandatory when perforation is seriously suspected or confirmed. Many confined perforations have been managed conservatively, with no oral intake, intravenous fluids or antibiotics—with or without placement of a sump tube across the perforation (with suction holes above and below it). The choice between surgical and conservative management (and the timing of surgical intervention if conservative management appears to be failing) are difficult decisions; review of the literature shows varied and strong opinions.

Achalasia

In establishing the diagnosis of achalasia, manometry provides the gold standard, but endoscopy is important to demonstrate the absence of mucosal disease at, or below, the cardia. Dysphagia can be relieved temporarily by simple dilatation using the techniques described above for reflux strictures. However, long-term benefit requires destruction of at least part of the sphincter either by surgery or by more forceful dilatation. Most physicians and informed patients prefer to try the endoscopic approach first. Long-term results (after one or more dilatation) are good in about 80% of patients; surgery is reserved for endoscopic failures (and complications).

Tools and techniques

For safety reasons, it is important to attempt to clear the oesophagus of fluid and food debris before performing dilatation. This is best done by keeping to a clear liquid diet for several days supplemented by naso-oesophageal suction overnight. When there is significant residue despite this, the endoscopist should remove the endoscope and personally perform lavage with a large (36 French gauge) tube with the patient in the head down position to minimize the risk of aspiration, preferably with an overtube.

Many different balloon systems have been used. Correct position can be checked radiologically, or under direct vision with the endoscope alongside the balloon shaft. However, we prefer to dilate under fluoroscopy using a balloon passed over a guidewire placed endoscopically (Fig. 5.8). Achalasia balloons are available with diameters of 30, 35, and 40 mm. Start with the smallest balloon, warning the patient that a repeat treatment will be necessary if symptoms persist or recur quickly.

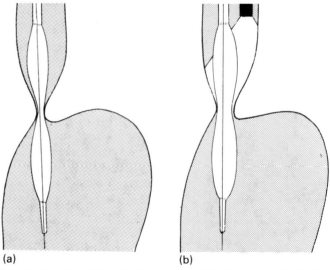

(a)   (b)

Fig. 5.8 Achalasia dilating balloons (before full inflation). (a) Checked fluoroscopically; (b) visualized endoscopically.

There are no validated guidelines for the length of time a balloon should be inflated. Traditionally this is for up to 2 min, and up to three times during a session. However, most patients become restless during the dilatation, and it is probable that shorter periods are equally effective. Most endoscopists stop inflating when the patient feels pain, and hold the dilatation for 1–2 min. It is usual to see some blood on the balloon after dilatation.

Recovery and risks

The risk of perforation after achalasia dilatation is greater than with dilatation of simple strictures, so close observation is mandatory for at least 4 hours after the procedure. Overnight admission is not usually necessary, but may be appropriate in selected cases. A chest X-ray and water-soluble X-ray contrast swallow should be done once the patient has recovered from sedation (at 1–2 hours). Nothing should be given by mouth until the patient and X-rays have been examined by the endoscopist personally. Admission should be arranged and surgical advice sought if the patient shows any discomfort.

The uncomplicated patient can return to a normal diet on the next day. A clinic appointment is arranged to assess the effect of dilatation and the need for repeat sessions.

Malignant oesophageal strictures

Endoscopy plays an important role in assessing the site and nature of oesophageal neoplasms, and endoscopic ultrasonography is proving useful in detecting degree of spread outside the mucosa and into nearby nodes. Barium studies are necessary in narrow strictures to document the length.

Unfortunately, many patients with malignant strictures of the oesophagus and cardia are unsuitable for major surgery because of advanced intercurrent disease or established metastases. In such cases, endoscopy can help to improve swallowing in several ways. The abrupt onset of severe dysphagia may be due to impaction of a food bolus, which can be removed endoscopically (see p. 72). The bulk of an exophytic tumour can be reduced by diathermy, lasers or injection of toxic agents such as alcohol. Like benign lesions, malignant strictures can be dilated using balloons or wire-guided bougies, but improvement is only short-lived and there is a higher risk of perforation. Recurrence of dysphagia after dilatation can be prevented by inserting an oesophageal tube/stent. The strengths and weaknesses of these methods are discussed below.

Stents in the oesophagus: indications

The best candidates for stents are patients with mid-oesophageal tumours who are not expected to survive more than a few months. Stents cannot be used when the tumour extends to within 2 cm of the cricopharyngeus, and stent function is less predictable with

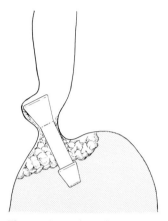

Fig. 5.9 Stents through angulated tumours at the cardia may not function well.

lesions at the cardia, since, because of angulation, the upper funnel of the stent may lie against the oesophageal wall (Fig. 5.9).

Stents are particularly useful in patients with a malignant tracheo-oesophageal fistulae (whether spontaneous or induced during dilatation).

Different types of stents

Some experts in this field make their own stents, since they wish to be able to tailor the length and shape precisely to the individual patient. However, satisfactory stents are available commercially from several sources. They are of broadly similar design, with a lumen of at least 10 mm, upper and lower flanges to prevent migration, and radio-opaque marking (Fig. 5.10). They must be sufficiently flexible for ease of insertion and comfortable 'seating', but not collapsible. Stents come in a variety of lengths, and narrower tubes are available for lesions which prove difficult to dilate.

A cuffed tube is available for use in patients with large fistulae.

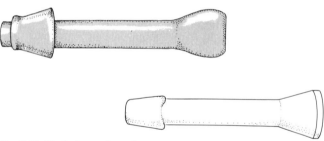

Fig. 5.10 Typical oesophageal stents.

Stent insertion

The stricture is first assessed carefully by radiology and endoscopy, and the patient informed about the aims and risks of the procedure, and available alternatives. The stricture is then dilated by standard methods, using wire-guided dilators, up to 50 French gauge (16 mm). Several sessions may be necessary to achieve this size. The process must not be hurried since there is a significant risk of perforation by splitting the tumour. Dilatation may be more difficult and perhaps more hazardous after radiation therapy.

The principle of stent insertion is simple once the stricture has been dilated adequately—the stent is slid down the oesophagus over an introducing tube riding on the guidewire originally used for dilatation, and advanced into the correct position with a 'pushing-tube'—but there are several variations. The practice is technically demanding, and requires a fine blend of dexterity, caution and force. This procedure is not for the inexperienced.

'*Over the dilator*' *method*. A popular method is to use an extra-long 10-mm dilator of standard bougie type. This is placed through the previously dilated stricture and into the stomach over the original guidewire. The shaft of the dilator is lubricated, and an appropriate stent simply slid down over the shaft with the pusher tube behind it (Fig. 5.11a). It is often necessary for the endoscopist to 'help' the stent around the pharynx, using his fingers. Correct positioning of the dilator and guidewire is maintained by an assistant, and monitored fluoroscopically. Usually it is easy to feel when the stent enters the stricture, and when the proximal funnel abuts its upper end. Rather than relying solely on feel, it is wise to place distance markers on the pusher tube shaft, having made the appropriate measurements (to the top and bottom of the tumour from the incisor teeth) at endoscopy after the final dilatation.

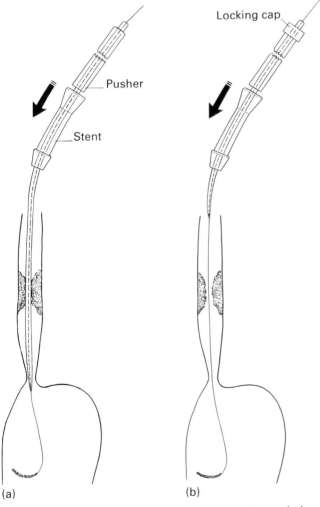

(a)   (b)

Fig. 5.11 'Over the dilator' methods for dilatation. (a) Stent pushed over the static dilator. (b) Stent and pusher tube locked onto dilator and move in together over the guidewire.

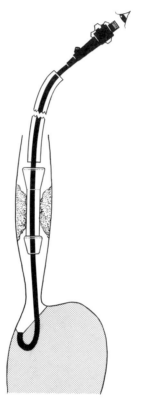
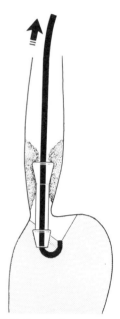
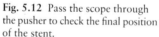

Fig. 5.12 Pass the scope through the pusher to check the final position of the stent.

Fig. 5.13 Use the hooked scope to pull back the stent—providing the tip is in the stomach.

When the stent appears to be in the correct position (by distance and fluoroscopy), the inner dilator and guidewire are removed leaving the pusher tube in place. The endoscope is re-inserted through the pusher tube (withdrawn about 2 cm to separate from the stent) (Fig. 5.12). The endoscopist views the upper flange of the stent and can pass through it to check that the distal tip is completely through the tumour and not abutting against the lateral wall of the oesophagus (or stomach). If the stent is not sufficiently far in, its position can be adjusted with the pusher advanced over the endoscope. If the stent appears to have been advanced slightly too far, it can be withdrawn (if the tip is in the stomach) by pulling back with the acutely angled endoscope (Fig. 5.13).

Some endoscopists routinely use the endoscope (over a guidewire) as the shaft over which to slide the stent, using the standard pushing tube. However, this may damage the endoscope, especially when extra force must be applied.

A slight variant to the 'over the dilator' method is to pass the dilator, stent and pusher as one unit, over the previously placed guidewire. The pusher tube can be locked onto the dilator with the Savary/Wilson–Cook stent system (Fig. 5.11b).

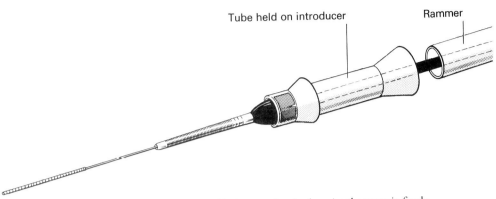

Tube held on introducer   Rammer

Fig. 5.14 'Nottingham introducer' system—the black expanding leader grips the stent tip firmly.

The 'Nottingham introducer' system (KeyMed Ltd). This method uses a flexible metal shaft with an expanding plastic holder which grasps the inside of the stent (Fig. 5.14). It is passed over a standard guidewire after the initial dilatation has been completed (Fig. 5.15). Once the stent has been placed correctly (as judged by distance markers and fluoroscopy) the lock is released and the inserting assembly (with guidewire) is withdrawn. Some like to use a 'rammer' (pushing tube) to hold the stent in place while the inner assembly is removed. This also allows re-insertion of an endoscope through the pushing tube to check the position before the procedure is completed (Fig. 5.15).

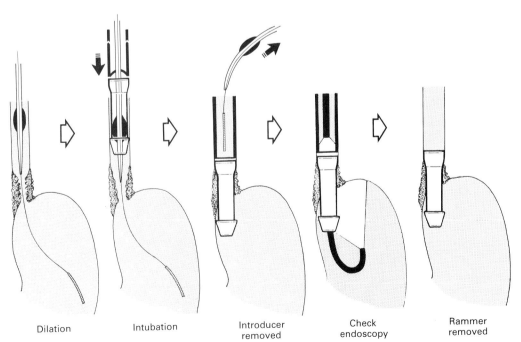

Dilation   Intubation   Introducer removed   Check endoscopy   Rammer removed

Fig. 5.15 Sequence of events for stent insertion using the 'Nottingham introducer' system.

None of these methods is clearly superior to another, and it is probably wise for the average endoscopist to become familiar with only one.

Stent removal

Complete removal of a stent can be difficult, especially if there has been tumour overgrowth. Theoretically, a balloon inflated within the stent will provide sufficient purchase for extraction, but this technique is not always effective. When a stent has migrated downwards, removal is easier if it is first pushed into the stomach, rotated and withdrawn with the distal tip leading. If the stent cannot be gripped by inflating a large TTS balloon within its lumen, a polypectomy snare may be employed (Fig. 5.16). Fortunately, stents which have migrated into the stomach rarely cause problems if left *in situ*.

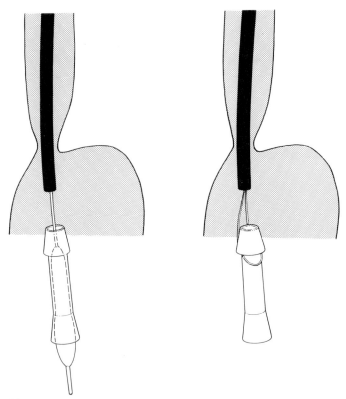

Fig. 5.16 Removing a stent—after rotation—using a TTS balloon or polypectomy snare.

Risks and precautions

Patients with large tumours may develop respiratory distress when the stent further compresses the trachea. Always be prepared to remove the stent rapidly if this occurs. Stent insertion carries a perforation risk of 5–10%. The patient should be monitored

A short *plastic tube* has been placed in the narrowing of your *oesophagus* (gullet) to help your swallowing. This leaflet has been prepared to help you look after your tube and gain maximum benefit from it. Don't hesitate to ask if you have any questions or worries.

Diet:

You can take any fluid or liquidized food. Some solid foods are allowed, but must be cut up well, and thoroughly chewed.

Avoid chunks, and all fibrous, pithy or stringy foods; they can block the tube. Common foods to avoid are: orange and grapefruit segments, celery, fruit skins, rhubarb, tough vegetables, lettuce and coarse cereals such as shredded wheat. All tablets should be broken up or crushed, and taken with fluid.

A talk with the hospital dietician may help you adjust to your new diet.

Do:

—Eat slowly—don't try to keep up with others.
—Chew your food for twice as long as normal. This reduces the bulk and prevents any blockage in the tube.
—If you have dentures, wear them. If they are uncomfortable see your dentist as soon as possible.
—Sit upright whilst eating; a straight backed chair will help.
—Drink plenty of water with your food and always have a fizzy drink after every meal, however small (e.g. sparkling mineral water).
—When in bed, always have 2–3 pillows to support you. This will stop acid coming back into your oesophagus from your stomach and causing heartburn. If you do suffer from this, contact your doctor who can prescribe some medicine to help it.

Don't:

—Do not rush any meal, however small.
—Do not swallow any chunks of food.
—Do not continue to eat if food is getting stuck. Stand up, take a small fizzy drink and walk about until you feel it clear.
—If you are having problems, don't struggle on. Get medical help.

Emergencies:

If you suddenly find it difficult to swallow it is likely that your tube has become blocked. Try to clear it by taking sips of a fizzy drink and walking about. If you cannot swallow any liquid for more than a few hours then:
—*Take no more food.*
—*Don't be alarmed.*
—*Get medical help*—Contact your own doctor, or the specialist team who inserted the tube.

Department: ....

Hospital: ....

Telephone Number: ....Ext: ....

Fig. 5.17 Instruction sheet for patients fitted with an oesophageal tube.
(Reproduced by kind permission of KeyMed Ltd.)

carefully (as after dilatation in achalasia) with frequent observation, and both a chest X-ray and water-soluble X-ray contrast swallow performed within 2 hours. Clear fluids can be given after 4 hours if there have been no adverse developments. Some experts give broad-spectrum antibiotics for about 24 hours, starting 1 hour before the procedure.

Patients must understand the limitations of the stent, and the need to maintain a soft diet with plenty of fluids during and after the meal. Written instructions should be provided (Fig. 5.17), and relatives counselled. Over-ambitious eating or inadequate chewing may result in obstruction. When this occurs, the food bolus can usually be removed or fragmented at endoscopy, using snares or biopsy forceps. Sometimes the whole stent must be removed and replaced.

Most patients treated with oesophageal stents are expected to survive for only a few weeks or months. However, it may be possible to remove stents in some patients where there has been a good response to chemotherapy and/or radiotherapy. Longer-term survivors with stents are at risk from tumour overgrowth. This can be managed by diathermy, laser photocoagulation, or placement of another small stent above the first. Benign reflux strictures have developed above stents, especially when they traverse the cardia. This risk can be minimized by standard medical measures including H_2-receptor antagonists. Some stents deteriorate with time, and may eventually disintegrate. It may be wise to consider stent exchange after about 6 months (if the patient survives that long), but stent removal may prove to be very difficult.

Tumour disobliteration

Laser treatment

The use of the neodymium YAG laser for tumour destruction in the oesophagus (and rectum) has been embraced enthusiastically by a few practitioners, particularly those already equipped with lasers which are no longer being used for the treatment of bleeding. The principle is simple, but the practice can be tedious and difficult for both endoscopist and patient. Repeated treatments are often required.

The best candidates for laser treatment are patients with relatively short exophytic tumours in a straight part of the oesophagus, and those with tumour recurrence at an oesophago-gastric anastomosis or above a stent. Laser treatment is more difficult to apply and potentially more dangerous when lesions are long, tortuous, high and submucosal.

Strictures are evaluated with X-rays and endoscopy in the usual way, and the patient fully informed about the aims, risks, and alternatives. Ideally, treatment should be applied from below upwards (Fig. 5.18), since treating from the top downwards may cause oedema and obscure the view completely. However, each patient is different, and it is often necessary to use both approaches.

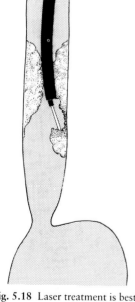

Fig. 5.18 Laser treatment is best performed from below upwards.

Treatment from below upwards usually requires prior dilatation of the stricture using standard wire-guided dilators. The endoscope is passed after the dilatation, and it may be convenient to use the same guidewire to follow the lumen. It is preferable to use an instrument with a large operating channel (or two channels) to be able to aspirate smoke and the excess insufflated gas, but sometimes that is not possible, and a small scope is used.

Most experts try to vaporize tumour tissue using high energies (80–100 W) in pulses of 2 seconds or more, attempting to keep about 1 cm away from the lesion. Treatment from a greater distance reduces the effect (through divergence of the beam); treating too close (which is often inevitable) causes intense drilling, and splatter of charred debris onto the endoscope lens. The tip of the instrument itself can be damaged if the laser fibre is inadvertently withdrawn too far into the channel before firing, or by reflected light energy absorbed by the black tip of standard endoscopes—which is why white-tipped endoscopes are sometimes used.

Judging when to stop laser treatment is a balance between achieving the desired result (passage of the endoscope through the lesion), the limits of the patient and operator tolerance, and the estimated risk of perforation.

It is usually necessary to re-treat after several days. Before the laser is applied again, any charred tumour debris is dislodged using the tip of the endoscope or wire-guided dilators.

After treatment, patients are observed carefully (as after insertion of a stent), and appropriate advice is given about diet. The effects of laser treatment rarely last more than a few weeks, and further sessions may be required. It may be necessary to place a stent if recurrence is rapid, or when laser treatment causes perforation.

The Bicap tumour probe

As in the treatment of bleeding, attempts are being made to replace laser techniques with cheaper and more portable methods. The Bicap tumour probe is basically a metal bougie with inbuilt electrodes, looking somewhat similar to an Eder–Puestow dilator (Fig. 5.19). This is passed through the stricture over a guidewire and under fluoroscopic control. Coagulation treatment is applied at several levels, the effect ideally being judged by viewing the upper margin of the tumour with an endoscope passed alongside the probe. Currently available probes apply treatment at 360°, so can be used only with circumferential tumours. More selective versions are being developed, and sophisticated probes may eventually also combine endoluminal ultrasound to determine the depth of treatment.

Other debulking techniques

Polypoid oesophageal tumours can be debulked by simple snare diathermy as primary palliation or prior to treatment with lasers or

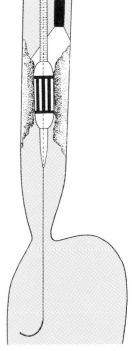

Fig. 5.19 Bicap tumour probe over a guidewire—the procedure monitored endoscopically.

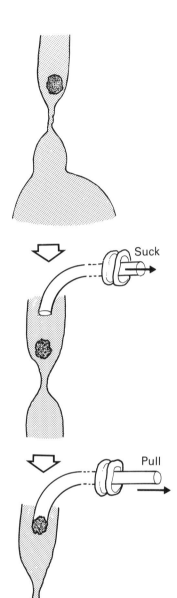

Suck

Pull

Fig. 5.20 Use an endoscopic over-tube (after removing the scope) with suction to remove a food bolus.

bipolar probes. Initial experience suggests that the simple injection of toxic agents (such as absolute alcohol) may also provide an effective and relatively safe method for palliation of dysphagia.

Management of foreign bodies and polyps

Objects impacted at, or above, the cricopharyngeus are best removed by surgeons, who may use flexible or rigid instruments. Below the cricopharyngeus, the flexible endoscope can be used in most instances, although great care must be taken with sharp objects. A rigid oesophagoscope is reasonably safe when used by an expert, and has the advantage that it allows better suction and the use of larger grasping tools; however, general anaesthesia is usually required and the technique is more hazardous in elderly patients with bent spines. Most advantages of the rigid oesophago-scope can be retained if a flexible endoscope is used in conjunction with an overtube; if this is (carefully) advanced to the obstruction, suction on the overtube itself (after removal of the endoscope) may trap the bolus and allow both to be removed together (Fig. 5.20). Alternatively, the presence of an overtube makes it easier to break up the bolus with biopsy forceps or the tip of a small-calibre fibrescope.

A full diagnostic examination should be performed after removing the bolus, and it may be appropriate to proceed directly to dilatation of any stricture.

Foreign bodies

Food impaction

Sudden severe dysphagia ('steakhouse syndrome') may be the first symptom of oesophageal disease, or can occur in patients with known strictures. Urgent removal of the food bolus is essential if the patient cannot swallow saliva. However, there is no urgency if the patient can swallow and is not distressed. Glucagon (0.5 mg given i.v.) may then help spontaneous passage of the bolus.

If endoscopy is performed soon after the food has been ingested, meat can be removed easily as a single piece, using a polypectomy snare, tripod grasper, or stone retrieval basket. However, meat begins to fragment within a few hours, after which it can usually be broken up further with a snare and the pieces pushed (with the tip of the endoscope) into the stomach. This must be done carefully, especially if there is any question of a bone being present. Sometimes it is possible to manoeuvre a small endoscope past the food bolus, and to use the endoscope tip to dilate the distal stricture; the food can then be pushed through the narrowed area. The endoscopist's task is not complete until the cause of the obstruction has been established and treated. Usually, dilatation can be performed at the time of food extraction, but should be delayed if there is considerable oedema or ulceration. Enzyme preparations (meat tenderizer) should *not* be used since severe complications have been reported.

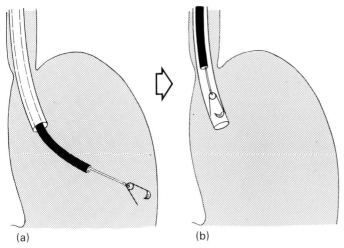

(a)   (b)

Fig. 5.21 Remove sharp foreign bodies with a protecting overtube.

True foreign bodies

Foreign bodies should always be removed if they are trapped in the oesophagus. Endoscopists have shown great ingenuity in designing ways to remove individual objects. It is essential to think ahead, preferably to perform a 'dry run' with a similar object outside the patient. Pointed objects (such as open safety pins) should only be withdrawn with the pointed edge trailing. Some sharp objects can be withdrawn into the tip of an overtube (Fig. 5.21); on occasions it is safer to use a rigid oesophagoscope.

Most objects entering the stomach will pass spontaneously, and there are few indications for early removal. Foreign bodies wider than 2 cm and longer than 5 cm are unlikely to pass the stomach and should be removed endoscopically if possible. Sharp and pointed objects have a 15–20% chance of causing perforation (usually at the ileocaecal valve) and should be extracted while still in the stomach or proximal duodenum.

There is urgency if a button battery impacts in the oesophagus, since leakage of its alkaline contents can cause major local complications. Once in the stomach batteries usually pass spontaneously; a purgative should be given to accelerate the process. Endoscopists should resist the temptation to attempt removal of condoms containing cocaine or other hard drugs since rupturing the containers can lead to massive overdose; surgical removal is the safe option.

Observe the golden rules for foreign body removal:
1 Be sure that your extraction procedure is really necessary.
2 Think before you start, and rehearse outside the patient.
3 Do not make the situation worse.
4 Do not be afraid to get surgical assistance.
5 Protect the oesophagus, pharynx and bronchial tree during withdrawal.

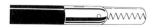

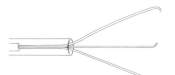

Fig. 5.22 Foreign-body extraction forceps.

Fig. 5.23 Triprong grasping device.

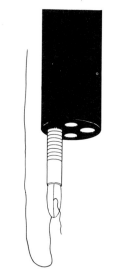

Fig. 5.24 Take a thread down with the forceps to pass through any object with a hole in it, e.g. ring or key.

The airway must be protected when removing objects which cannot be firmly grasped in their entirety; use an overtube or general anaesthesia with an endotracheal tube.

The endoscopist should have several specialized tools available, in addition to the overtube. There are forceps with claws or flat blades designed to grasp coins (Fig. 5.22), and a triprong extractor is useful for meat (Fig. 5.23). Many objects can be grasped with a polypectomy snare or stone retrieval basket. Any object with a hole (such as a key or ring) can be withdrawn by passing a thread through the hole. The endoscope is passed into the stomach with biopsy forceps or a snare closed within its tip, grasping a thread which passes down the outside of the instrument (Fig. 5.24). It is then simple to pass the thread through the hole in the object by advancing the forceps, dropping the end, and picking it up on the other side.

Gastric bezoars

Bezoars are aggregations of fibrous animal or vegetable material. They are usually found in association with a lesion which prevents gastric emptying. Most of these masses can be fragmented with biopsy forceps or a polypectomy snare. More distal bolus obstruction may result if fragmentation is inadequate. Various enzyme preparations have been recommended to facilitate disruption, but these are rarely necessary or effective. Large gastric bezoars are best disrupted and removed by inserting a large bore (36 French gauge) lavage tube, and instilling and removing 2–3 litres of tap water with a large syringe. The gastric outlet can then be evaluated endoscopically.

Polypectomy and snare loop biopsy

There are very few indications for polypectomy in the oesophagus, and fewer in the stomach than in the colon. The principles of polypectomy are the same, and are discussed in Chapter 10. The risk of bleeding may be higher with gastric polypectomy. We usually inject the base of gastric and duodenal polyps with adrenaline (1:10 000) prior to standard diathermy removal; using saline (rather than aqueous) adrenaline solution slows its dispersal.

When the gastric mucosa is clearly thickened, and standard biopsy specimens have failed to provide a diagnosis (e.g. suspicion of Ménétrièr's disease or lymphoma), deeper tissue can be removed by using a snare loop to 'construct' a broad-based polyp. This technique carries a significant risk of bleeding and perforation, and should be perfomed only after due consideration of the alternatives and with an adrenaline/saline submucosal injection beforehand. The tendency is to snare too large a portion. Check the size of specimen against the snare sheath diameter, and move the closed snare to and fro to ensure that the mucosal specimen is mobile over the stomach wall. If in doubt, release it and take a smaller bite. The snare loop is used to retrieve the specimen.

An ulcer is present for 2 or 3 weeks after gastric polypectomy and snare loop biopsy. It is probably wise to prescribe anti-ulcer treatment for this period.

Bleeding

Endoscopy is now the standard method for defining the source of upper gastrointestinal bleeding, and many haemostatic methods are in routine use.

Treatment of varices

Injection sclerotherapy

Sclerotherapy was originally applied with rigid oesophagoscopes— which do have the advantage of allowing good suction. However, flexible instruments are now used routinely. Many adjuvant tools have been described, including overtubes with a lateral window, and the use of balloons, either in the stomach to compress distal varices, or on the scope itself to permit tamponade if bleeding occurs. Most experts use a simple 'free-hand' method, with a standard 'operating' (large-channel) endoscope and a flexible retractable sclerotherapy needle (Fig. 5.25). Injections are given directly into the varices, starting close to the cardia, and working spirally upwards for about 5 cm. Each injection consists of 1–2 ml of sclerosant, to a total of 15–30 ml.

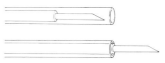

Fig. 5.25 Retractable sclerotherapy needle.

Precise placement of the needle within the varix (as guided by co-injection of a dye such as methylene blue, or by simultaneous manometric or radiographic techniques) may improve the results and reduce the complications. However, some experts believe that paravariceal injections are also effective, and it is often difficult to tell which has been achieved.

Sclerosants

Several sclerosants are available. Most commonly used in the USA are sodium morrhuate (5%) and sodium tetradecylsulphate—STD (1–1.5%). Polidocanol, ethanolamine oleate (recently available in the USA) and STD are widely used in Europe. Efficacy, ulcerogenicity and the risk of complications run together, since it is the process of damage and healing by fibrosis which eradicates or buries the communicating veins, but may equally result in stricture. In general excessive volumes, especially if given paravariceally, increase the risk of ulceration or stricture, whereas higher concentrations of stronger agents (e.g. 3% STD) increase the likelihood of perforation.

Sclerotherapy is more difficult to perform during active bleeding. In these circumstances it may be helpful to place the patient slightly head-up, or to apply traction on a balloon previously placed in the stomach. In some cases it may be wiser to defer endoscopy for several hours and temporize with a Sengstaken–Blakemore tube or other method for temporary control of bleeding (including pharmacological agents such as vasopressin and metoclopramide).

Sclerotherapy must be repeated (initially every 5–7 days and then every 2–3 weeks) until varices are obliterated. Thereafter, follow-up examinations are performed every 6–12 months.

Sclerotherapy of gastric varices is technically more difficult and less rewarding. There is some encouraging preliminary experience using cyanoacrylate glue injection, the risk of also glueing up the endoscope being largely removed by liberally coating it with silicone oil.

Rubber-banding

A device has been developed for placing rubber bands on varices–akin to the technique used with haemorrhoids. The relative value of this technique has not yet been established.

Complications of endoscopic treatment of varices

The risks of sclerotherapy include all of the complications of emergency endoscopy (especially pulmonary aspiration). In addition, sclerotherapy can cause immediate or delayed oesophageal perforation and later severe ulceration and stricturing. Patients are often given medications designed to 'protect the mucosa' during the healing phase, but efficacy is unproven. Sclerotherapy-induced strictures are dilated in the standard fashion.

Treatment of ulcers

Many endoscopic methods have been applied to actively bleeding ulcers, or ulcers with stigmas (e.g. 'visible vessel') thought to indicate a high risk of re-bleeding. The preferred equipment has become simpler and cheaper over recent years. Initially it was believed that simple diathermy was dangerous (the depth of injury is certainly not predictable), and a 'no touch' laser technique was assumed to be ideal. The consensus of many randomized trials was that neodymium YAG laser therapy is indeed effective.

However, it has become obvious that the same results can be achieved with simpler tools, and that *touching* the lesion may have advantages. The first advantage is that the probe impacting on the lesion is more or less fixed in position during the application of treatment (whereas precise aiming with the laser may be difficult). Secondly, a pressure tamponade effect can be achieved with some probes. As a result the heat probe and bipolar (Bicap) electro-coagulator have become popular (Figs 5.26 and 5.27). These have now been challenged by an even simpler technique—injection therapy. Ethanol, variceal sclerosants and adrenaline (with or without sclerosants) have all been used.

Technical points common to all of the methods are discussed below.

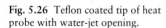
Fig. 5.26 Teflon coated tip of heat probe with water-jet opening.

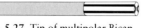
Fig. 5.27 Tip of multipolar Bicap probe with central water-jet.

Experience and safety

Emergency endoscopy is a challenging task. There is considerable potential for benefit—but also risk. These techniques require experience, nerve, and judgement. The endoscopist should be expert, must know the equipment, and should be assisted by an experienced GI nursing team.

Safety considerations are paramount. Sedation should be given cautiously in unstable patients, and every precaution must be taken to minimize the risk of pulmonary aspiration. Gastric lavage, even when performed personally with a large tube, rarely empties the stomach. Actively bleeding patients are often best examined under general anaesthesia with the airway protected by a cuffed endotracheal tube.

Provide good visualization of the bleeding point

Major bleeding rarely originates from the greater curvature of the stomach, so that the standard left lateral position provides the best chance of seeing the lesion. Sometimes the patient must be rotated onto the right side to see the greater curvature (with due protection of the airway). A large-channel endoscope should be used, to allow suction of fluid blood. A saline jet can be applied under considerable pressure through the instrument channel using a syringe or Water-Pik pump, or with the heat probe or Bicap which incorporate a flushing channel. Adherent clots should be removed (with a snare or basket) but only after due consideration and when ready to apply treatment. Thermal coagulation or injection sclerotherapy can be commenced around the base of a clot before it is removed.

Treat the feeder before the bleeder

Direct application of a treatment probe to a 'visible vessel' (often an aneurysm of the arterial wall) may provoke uncontrollable bleeding. It is wise first to 'rim' around the visible vessel with coagulation or injections (Fig. 5.28). When a vessel is actively spurting, and a direct attack is needed, pressure with the heat probe or Bicap onto it may reduce the flow and increase the effectiveness of coagulation.

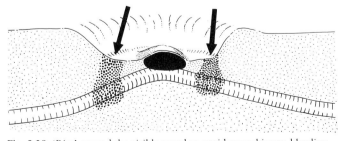

Fig. 5.28 'Rim' around the visible vessel to avoid provoking re-bleeding.

Know your equipment and doses

Lasers. Lasers are potentially dangerous to the operators and assistants. Appropriate safety measures must be employed at all times. Neodymium YAG laser energy is best applied face-on (where this is possible) with the probe tip about 1 cm from the lesion. Most experts recommend 60–90 W of energy given in pulses lasting about 0.5 seconds. A co-axial flow of gas is used to cool the fibre and to blow blood away from the tip. The treatment will become less effective as the fibre tip is discoloured or damaged. The probe should be withdrawn and inspected if the desired effects are not being achieved.

Heat probe. Use the largest available probe, at about 30 J, with a high-power water jet. Attempt to occlude the vessel with pressure whilst coagulating.

Injection. Treatment is applied with a standard sclerotherapy needle. Noradrenaline/adrenaline (1 : 10 000 dilution) is probably the most popular solution. This is injected in 0.2–0.5 ml aliquots around the base of the bleeding site, up to a total of 10 ml; using it in 0.9–1.8% saline solution gives a more localized bleb. Other experts have used absolute alcohol in much smaller volumes (a total of 1 ml in 0.1 ml aliquots), or combinations of noradrenaline with alcohol or the sclerosants used for treatment of varices.

Know when to stop treatment—and when not to start

Treatment attempts should not be protracted if major difficulties are encountered; the risks rise as time passes. There are some patients and lesions in which endoscopic intervention may be foolhardy, for example, large posterior wall duodenal ulcers which probably involve the gastroduodenal artery. Coagulation and injection treatment of bleeding ulcers in the oesophagus may be dangerous, because of the risk of full thickness damage.

Follow-up and carry-through

A single endoscopic treatment is not an all-or-none event. It is necessary to continue other medical measures, to maintain close monitoring, and to plan ahead for further intervention (endoscopic, radiological or surgical) if bleeding continues or recurs. The job is not complete until the lesion is fully healed.

Complications of ulcer haemostasis

The two most important hazards of ulcer haemostasis are pulmonary aspiration and provocation of further bleeding. It is difficult to know how often endoscopy causes re-bleeding which would not have occurred spontaneously, but major immediate bleeding is unusual, and can usually be stopped. The risk of pulmonary aspiration is minimized by protecting the airway—using pharyngeal suction and a head-down position, or a cuffed endotracheal tube. Perforation can be induced with any of the treatment methods if used too aggressively, especially in acute ulcers which have little protecting fibrosis.

Treatment of mucosal lesions

All of the modalities described above can be used to treat vascular malformations such as angiomas and telangectasia. The risk of full thickness damage and perforation is greater in organs with thin walls (e.g. small bowel) than in the stomach. Lesions of diameter > 1 cm should be approached with caution, and from the periphery inwards to avoid provoking haemorrhage.

Feeding tubes and gastrostomy

Intubation

Tubes for relatively short-term feeding (and gastric decompression) are normally placed under fluoroscopy. Only when this fails is it necessary to employ an endoscopic method. Tubes can be placed through the pylorus (or other stoma) under direct vision, having been carried down alongside the endoscope, or passed through the channel.

Through-the-channel method

The simplest technique is to use a 'therapeutic' large-channel endoscope, and to advance a 7 French gauge tube through the channel, over a standard (400-cm long) 0.035-in. diameter guidewire (Fig. 5.29). The tube can be of polyurethane or polyethylene. The tube and guidewire are advanced through the pylorus under direct vision, and subsequent passage checked by fluoroscopy. When the tip is in the correct position, the endoscope is withdrawn (by further advancing the tube and guidewire through it). Finally, the guidewire is removed, and the tube is re-routed through the nose (see Chapter 7).

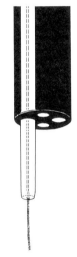

Fig. 5.29 Feeding tube and guidewire passed through large-channel scope.

Alongside-the-scope method

This technique allows placement of a tube larger than the endoscope channel, and is appropriate when a therapeutic instrument is not available—or when there is need to pass a large decompression tube. A short length of suture material is attached to the end of the tube, and grasped within the instrument channel by a pair of biopsy forceps or snare (Fig. 5.30). This assembly is passed down to the pylorus, and the tube then advanced through it using the forceps or snare. Once in position (checked by fluoroscopy) the thread is released, and the endoscope is withdrawn. Take care not to dislodge the tube during endoscope withdrawal. To avoid this it

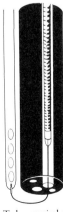

Fig. 5.30 Tube carried alongside the scope by a thread grasped with biopsy forceps.

is helpful to make the tube stiffer with a large-gauge guidewire. Finally, the position should be checked by fluoroscopy.

Percutaneous endoscopic gastrostomy (PEG)

Naso-enteric feeding can be used for several weeks but is less convenient in the longer term, and in confused patients who may pull out the tube. Percutaneous endoscopic gastrostomy is an alternative long-term feeding method which has become popular in the USA, particularly to permit transfer of patients with chronic neurological disability from acute care hospitals into nursing homes. The technique can be extended into a feeding jejunostomy by the use of appropriate tubes, in an attempt to reduce the risk of gastro-oesophageal reflux and pulmonary complications.

Studies comparing PEG with operative gastrostomy have shown some advantages for the endoscopic technique, but the surgical options should always be considered, especially in circumstances (e.g. ascites) where the endoscopic approach may be more difficult and more hazardous.

The risk of skin sepsis may be reduced by using prophylactic antibiotics, and some experts recommend disinfectant mouth-washes.

Although many variants have been described, there are two major methods for PEG—the 'pull' technique and the 'push' method.

'Pull' techniques

The 'pull' technique was the one originally described, and probably remains the most popular.

The patient is sedated and the endoscope passed into the stomach and a check made that the gastric outlet is patent. The patient is rotated onto the back, the stomach distended with air, and the room darkened. Darkening is particularly important if a video-endoscope is used, since the illumination provided is less. The tip of the endoscope is directed towards the anterior wall of the stomach, and the abdomen observed for transillumination. When this is seen, an assistant indents the anterior abdominal wall with a finger; the endoscopist checks that the indentation can be seen, and that it is in an appropriate part of the body of the stomach. The assistant marks this spot on the anterior abdominal wall, and then applies disinfecting solutions to the skin. Local anaesthetic is infiltrated into the skin, subcutaneous tissues and fascia, and a short (about 5 mm) skin incision is made with a pointed blade, extending into the subcutaneous fat. An 18 gauge intravenous catheter is then pushed through the anterior abdominal wall and its entrance into the stomach is observed by the endoscopist, who has meanwhile placed an opened polyp snare under the area of inden-tation and maintained gastric distension (Fig. 5.31a). The needle is removed from the intravenous catheter, and a silk suture (at least 150-cm long) is passed through it, and grasped with the snare

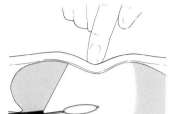

(a) Scope inflates and transillumin-ates stomach wall (and finger in-dentation can be seen) . . .

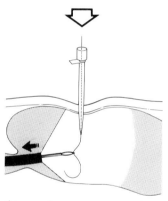

(b) . . . polypectomy snare catches and withdraws suture introduced by intravenous catheter . . .

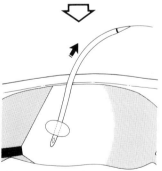

(c) . . . suture used to pull PEG catheter back from the mouth, through the abdominal wall—checked endoscopically.

Fig. 5.31 Stages in percutaneous endoscopic gastrostomy tube place-ment.

(Fig. 5.31b). The endoscope and snare are withdrawn through the mouth, carrying the suture loop, ensuring that the free end of the suture remains outside the abdominal wall.

The suture at the mouth is then tied to the PEG catheter, which is pulled down the oesophagus, and through the anterior abdominal wall. It should not be pulled tight, since compression necrosis of the gastric wall has been described. The cross bumper of the PEG tube should be left about 5 mm from the gastric wall. This is checked visually, having re-inserted the endoscope (Fig. 5.31c). The tube is best anchored at the skin with a special disk. Some experts believe that sutures increase the risk of local tissue reactions.

The tube can be used for feeding on the day after the procedure if there are no complications.

A simplified 'pull' technique. A variation of the above technique eliminates the necessity to pass the endoscope twice. When the endoscope is inserted originally, the long suture is pulled down alongside it (holding the tip with forceps in the channel—as Fig. 5.24). This suture is grasped using a polyp snare (without the sheath) passed by the assistant through the intravenous cannula traversing the abdominal wall. The snare loop is withdrawn with the suture, and the PEG tube pulled down through the mouth and monitored endoscopically into correct position.

The 'push' technique

This inherently simpler method involves pushing the feeding tube through the abdominal wall (rather than pulling it down from the mouth). The stomach is distended and an appropriate position chosen by transillumination and finger indentation, as with other methods. The skin and subcutaneous tissue must be thoroughly infiltrated with local anaesthetic, to allow a wider and deeper skin incision. A needle is then inserted through this incision into the stomach, and a guidewire passed through the needle (Fig. 5.32a). The needle is withdrawn, and a larger trochar with a plastic 'peel away' catheter over it inserted (over the guidewire) with pressure and rotation. The trochar is withdrawn once the catheter enters the stomach, and the feeding tube is inserted through the catheter (Fig. 5.32b). The outer 'peel-away' catheter is then removed, and the tube fixed to the abdominal wall. This push method eliminates contamination of the feeding tube by passage through the mouth, and requires only one insertion of the endoscope. Indeed it can be performed (by radiologists) without the need for endoscopy at all. However, it sometimes proves difficult to push the trochar and catheter through the abdominal and gastric walls.

Problems and risks

PEG placement cannot be performed in patients with oesophageal strictures too tight to permit passage of an endoscope. Technical

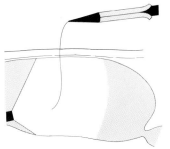

(a) Trochar and peel-away sheath follow over the catheter-inserted guidewire.

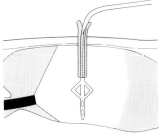

(b) Feeding catheter placed through the peel-away sheath.

Fig. 5.32 Push method for PEG.

difficulties and risks are higher in patients who have previously undergone abdominal surgery, particularly with partial gastric resection, and in patients with ascites or obesity.

Local infection can occur (even spreading fasciitis), particularly if the skin incision was too small, or if the tube has been pulled too tight against the gastric wall. A small pneumoperitoneum is not uncommon and usually benign, but major and persisting leakage will require operative correction. Injury to the transverse colon may result in gastrocolic fistula.

Tube dislodgement was distressingly frequent with original Foley catheter-type tubes, but should occur only rarely with other commercial devices unless the patient pulls on them. Early dislodgement usually results in peritonitis, requiring surgical repair. Tube blockage occurs rarely if commercial liquid diets are employed. A blocked or displaced tube can be replaced once a fibrous tract has formed (after a few weeks) by simple insertion of a Malecot-type catheter, or one of the 'buttons' available commercially.

Percutaneous endoscopic jejunostomy (PEJ)

Jejunal feeding is often recommended in patients with gastro-oesophageal reflux, in an attempt to reduce the risk of pulmonary aspiration. Current evidence suggests that this hope may not always be realized.

The jejunostomy tube may be inserted (under endoscopic guidance) through an established gastrostomy tract, or using special commercial kits at the time of the original PEG puncture.

Further reading

Oesophageal strictures

Chung, R. S. (1987) 'Dilation of strictures', in *Therapeutic Endoscopy in Gastrointestinal Surgery*, pp. 181–208 and 209–226. Churchill Livingstone, Edinburgh.

DeMeester, T. R. (1986) 'Perforation of the esophagus'. *Annals of Thoracic Surgery*, **42**, 231–232.

Earlam, R. and Cunha-Melo, J. R. (1982) 'Malignant oesophageal strictures: A review of techniques for palliative intubation'. *British Journal of Surgery*, **69**, 61–68.

Fleischer, D. E. (1989) 'Lasers and tumor probes', in *Annual of Gastrointestinal Endoscopy*. Current Science, London.

Fleischer, D. E. (1989) 'Laser and treatment of esophageal cancer'. *Lasers in Medicine and Surgery*, **9**, 6–16.

Hartog Jager D. F. C. A., Bartelsman, J. F. F. and Tytgat, G. N. J. (1979) 'Palliative treatment of obstructive oesophago-gastric malignancy by endoscopic positioning of a plastic prosthesis'. *Gastroenterology*, **77**, 1008–1014.

Kozarek, R. A. (1987) 'Esophageal dilation and prostheses'. *Endoscopy Review*, **4**, 8–20.

Moghissi, K. (1988) 'Instrumental perforations of the esophagus'. *British Journal of Hospital Medicine*, **39**, 231–236.

Tytgat, G. N. J. (1989) 'Dilation therapy of benign esophageal strictures'. *World Journal of Surgery*, **13**, 142–148.

Tytgat, G. N. J. (1989) 'Endoscopy of the oesophagus', in *Annual of Gastrointestinal Endoscopy*. Gower Scientific Publications, Current Science.

Tytgat, G. N. J. *et al.* (1986) 'Endoscopic prosthesis for advanced oesophageal cancer'. *Endoscopy*, **18** (Suppl. 3), 32–39.

Vantrappen, G. and Hellemans, J. (1980) 'Treatment of achalasia and related disorders'. *Gastroenterology*, **79**, 144–154.

Webb, W. A. (1988) 'Esophageal dilation: personal experience with current instruments and techniques'. *American Journal of Gastroenterology*, 471–475.

Foreign-body removal

Chung, R. (1987) 'Removal of foreign bodies', in *Therapeutic Endoscopy in Gastrointestinal Surgery*, pp. 227–242. Churchill Livingstone, Edinburgh.

Webb, W. (1988) 'Management of foreign bodies of the upper gastrointestinal tract'. *Gastroenterology*, **94**, 204–216.

Haemostasis

Cello, J. P., Grendell, J. H., Crass, R. A., Weber, T. E. and Trunkey, D. D. (1987) 'Endoscopic sclerotherapy versus portocaval shunt in patients with severe cirrhosis and acute variceal hemorrhage'. *New England Journal of Medicine*, **316**, 11–15.

Hosking, J. W., Robinson, P. and Johnson, A. G. (1987) 'Usefulness of manometric assessment of varices in maintenance sclerotherapy: a controlled trial'. *Gastroenterology*, **93**, 846–851.

Kitano, S., Noyanagi, N., Iso, Y., Iwanaga, T., Higashi, H. and Sugimachi, K. (1987) 'Prospective randomized trial comparing two injection techniques for sclerosing oesophageal varices: Overtube and free hand'. *British Journal of Surgery*, **74**, 603–606.

Larson, A. W., Cohen, H., Zweiban, B., Chapman, D., Gourdji, M., Korula, J. and Weiner, J. (1986) 'Acute esophageal variceal sclerotherapy'. *Journal of the American Medical Association*, **255**, 497–500.

Piai, G., Cipolletta, L., Claar, M. *et al.* (1988) 'Prophylactic sclerotherapy of high-risk esophageal varices: Results of a multicentric prospective controlled trial'. *Hepatology*, **8**, 1495–1500.

Prindiville, T. and Trudeau, W. (1986) A comparison of immediate versus delayed endoscopic injection sclerosis of bleeding esophageal varices. *Gastrointestinal Endoscopy*, **3**, 385–388.

Sanowski, R. A. and Waring, J. P. (1987) 'Endoscopic techniques and complications in variceal sclerotherapy'. *Journal of Clinical Gastroenterology*, **9**, 504–513.

Santangelo, W. C., Dueno, M. I., Estes, D. L. and Krejs, C. J. (1988) 'Prophylactic sclerotherapy of large esophageal varices'. *New England Journal of Medicine*, **318**, 814–818.

Schuman, B. M., Beckman, J. W., Tedesco, F. J., Griffin, J. W. and Assid, R. T. (1987) 'Complications of endoscopic injection sclerotherapy: A review'. *American Journal of Gastroenterology*, **82**, 823–830.

Trudeau, W. and Prindiville, T. (1986) 'Endoscopic injection sclerosis in bleeding gastric varices'. *Gastrointestinal Endoscopy*, **32**, 264–268.

Westaby, D., MacDougall, R. R. D. and Williams, R. (1985) 'Improved survival following injection sclerotherapy for esophageal varices: Final analysis of a controlled trial'. *Hepatology*, **5**, 827–830.

Non-variceal haemostasis

Chung, R. S. (1987) 'Management of upper gastrointestinal bleeding', in *Therapeutic Endoscopy and Gastrointestinal Surgery*, pp. 5–38. Churchill Livingstone, Edinburgh.

Chung, S. C. S., Leung, J. W. C., Steele, R. J. L., Crofts, T. S. and Li, A. K. C. (1988) 'Endoscopic injection of adrenaline for actively bleeding ulcers: A randomized controlled study'. *British Medical Journal*, **296**, 1631–1633.

Fleischer, D. (1986) 'Endoscopic therapy of upper gastrointestinal bleeding in humans'. *Gastroenterology*, **90**, 217–234.

Johnston, J. (1985) 'Endoscopic thermal treatment of upper gastrointestinal bleeding'. *Endoscopy Review*, **3**, 12–26.

NIH Consensus Development Conference Statement. (1989) *Therapeutic Endoscopy and Bleeding Ulcers*. Office of Medical Applications of Research, NIH Building 1, Room 260, Bethesda, MD 20892, USA.

Soehendra, N., Grimm, H. and Stenzel, M. (1985) 'Injection of nonvariceal bleeding lesions of the upper gastrointestinal tract'. *Endoscopy*, **17**, 129–132.

Swain, C. P. (1989) 'Endoscopy of upper gastrointestinal bleeding', in *Annual of Gastrointestinal Endoscopy*. Current Science, London.

Tubes and gastrostomy

Chung, R. S. (1987) 'Intubations', in *Therapeutic Endoscopy in Gastrointestinal Surgery*, pp. 243–259. Churchill Livingstone, Edinburgh.

Larson, D. E., Burton, T. D., Shroeder, K. W. and DeMagno, E. P. (1987) 'Percutaneous endoscopic gastrostomy: Indications, success, complications and mortality in 314 consecutive patients'. *Gastroenterology*, **93**, 48–52.

Ponsky, J. L. and Gauderer, M. W. L. (1989) 'Percutaneous endoscopic gastrostomy: Indications, limitations, techniques and results'. *World Journal of Surgery*, **13**, 165–170.

Russell, T. R., Brotman, M. and Norris, F. (1984) 'Percutaneous gastrostomy; a new simplified and cost-effective technique'. *American Journal of Surgery*, **148**, 132.

Schuman, B. H. (1989) 'Endoscopy of the stomach', in *Annual of Gastrointestinal Endoscopy*. Current Science, London.

Solomon, S. M. and Kirby, D. F. (1988) Percutaneous endoscopic gastrostomy; a matter of choice. *Endoscopy Review*, **5**, 36–45.

Endoscopic Retrograde Cholangio-Pancreatography (ERCP)

6

ERCP has many applications in patients with suspected biliary and pancreatic problems. The techniques are complex, and carry some risk. Optimal results require the co-operation of a skilled endoscopist, trained GI nurse/assistants, and an interested radiologist—all using appropriate equipment.

The experience needed for training and to maintain competence thereafter is such that not all endoscopists should expect to perform ERCP. The therapeutic developments (e.g. sphincterotomy, stenting) have become as (or more) important than the purely diagnostic studies. Furthermore, there are risks in performing a diagnostic ERCP in the presence of biliary or pancreatic obstruction without providing immediate treatment by endoscopic drainage techniques. Thus, ERCP and its therapeutic applications should be considered together. Training in diagnostic ERCP *alone* is no longer appropriate.

Equipment

Endoscopes

Cannulation is performed with side-viewing duodenoscopes. These allow face-on views of the papilla which cannot be achieved with standard forward-viewing endoscopes (Fig. 6.1). There is little to choose between the duodenoscopes of different companies. All have wide-angle lenses to facilitate orientation, and a working channel of at least 2.8 mm. Larger channel endoscopes are used for stenting (see Chapter 7). As in other areas, video-endoscopes are

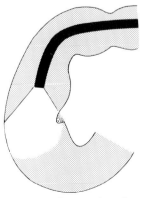 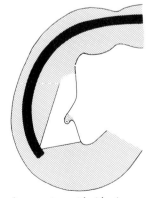

Fig. 6.1 Inadequate view of papilla with forward-view endoscope . . .   . . . face-on view with side viewer.

supplanting fibreoptic duodenoscopes. Videoscopes provide excellent images and working conditions for ERCP. The slightly longer tips of some first-generation videoscopes can occasionally be a slight disadvantage (e.g. when attempting to cannulate from within a diverticulum).

Catheters (Fig. 6.2)

Standard catheters are simple Teflon tubes of 5 French gauge (1.7 mm), with a slight rounding of the distal tip, and markings to help judge the depth of insertion. A radio-opaque metal tip is helpful for orientation during fluoroscopy, and some experts believe that the 'bullet shape' facilitates cannulation. We only use catheters through which a standard 0.035-in. guidewire can be passed.

The proximal end of the catheter has two orifices: one for a stiffening metal stilette (to prevent kinking) and one for a luer fitting at the side for attachment of the syringe of contrast (Fig. 6.3).

There are also many variants of taper-tipped catheters, which some endoscopists use when cannulation proves to be difficult. We rarely use them (except for the accessory papilla—see below) since they can easily cause a false passage leading to submucosal injection of contrast.

Disinfection

ERCP—more than any other endoscopic technique—carries a significant risk of introducing infection into closed spaces (i.e. ducts, pseudocysts, etc.). There have been many reported outbreaks of serious nosocomial infections (especially of *Pseudomonas*), traced to the use of contaminated equipment. Disinfection procedures are therefore of paramount importance. Everything that can be autoclaved or gas-sterilized should be, including all catheters, guidewires, and the water bottle. We use a newly autoclaved water bottle for each case, and sterile water. The endoscopes are disinfected in the standard manner (Chapter 12) on the same day and *before each case*.

X-ray facilities

ERCP is fundamentally a radiographic procedure, although initiated by an endoscopist. It is essential to use optimal X-ray equipment, which usually means a standard fluoroscopy or 'barium' suite. Some endoscopy units are fortunate enough to have their own radiology facilities. Those who have to borrow a room in the X-ray department know of the potential problems this can bring.

It is essential to ensure that there is enough room for the endoscopist, radiologist (and/or technician), and nurse assistants (and their equipment), and also that the endoscopist can see the fluoroscopy monitor easily. Most X-ray tables are installed close to one wall. If the patient is put on the table in the standard position

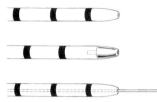
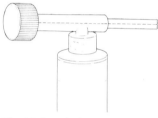

Fig. 6.2 Catheters in routine diagnostic use: standard (above); metal tip (centre); catheter with 0.035-in. guidewire (below).

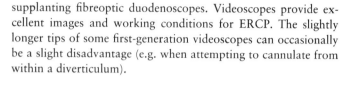

Fig. 6.3 Luer-lock syringe attachment to ERCP catheter with stiffening stilette.

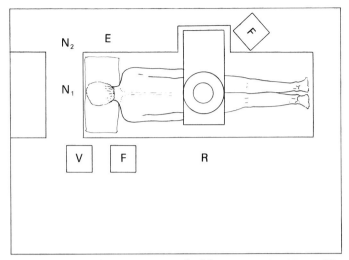

Fig. 6.4 *Do not use* X-ray room in standard 'barium' position. Nurses (N) and endoscopist (E) are cramped, only the radiologist (R) has space and can see fluoromonitor (F) in usual positions; the endoscopist needs an extra fluoromonitor. Radiologist cannot see video-monitor (V).

(as for a barium examination), the endoscopist and his assistants are cramped into a corner (Fig. 6.4). Therefore, it is usually better to work with the patient's position reversed. As a result, the endoscopist and radiologist are on the same side of the table, and both can see the fluoroscopy (and video) monitor placed across from them (Fig. 6.5). When working in this position, check that the table top can travel far enough so that the patient's upper abdomen can be brought into fluoroscopic view; and also that the X-ray image can be reversed. The table should be capable of tilting at least 30° feet and head down.

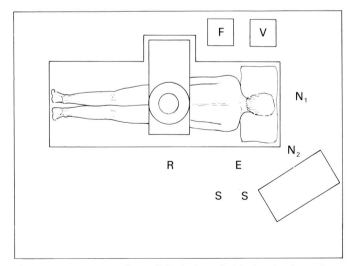

Fig. 6.5 Turn patient so that radiologist (or technician) and endoscopist work side by side. They, and the assisting nurse (N₂), can easily see both monitors. More space for gear and students (S).

Patient preparation

ERCP can be performed as an out-patient procedure, but post-examination observation may need to be more prolonged than after other endoscopies, to detect the earliest signs of complications such as pancreatitis.

The indication is carefully reviewed, and the procedure discussed with the patient. It is helpful to give patients a standard explanation sheet, which includes the potential hazards, as part of the education and consent process (see Chapter 13).

The patient should be asked about allergy to iodine. Despite the fact that there have been no published reports of anaphylactic reactions to contrast agents at ERCP, and that there is little evidence that specific precautions are helpful, a patient's history of contrast 'allergy' should not be ignored. In such circumstances we use non-ionic contrast agents, and pretreat with steroids for 12 hours prior to the procedure. Some radiologists also recommend giving antihistamines (H_1- and H_2-blockers) intravenously, 1 hour beforehand.

Antibiotics should be given intravenously 1 hour prior to the procedure in any patient with evidence or suspicion of duct obstruction or pseudocyst. We use gentamicin with ampicillin (or vancomycin if the patient is penicillin-sensitive).

The patient is kept 'nil by mouth' for at least 4 hours, usually overnight. An intravenous line is established, preferably in the right arm (since the patient will lie partially on the left arm).

The procedure

The patient lies on the X-ray table with the left arm behind the back, to facilitate rotating into the prone position (Fig. 6.6). A plain radiograph is taken (in the prone position) to check exposures, to document any soft-tissue shadows, and to ensure that the field is clear of previous contrast.

Standard sedation is given, usually diazepam and Demerol

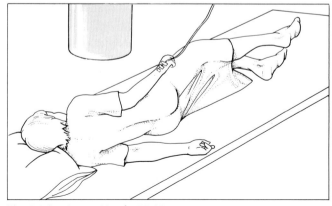

Fig. 6.6 Starting position for ERCP.

(pethidine). Once the duodenum has been entered, it is necessary to suppress duodenal and sphincter muscle activities. Buscopan (hyoscine butylbromide) is effective given in increments of 20 mg i.v. Where this agent is not available, glucagon is a reasonable alternative, if more short-lived, given in increments of 0.25 mg.

Gastro-duodenoscopy en route *or not?*

It is not difficult to examine the entire stomach and proximal duodenum with a side-viewing duodenoscope, and good views can be obtained of the distal oesophagus with care if the instrument tip is angled down and air insufflated. The endoscopist should be clear in his mind before starting an ERCP examination whether or not an endoscopic survey is indicated, and must make it clear in his report whether or not it has been performed. It is remarkably easy to miss substantial lesions in the stomach and proximal duodenum when hurrying to the papilla. For the beginner, who is likely to be rather slow, there are disadvantages in attempting to be comprehensive. Prime cannulating time and conditions will be lost. However, an expert should be able to provide a complete survey, and will usually wish to do so.

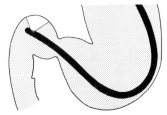

Fig. 6.7 The initial view is of the superior duodenal wall.

Entering the descending duodenum

The technique for passing a side-viewing endoscope through the pylorus and duodenal bulb has been described (Chapter 3). Remember that the lens faces in the same direction as the buttons on the instrument head (when the shaft is reasonably straight). With the patient in the usual left lateral position, the tip passes through the pylorus with the lens facing up towards the liver (Fig. 6.7). Examination of the duodenal bulb involves angling the tip down, withdrawing the endoscope considerably to hook it behind the pylorus, and insufflating some air (Fig. 6.8). This is the time to give injections (Buscopan or glucagon) to paralyse the duodenum. The next task is to enter the second part of the duodenum, and to find the papilla.

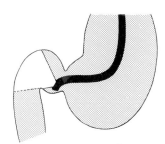

Fig. 6.8 Hook down in the cap to examine the cap and first part.

Straightening the scope

Most beginners simply push, steer and rotate as appears visually appropriate to advance over the superior duodenal angle, and into the second part of the duodenum. This technique is known as the *long route* (Fig. 6.9), and is commonly used by the inexperienced; it obviates the risk of falling back into the stomach, but is unpleasant for the patient, and control of the distal tip is greatly reduced.

The key to cannulation is to straighten the instrument to achieve the short route. The manoeuvre is very similar to straightening the sigmoid colon with the colonoscope by hooking in the descending or around the splenic fixture. The tip of the duodenoscope is hooked beyond the superior duodenal angle. Straightening the endoscope involves a sequence of moves, which should become combined and automatic with practice.

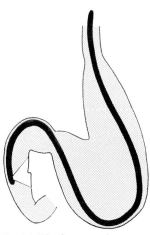

Fig. 6.9 The 'long route'.

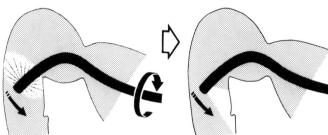

Fig. 6.10 Tip down over the superior duodenal angle.

Fig. 6.11 Rotate right and angle right . . .

Fig. 6.12 . . . to see the papillary region.

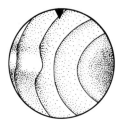

Fig. 6.13 A tunnel view of papillary region from above.

1 Advance the tip to engage the superior duodenal angle.

2 Pass the tip over the angle, steering under direct vision (Fig. 6.10). This will usually involve rotating the scope somewhat to the right, and also angling the tip to the right (Fig. 6.11). The endoscopist usually also rotates himself to the right, thus facing somewhat away from the patient. As the tip passes over the angle (Fig. 6.12), a partial tunnel view of the descending duodenum will be achieved from its apex (Fig. 6.13).

3 Straighten the endoscope. Angle the instrument tip sharply to the right and fix it with the brake. Then withdraw the instrument slowly, whilst angling the tip sharply up (using the left thumb on the up–down wheel) to see the papilla face-on (Fig. 6.13). The instrument shaft will be straight in the 'short route' position (Fig. 6.14a) when the 60–70 cm mark is at the mouth (Fig. 6.14b).

4 Once the shaft is straight, the up–down and left–right control wheels can usually be released into a neutral position, and the patient rotated prone. The endoscopist can then turn back slightly to his left, so as to face more towards the patient.

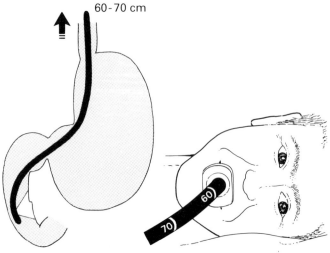

60-70 cm

Fig. 6.14 (a) Withdraw and angle up to see the papilla . . .

(b) . . . at 60–70 cm—the 'short route'.

Finding the papilla

With the *short route* (Fig. 6.14), the papilla is almost always directly in view when the straightening manoeuvre is completed. The lens automatically faces the medial wall of the descending duodenum if the patient is prone, and the endoscopist is facing the patient. If the papilla is not in view, the tip is usually too far distally, in the third part of the duodenum (Fig. 6.15). If in doubt, check with fluoroscopy. The shaft is withdrawn slowly (and rotated slightly from left to right) to scan the medial wall. Coming up from below the papilla, the first landmark is the angle dividing the second and third parts of the duodenum (Fig. 6.16). Above this is a bare shelf of mucosa, without transverse folds. A longitudinal fold, or several oblique folds of differing size, lead over the shelf directly up to the papillary structure (Fig. 6.17).

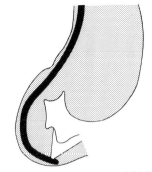

Fig. 6.15 Tip in entrance of third part of duodenum.

The normal papilla varies considerably in size, shape and appearance. Its colour (often pinker than its surrounds) and surface characteristics (usually rough or matt compared to the shiny duodenal mucosa) make it stand out to the trained eye. It is most commonly an elongated hemisphere approximately 8 mm wide and 10–12 mm long, tailing off below into the longitudinal fold (Fig. 6.17). The course of the bile duct may be obvious as a longitudinal bulge for 1–2 cm above it. Often a horizontal 'hooding' fold crosses just above the papilla, and may sometimes hide the orifice. The orifice is at the apex of the papillary nipple. It may be patulous, with several fleshy 'fronds' of protruding mucosa, or quite obscure.

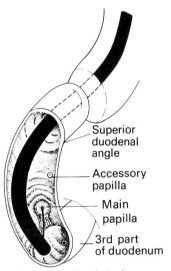

Fig. 6.16 Landmarks in the duodenal loop.

Although anatomy books record the papilla as occurring in any part of the duodenal loop (and even in the stomach), it is very rarely seen outside the second part of the duodenum, and occasionally just into the third part. If in difficulty finding the papilla, go back to first principles with the endoscope straight. Start with the tip at the junction of the second and third parts of the duodenum (check with fluoroscopy) and then withdraw slowly again. Often withdrawal is insufficient for fear of falling back into the stomach. If the instrument does spring back into the stomach, it may be easier to re-pass the pylorus by temporarily returning the patient to the left lateral position.

Cannulation of the papilla

Duodenal conditions must be ideal. If there are any air bubbles, inject 5–10 ml of water containing a few drops of an antifoaming solution down the instrument channel, and suck it back again. Further increments of Buscopan or glucagon should be given intravenously if peristalsis is a problem.

Cannulation should *never* be attempted until the papilla is seen properly *face on*. The aim is to pass the catheter through the papillary orifice in the same horizontal and vertical axis as the required duct system. Tangential thrusts are certain to fail. Only when a reasonable face-on position has been achieved with the

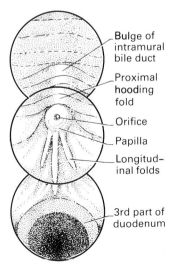

Fig. 6.17 The medial wall.

patient prone and the duodenum relaxed is the catheter passed through the instrument. To avoid injecting air up the ducts, the catheter should be pre-flushed with contrast, and attached to a large syringe reservoir (20–50 ml). Flushing contrast into the duodenum should be avoided because it stimulates peristalsis.

Sometimes it may be difficult to pass the catheter tip over the elevator, especially when using the long route (when the control wires are stretched). If in difficulty, straighten the instrument, and insert the catheter initially with the elevator *raised*. The catheter is advanced until it abuts against the elevator; this is then gradually lowered (using the left thumb to roll the control wheel towards the operator), and gentle forward pressure should allow the catheter tip to pass into the field of view.

It is unusual to see an actual hole in the papilla (except after surgery or stone passage), but the orifice is *always* at the apex of the nipple. Excessive fronds may make it difficult to judge the central axis of the structure. Occasionally the nipple and orifice are partly hidden by the proximal transverse fold. Then the catheter tip should be used to lift the fold away.

Before poking the papilla, the instrument tip should again be manoeuvred face on, looking directly up the papillary axis. It is helpful to fix the left–right angling wheel in a neutral position. Minor adjustments of left–right are achieved by rotating the instrument (in the left hand). The left hand also controls the up–down wheel, and the elevator.

The cannula is placed within the orifice of the papilla, but not pressed too hard. Unless it is precisely in the correct axis, undue pressure will distort the structure and increase the resistance to flow during contrast injection.

Concentrate on trying to imagine the axes of the required duct, and swing the endoscope tip around (and advance and withdraw it slightly) so as to cannulate in this axis (Fig. 6.18). Pushing the catheter may actually lose the axis due to exaggerating the curve in it (Fig. 6.19).

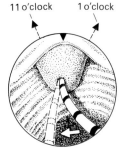

Fig. 6.18 Imagine the *axis* of the ducts and swing the tip around as necessary.

Selective cannulation

The most difficult part of ERCP is learning to select the relevant duct (or ducts), and to change where necessary from one to the other. Most endoscopists find pancreatography significantly easier to achieve than cholangiography, but success should be reached in at least 95% with practice.

Almost all patients have a single orifice for the pancreatic and biliary ductal systems, with a length of common channel which may vary from 1 to 10 mm. Often both ducts may opacify simultaneously if contrast is injected with the catheter tip only just within the orifice. However, in this position, contrast also refluxes back into the duodenum, and better radiographs are obtained with deep selective cannulation. Selective cannulation depends on finding the *correct axis*, so that the catheter tip does not impact within the papilla in a fold of mucosa (Fig. 6.19).

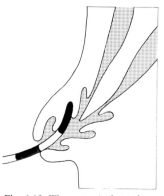

Fig. 6.19 Wrong vertical axis for deep cannulation.

Pancreatography is more likely to result if the catheter enters the orifice perpendicular to the duodenal wall, or pointing only slightly upwards and at 12 o'clock (Fig. 6.20). When aiming for the bile duct, the orifice should be approached from below, and slightly from the right (aiming the catheter towards the 11 o'clock axis) (Fig. 6.20). Just as important as these directional changes is the need to follow the correct plane, entering the correct segment of the orifice. The idea is to enter the roof of the orifice (and common channel) when aiming for the bile duct, and to enter the floor of the orifice when seeking the pancreatic duct. Thus, once the catheter tip has just entered the orifice, it should be lifted (or lowered) to achieve this aim (Fig. 6.21).

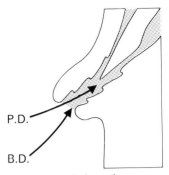

Fig. 6.20 Vertical axes for selective cannulation.

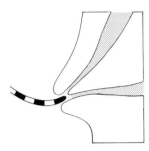

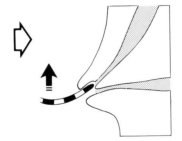

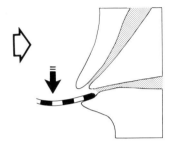

Fig. 6.21 Central catheter position.　　Lift up for the bile duct . . .　　. . . drop down for the pancreatic duct.

The commonest problem is changing from the pancreatic duct to the bile duct. Once a pancreatogram has been obtained, any septum between these ducts within the papilla has presumably been deflected upwards. The catheter tip should be removed and re-inserted within the roof of the orifice, and then lifted sharply with the elevator so as to lie firmly in the roof of any common channel. There should be more emphasis on *lifting* the catheter tip in the vertical axis rather than exaggerated attempts to approach the papilla from too far below (Fig. 6.22). Once the catheter tip is in the roof of the orifice, it may be helpful to pull back the endoscope slightly to straighten out the route from the orifice to the bile duct (Fig. 6.23). Often it is also necessary to swing the scope tip to the left at the same time. Advancing the catheter while maintaining the lift gives the best chance of sliding above the common septum into the bile duct. Initial catheter advance may best be achieved by up-angulation of the scope tip. The only way to check whether bile-duct cannulation has been achieved is to inject more contrast. This should be done carefully, since re-peated injections into the pancreatic duct may increase the risk of pancreatitis.

If a radio-opaque catheter (or metal-tipped catheter) is used, it should be possible to tell by fluoroscopy which duct has been entered. Movements of the catheter tip will move the pancreatic duct (visible if contrast is still present). Alternatively, if the catheter is in the bile duct, it can be freely inserted 5 or 10 cm. Occasionally

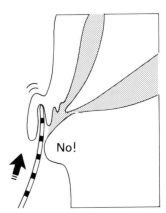

Fig. 6.22 Too much emphasis on pushing up from below is counterproductive.

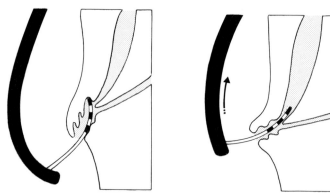

Fig. 6.23 Pull the scope back to correct the axis for bile duct cannulation.

a catheter will pass deeply into the pancreatic duct without resistance. This should be avoided since a branch duct may be entered, resulting in local duct disruption when contrast is injected.

The difficult bile duct cannulation

What should be done if the standard techniques are not effective? If the procedure has been prolonged and pancreatography repeated, it may be wise to admit defeat and return on another occasion—or refer the patient to another endoscopist.

However, there are some other tricks which may prove effective. Sometimes it is easier to cannulate with a sphincterotome, and an attempt to do so is certainly appropriate if it is suspected that sphincterotomy will be necessary. The use of the sphincterotome allows changes in direction of the tip (by bowing the sphincterotome) to change the angle of approach (Fig. 6.24). In addition, the sphincterotome is somewhat stiffer than a standard catheter, and the 'lifting' manoeuvre may be more easily achieved. However, since there are holes where the diathermy wire enters and leaves the catheter, contrast will spill into the duodenum unless the sphincterotome is inserted deeply into the duct.

An alternative cannulation method involves the use of a standard guidewire (0.035 in.) protruding from the tip of a catheter (preferably a metal-tipped catheter or the inner 'guiding' catheter of a stent set) which can be seen on fluoroscopy. The tip of a

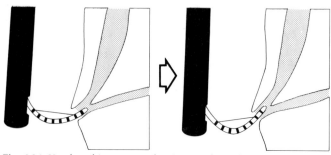

Fig. 6.24 Use the sphincterotome bowing to achieve the correct axis.

guidewire is probably more traumatic than a standard catheter, and should be used with care. However, we find that a guidewire sometimes slips into the bile duct when all else fails. This technique is used once contrast has been injected in the pancreatic duct. The guidewire is held protruding about 6 mm from the tip of the catheter (Fig. 6.25). The roof of the common channel is probed gently, using fluoroscopy to check whether the pancreatic duct moves. As soon as the bile duct is entered, the guidewire is advanced (by the nurse/assistant), and then the catheter over the wire. The wire is withdrawn and bile aspirated to empty the catheter of air. Contrast can then be injected.

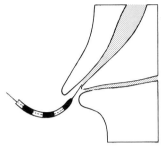

Fig. 6.25 Cannulating with a guidewire.

In some circumstances (related most specifically to sphincterotomy and stenting), cannulation may be achieved by a combination of the sphincterotome and guidewire methods, using the type of sphincterotome which accepts a (central) guidewire (Chapter 7).

Sometimes it is difficult to get a good position in front of the papilla (looking up the biliary axis), with the endoscope in the standard straight position. If the endoscope is advanced with the tip angled sharply upwards, the lateral wall of the duodenum may be distorted slightly to advantage (Fig. 6.26). Rarely it may be necessary to push the instrument into the long route.

Taper-tipped catheters may occasionally succeed where other methods fail. However, the sharpness of these catheters also increases the risk of submucosal injection (Fig. 6.27). This may give alarming endoscopic and radiological appearances. It is not dangerous, but makes completion of the procedure much more difficult, at least for several days.

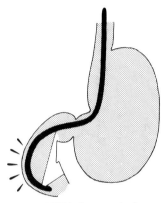

Fig. 6.26 With the scope in the straight position, angle the tip up and push further to gain a better bile duct axis.

The difficult pancreatic duct cannulation

Again, remember the importance of the correct ductal *axis*. Place the catheter tip at the lower margin of the orifice, and then press it downwards somewhat, by lowering the elevator during injection. If standard techniques fail, consider the possibility of a congenital anomaly. Take radiographs during contrast injection even when nothing can be seen entering the duct on fluoroscopy. Often a small ventral pancreas can be identified (Fig. 6.28). If so—and when no duct system is identified—it is mandatory to attempt cannulation of the accessory papilla when there is an indication for pancreatography.

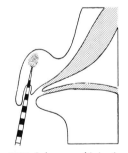

Fig. 6.27 Submucosal injection is too easy with a sharp taper-tipped catheter.

Cannulation of the accessory (minor) papilla

It is necessary to attempt cannulation of the accessory papilla (which drains Santorini's duct) when contrast injection through the main papilla does not provide a pancreatogram, and when it shows a congenital anomaly of a separate ventral pancreas. The minor papilla can be identified in virtually all patients, approximately 2 cm above and slightly to the right of the main papilla (as seen at endoscopy), lying just below (distal to) the superior duodenal angle. Its size varies enormously, from a tiny blind nodule to

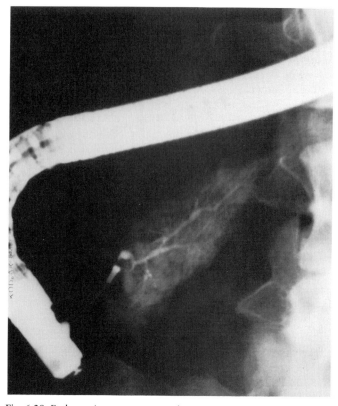

Fig. 6.28 Endoscopic pancreatogram showing a tiny ventral pancreas.

Accessory papilla

Main papilla

Fig. 6.29 Position of accessory and main papilla.

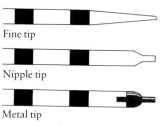

Fine tip

Nipple tip

Metal tip

Fig. 6.30 Specialized cannulas for the accessory papilla.

a major structure which can be mistaken for the main papilla. Unlike the main papilla, it does not have any distinct longitudinal structure, being solely a hemispherical nipple. It is found characteristically at the junction of two transverse folds (Fig. 6.29). A face-on position for cannulation of the minor papilla is best achieved using a 'semi-long' route, in order to push the endoscope tip against the outer wall of the duodenum and leave more room in which to move the catheter. Bring the endoscope back into the duodenal bulb, with the shaft straight. Then advance over the superior duodenal angle, whilst angling the tip sharply upwards, and maintaining some left rotation.

Cannulation is attempted with fine-tipped catheters, and should succeed in over 80% of cases. We prefer a metal tip or a short 'nipple' tip (Fig. 6.30). Catheters with long tapered tips tend to kink. The papilla can be made more prominent and the orifice visible if the pancreas is stimulated with secretin (give 25–50 units i.v., and wait 3 min). A problem with using secretin is that contrast must then be injected against a flow of juice. Whilst this does not appear to be dangerous, it may prove difficult to outline the entire duct system without using excessive pressure. Probably the easiest cannulation method for the minor papilla is to use a 0.018-in. guidewire protruding from a taper-tipped catheter, and secretin injection. Once the guidewire is inserted, the catheter tip is slid into the orifice. The guidewire is removed and contrast is injected. Unfortunately, there will be air in the catheter after removal of the guidewire, so that the pancreatogram may be incomplete.

A diagnosis of pancreas divisum can be made (or at least of dominant Santorini drainage, whether congenital or acquired) when secretin injection results in a visible flow of clear juice (rarely a fountain) after cannulation of the main papilla has failed.

Selective cannulation comes easier with practice and manipulative co-ordination increases. ERCP is always easier the quicker it is performed, before the staff, endoscopist, patient, duodenum and papilla all become tense. Clumsily-directed pokes probably induce papillary muscle spasm, as well as oedema. Further small increments of Buscopan or glucagon may help, but medication is no substitute for thoughtful gentle manipulation, and, especially, remember to *get the catheter into the correct axis*.

Radiographic technique

The degree of involvement of radiologists with ERCP varies considerably between units. Few endoscopists achieve the ideal of having a radiologist present throughout the procedure, but some collaboration with radiology staff is essential. The slickest cannulation is of no avail (and may be a disservice to the patient), without good radiological technique. If a radiologist is not involved 'hands on', it is essential to have a designated and specially-trained technician who understands what is being attempted, and can help achieve that goal.

Factors involving an appropriate X-ray layout and the issues of contrast allergy have already been discussed. Standard water-soluble contrast agents are used, as for urography (e.g. Renografin, Urografin, Conray, Angiografin). We start with 50% strength (in a 50-ml syringe attached to a pre-flushed catheter), but it is wise to change to a less dense mixture (15–25%) when filling dilated ducts. Unless this is done it is easy to miss small stones (or even quite large stones in a very dilated system), and much more difficult to see catheters and guidewires.

The volume of contrast used is irrelevant—this depends upon the system being filled, and the amount spilled into the duodenum. The correct amount is judged solely by fluoroscopy and intermittent radiographs; injection continues until the relevant ducts are fully outlined, without overdistension.

Radiographs always show more detail than fluoroscopy. By the time the pancreatic duct tail can be seen on most fluoroscopic monitors, radiographs will show filling of all major branches. Opacification of the parenchyma (acinarization) should be avoided. The appearance of a urogram during ERCP is a sign that excessive contrast has been injected (and absorbed); there is then an increased risk of pancreatitis.

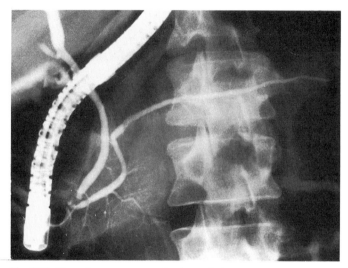

Fig. 6.31 Normal pancreatogram (and part cholangiogram) with the instrument in the 'short scope' position.

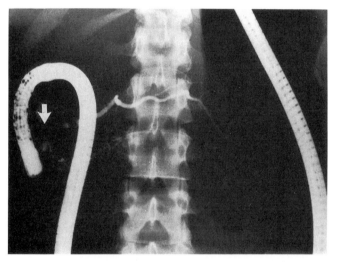

Fig. 6.32 Instrument with a long loop in the stomach ('long route'). The papilla of Vater is arrowed.

Contrast leaves the normal pancreatic duct system rapidly, and is often completely cleared within 5 min. Radiographs should therefore be taken during contrast injection, with the instrument and catheter in place. The prone position is convenient, and a 'straight scope' does not overlie the pancreas (as would a long scope) (Figs 6.31 and 6.32). Oblique films may be necessary to clarify local duct changes, and to separate areas of interest from the vertebral column. Lateral views are rarely necessary, and often confusing.

Techniques in cholangiography

Many cholangiograms produced by beginners at ERCP are inadequate for interpretation. The whole biliary tree (and gallbladder when present) must be filled, and views taken in appropriate positions. In the prone position the right intrahepatic ducts
fill last (because they are 'uphill') (Fig. 6.33), and the gallbladder
fundus may not be seen.

After cholecystectomy the biliary tree may be completely 'full'
with bile. Contrast injection may result in pain through over-
distension, even before adequate opacification is achieved. Thus, it
is good practice to aspirate bile once deep biliary cannulation has
been achieved. We try to *exchange* contrast for bile. This is
particularly important in the presence of infected bile, since increasing the biliary pressure can provoke septicaemia.

When the gallbladder is present, it acts as a reservoir, and may

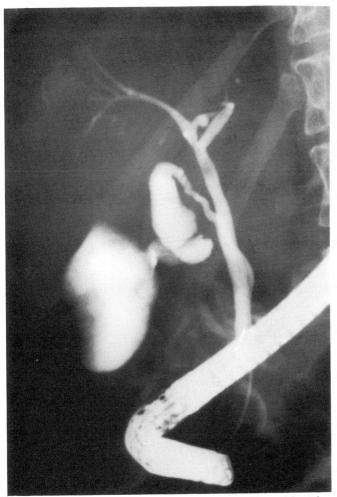

Fig. 6.33 Retrograde cholangiography showing poor filling of the right
intrahepatic ducts during injection in the prone position.

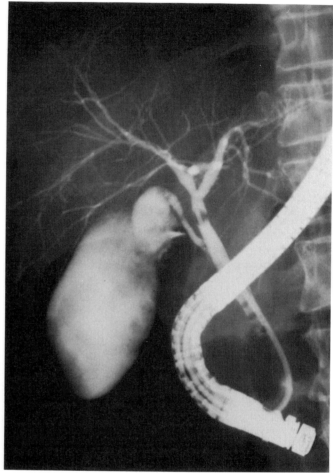

Fig. 6.34 Further injection after occluding the common hepatic duct with a balloon gives better intrahepatic filling.

(because it fills preferentially) prevent adequate views of the upper biliary tree. To provide good intrahepatic cholangiograms it is usually necessary to inject when the tip of the catheter is above the cystic duct orifice. Even better and selective filling can be achieved by the *balloon occlusion technique*. A balloon-tipped catheter (as used for stone retrieval) is placed, if necessary with use of a guidewire, in the common hepatic duct. Contrast is injected after the balloon is inflated (Fig. 6.34).

To obtain good views of the whole biliary tree it is often necessary to rotate the patient somewhat (to the right), to tip the table 20–30° feet down (less often head down), and temporarily to push the endoscope in deeper to form a loop in the stomach, so as to expose the mid-duct which is otherwise overlain by the catheter (Fig. 6.35). It is also necessary to take radiographs after the scope has been removed, with the patient supine—usually tilted 20–30° feet down, and rotated slightly to the right (to separate the bile

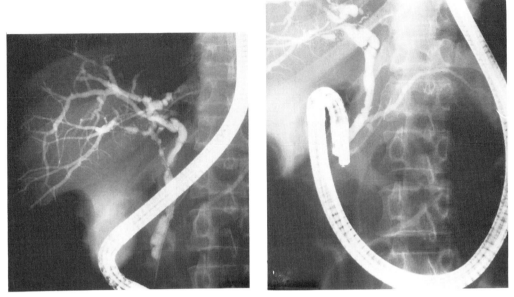

Fig. 6.35 Changing the position of the endoscope to provide better views of the bile duct.

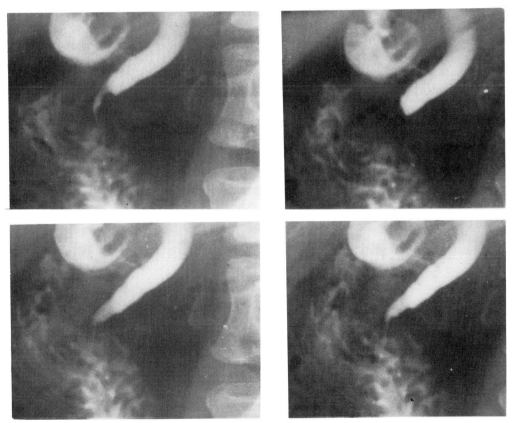

Fig. 6.36 Sequential views of the bile duct termination during relaxation and contraction.

duct from the vertebral column). These and other views are necessary to provide a full perspective of the gallbladder (when present), facilitate study of the sphincter zone in contraction and relaxation (Fig. 6.36), and help differentiate stones from air bubbles.

Drainage times should be documented in patients who have previously undergone cholecystectomy if 'papillary stenosis' is suspected. We take films at 5, 15, 30 and 45 min after withdrawal of the biliary catheter, with the patient supine. The radiographs are marked, and the degree of drainage is recorded on a scale of 1–5 (1 = no drainage, 2 = slight, 3 = approximately half, 4 = most, 5 = complete drainage of contrast). These numbers are recorded at

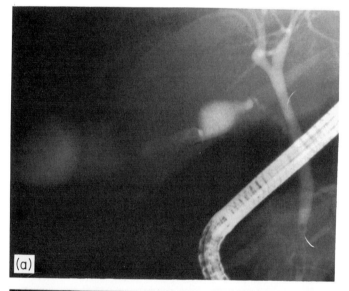

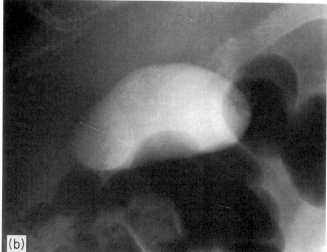

Fig. 6.37 (a) Initial filling of the gallbladder at retrograde cholangiography. (b) Inadequate emptying and asymmetric shape of gallbladder after injection with CCK.

each time, and no further radiographs are taken after a score of 4 is achieved. More control data are required, but we consider anything less than a score of 4 at 45 min to be suspicious of biliary obstruction.

When gallbladder disease is suspected, delayed radiographs should be taken at 1–2 hours when the patient can be moved around more easily, and contrast mixing is more complete. Small gallstones can be detected in the fully erect position and compression views may also be helpful. Abnormalities of gallbladder emptying can be detected by serial films taken at 30 and 60 min after i.v. injection of CCK (25–50 units) (Fig. 6.37).

Problems of access to the papilla

Diseases of the duodenal mucosa and papilla

In the context of ERCP, the commonest major lesion involving the descending duodenum is cancer of the pancreas. Pancreatic tumours may simply distort the anatomy, or ulcerate through the floor of the bulb or the medial wall of the descending duodenum. There is a differential diagnosis, but the endoscopic appearances of ulcerating malignancy are fairly characteristic, and biopsy specimens should confirm the diagnosis. When the tumour remains submucosal, the endoscopic appearances of oedema and irregularity are similar to those seen in patients with advanced and active pancreatitis. A mass lesion in the pancreas (tumour or pseudocyst) often makes it more difficult to straighten the endoscope.

Most primary tumours of the papilla are obvious endoscopically, and the diagnosis is easily confirmed by biopsy and/or brush cytology. Sometimes it is appropriate to take a larger specimen with a snare loop, or to use forceps biopsy within the papilla after endoscopic sphincterotomy of the tumour. The orifice is usually in the centre of the tumour mass. Look carefully for clues (especially for any trace of bile) before touching the papilla, which often bleeds easily.

The apex of the papilla may also appear lumpy, oedematous and congested in the absence of tumour or previous surgery. Such changes are often seen in patients with biliary-tract diseases, and the orifice may be lax and ragged soon after passage of a stone. Impacted stones cause a prominent oedematous papilla, and the orifice may be obscured below it. Cannulation is often most easily achieved with a sphincterotome, used to 'hook' it upwards. Impacted stones may cause a false orifice at the apex of the oedematous papilla (above the normal orifice), as may surgically and percutaneously placed catheters.

Peripapillary diverticula

Diverticula close to and surrounding the main papilla are very common, especially in elderly patients with duct stones. Small

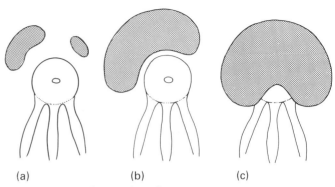

Fig. 6.38 Diverticula around papilla.

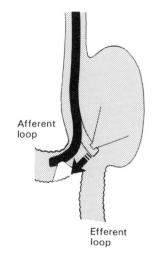

Fig. 6.39 Usual orientation in Billroth II and gastroenterostomies.

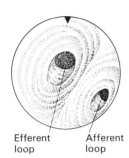

Fig. 6.40 'Backing in' to the afferent loop.

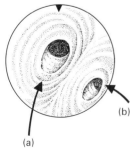

Fig. 6.41 (a) Usual approach. (b) Approach for access to afferent loop.

diverticula are shallow caves, most frequently seen above the papilla at 9–11 or 1–3 o'clock, when seen face on (Fig. 6.38). Larger diverticula may override the papillary mass, and eventually swallow it, so that the orifice lies within the diverticulum. The papilla can sometimes be persuaded out of the diverticulum by probing the folds radiating towards it with the cannula, and using a combination of endoscope tip manipulation and suction. Once the orifice is visible, it is often helpful to 'hook' the papilla out of the diverticulum using the tip of a sphincterotome (with or without a guidewire). Diverticula are sometimes seen around the accessory papilla.

Gastroduodenal surgery and Billroth II gastrectomy

ERCP techniques are not significantly affected by pyloroplasty or Billroth I gastrectomy. Gastroenterostomy should not interfere if the pylorus is patent, although it may sometimes be difficult to slide around a large stoma to enter the antrum.

Billroth II gastrectomy is the commonest anatomical difficulty encountered by an endoscopist attempting ERCP. However, it should be possible to achieve a success rate of at least 80%.

The first problem is to identify the afferent loop; unfortunately, the efferent and afferent loops look the same. The orifice to the afferent loop is usually less obvious than that for the efferent loop, and more difficult to enter. The correct orifice is usually (but not always) found in the 2–5 o'clock sector when viewing the stoma (Fig. 6.39). Entry to this loop can often be achieved by 'backing in' (Fig. 6.40), a technique often used at colonoscopy. The tip of the endoscope is placed over the orifice, angled sharply downwards and gently withdrawn. It may also be helpful to approach the stoma from about 3 o'clock, rather than the usual 6 o'clock position (Fig. 6.41).

Once in a loop, there are no useful landmarks until the papilla is recognized. To see increasing amounts of bile (or resulting bubbles) whilst advancing is encouraging. Fluoroscopy is somewhat helpful, but only in the sense of being sure the scope is in the

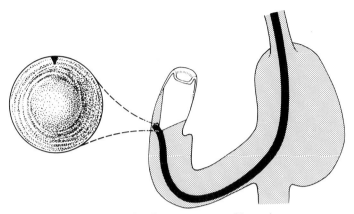

Fig. 6.42 Invaginated duodenal stump may resemble a polyp.

'wrong' (efferent) loop when fluoroscopy shows the endoscope tip to be deep within the pelvis. When confident of being in the *wrong* loop, it may be helpful to take a few biopsies just below the stoma, to leave a little blood as a marker of the wrong route.

Once in the afferent loop, it may be possible to recognize the bare shelf below the papilla in the distal half of the second part of the duodenum. The other landmark is the blind termination of the duodenal loop, which (because invaginated) may resemble a smooth polyp (Fig. 6.42).

The problem for cannulation is that everything is upside down, and specifically that the natural curl of standard catheters is counterproductive (Fig. 6.43). For the same reason, cholangiography is much more difficult to achieve than pancreatography. Several techniques are helpful in trying to overcome this problem of orientation.

A 'new' catheter tends to go straighter than an old one (Fig. 6.44). Pulling the scope back to the junction of the second and third parts of the duodenum can change the angle of attack appropriately, but it may then be necessary to attempt cannulation from a distance

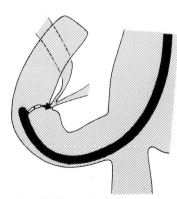

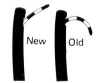

Fig. 6.43 Natural curl of catheter unhelpful.

Fig. 6.44 A new catheter tends to curl less than an old one.

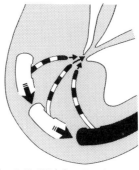

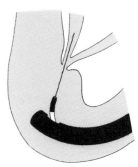

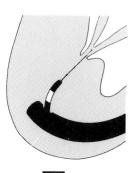

Fig. 6.45 Withdrawing the scope produces a better catheter axis but a more distant approach.

Fig. 6.46 Cannulating with a guidewire.

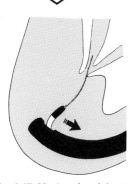

Fig. 6.47 Having placed the tip of the guidewire in the orifice, its direction can be changed by altering the catheter direction with the elevator.

(Fig. 6.45). Our favoured method involves the use of a 0.035-in. guidewire, protruding from the tip of a standard catheter or inner 'guiding' catheter of a stent set. The guidewire travels in a straight line (until it reaches the papilla). Its angle of approach can be altered by changing the length of guidewire protruding from the catheter, as well as by use of the elevator (Fig. 6.46). Once the tip of the guidewire has been impacted in the orifice of the papilla, its direction can be altered somewhat by looping manoeuvres (Fig. 6.47).

Some experts favour an end-viewing instrument for Billroth II cannulation. In theory, the lens looks directly into the axis of the papilla (Fig. 6.48). However, the lack of an elevator often makes detailed cannula movements more difficult, and we prefer the standard side-viewing duodenoscope. A long floppy (paediatric) colonoscope may be helpful in patients with a very long afferent

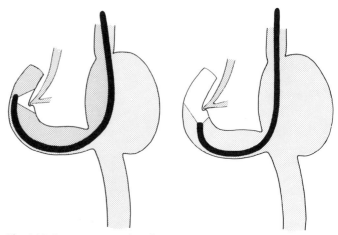

Fig. 6.48 Some experts prefer a forward-viewing scope to obtain better alignment at the papilla, especially for the bile duct.

limb, or when attempting cannulation up a Roux-en-Y loop. Cannulation in the latter situation is almost impossible without a combined percutaneous–endoscopic approach (see Chapter 7).

After surgery to the papilla, pancreas and biliary tree

Duodenotomy performed at surgery for access to the papilla results in a puckered scar on the lateral wall of the duodenum, which may slightly reduce its lumen and affect endoscopic manoeuvrability; these scars can be misdiagnosed as polyps and tumours by the unwary. Papillary appearances after surgical 'sphincterotomy' vary from normality to a wide-open biliary orifice. Standard surgical sphincteroplasty results in a gaping hole, dribbling bile and blowing bubbles; the pancreatic duct orifice is usually visible in the floor of the sphincteroplasty (Fig. 6.49).

A small biliary fistula is sometimes seen above the papilla (Fig. 6.50). This can arise spontaneously after stone impaction, or, more commonly, when dilators have been forced through the roof of the papilla during surgical exploration. A similar fistula can also be caused by percutaneous transhepatic catheters. The presence of a fistula should be suspected (especially when biliary cannulation proves difficult through the main papillary orifice) when there is air in the biliary tree on plain radiology, and when 'biliary bubbles' appear above the papilla.

Air in the biliary tree is also seen after a choledochoduodenostomy. The stoma is usually easy to find in the roof or left lateral wall of the duodenal bulb, but can escape detection when stenosed. Cannulation of a tight stoma may require a guidewire. When the orifice is widely patent, a balloon occlusion catheter technique will provide quality radiographs. It may be necessary to use a guidewire to facilitate selective cannulation of upper and lower limbs.

Most operations on the pancreas do not involve the papillary region, and cannulation is unaffected. The standard Whipple procedure usually takes the biliary and pancreatic duct orifices out of endoscopic reach. The site of a pseudocyst-gastrostomy looks like a ragged pale gastric ulcer. These stomas always close completely within a few weeks.

ERCP in children

There are few indications for ERCP in children, but several series have indicated success and value in the context of recurrent pancreatitis and obscure jaundice. There are experimental small paediatric instruments, but the standard duodenoscope can be used (with the straight scope technique) down to the age of about 1 year. Success in neonates has been reported. Small-diameter flexible taper-tipped catheters pre-formed with a tight distal curve are easier to manoeuvre in the confines of the infant duodenum. Actual cannulation is usually easy, often with simultaneous filling of both duct systems.

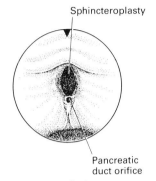

Fig. 6.49 Standard sphincteroplasty.

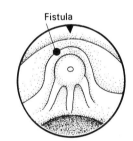

Fig. 6.50 Biliary fistula due to stone or instrumentation.

We use general anaesthesia up to the mid-teens, since it is essential for the patient to remain still. General anaesthesia eliminates normal warnings of discomfort, and care must be taken to avoid unnatural manipulations, and the excessive use of air and contrast.

Radiographic interpretation and artefacts

Cholangiograms are relatively familiar, and retrograde studies resemble those obtained by other techniques. Specific artefacts caused by layering and streaming of contrast, and also by the introduction of air bubbles, can be recognized and eliminated by good technique. There should be relatively few problems of interpretation. Bile-duct size remains a controversial issue (especially after cholecystectomy). There is little evidence that the bile duct increases in size after cholecystectomy (unless there is pathology), and a 'dilated' duct (unless more than about 12 mm) cannot be interpreted as indicating obstruction unless it is known that the bile duct was smaller at the time of surgery. The appearances of the terminal bile duct are very variable, and overinterpretation is more common than the reverse. Numerous views taken during emptying may resolve diagnostic problems (Fig. 6.36). It can be difficult to decide whether a distal biliary stricture is due to pancreatitis or carcinoma, but coincident pancreatography may help. The radiographic distinction between sclerosing cholangitis and cholangiocarcinoma may be impossible, and the diagnostic specificity of changes in the intrahepatic biliary tree remains controversial. Beginners are often struck by low insertion of the cystic duct, but this finding is very common. Failure to fill the cystic duct and gallbladder indicates pathology if sufficient contrast has entered the biliary system to demonstrate the entire intrahepatic tree.

Pancreatograms are less familiar than cholangiograms, and are often more difficult to interpret than to obtain. The course of the main duct varies considerably. It usually ascends almost vertically in the head; after a sharp turn or loop at the neck it crosses the vertical column horizontally or slightly upwards towards the tail. No diagnostic significance can be attributed to odd shapes of the pancreatic duct. The mean diameters of the main duct in the head, body and tail of the normal pancreas are approximately 4, 3 and 2 mm, respectively, but the upper limits of normality are closer to 6, 4 and 3 mm, respectively. These figures are corrected for the radiographic magnification (usually about 30%), by checking the apparent endoscopic diameter on the radiographs. There is some increase in pancreatic duct diameter beyond middle age. First- and second-order branches are usually visible throughout the gland (with good technique), but the distribution and course of these branches is variable (Fig. 6.51). There are fewer branches over the vertebral column where the pancreas is thinner. Congenital variations in the duct relationships in the head of the pancreas are predictable from their embryological derivation. There is often a narrowing in the main duct close to the junction with Santorini's

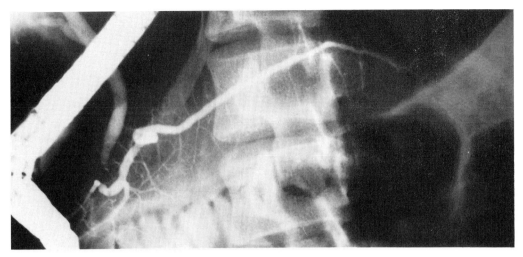

Fig. 6.51 Good quality normal pancreatogram.

duct—an appearance which should not be misinterpreted as pathological. The absence of upstream dilatation should provide reassurance. Complete non-union of the ventral and dorsal segments gives rise to 'pancreas divisum' (Fig. 6.52). Cannulation of the main papilla then shows only a small ventral pancreas (Fig. 6.28), which may be rudimentary (or even absent). The dorsal duct becomes dominant and drains the bulk of the pancreas, through Santorini's duct and the accessory papilla (Fig. 6.53). Santorini's duct may be dominant even when union occurs—the 'partial pancreas divisum' (Fig. 6.54).

Pancreatograms are usually grossly abnormal in patients with ductal adenocarcinoma, showing complete obstruction or a tight stricture with upstream dilatation. Tumours which do not arise in the ductal system are less apparent, and tumours of the uncinate process can be missed. A normal pancreatogram (of good quality, i.e. showing branches throughout the gland) has a specificity of about 95% in ruling out pancreatic cancer.

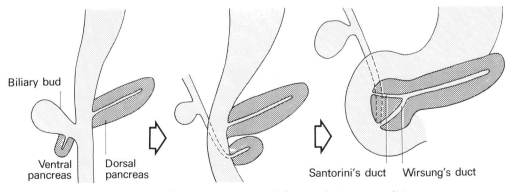

Fig. 6.52 Embryonic development of pancreas. Arrest at mid-phase results in pancreas divisum.

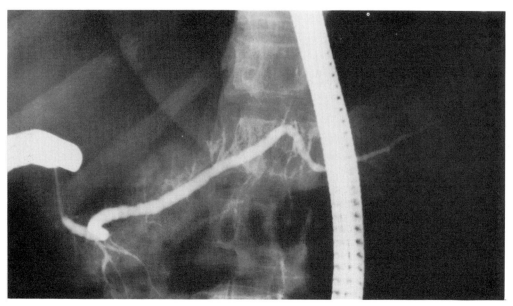

Fig. 6.53 Normal dorsal pancreatogram achieved by cannulating the accessory papilla and filling the body and tail of the pancreas through Santorini's duct.

The pancreatogram is often normal in patients with recurrent attacks of acute pancreatitis. In severe chronic pancreatitis, the main or branch ducts are usually diffusely and irregularly dilated (Fig. 6.55), and often contain filling defects which eventually calcify and cause duct obstruction. Without calcification, the radiographic appearances of duct obstruction due to pancreatitis may resemble those seen in cancer—indeed the two diseases may occasionally co-exist.

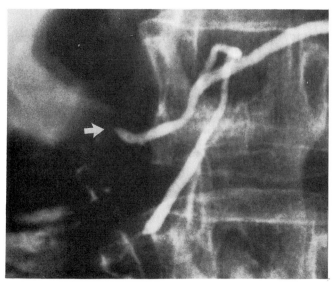

Fig. 6.54 Dominant Santorini duct discharging at the accessory papilla (arrowed).

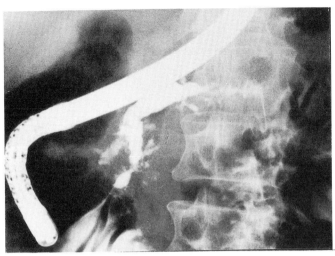

Fig. 6.55 Chronic pancreatitis with disorganization of the duct system, multiple strictures and areas of dilatation.

Radiographically, 'moderate' pancreatitis is characterized by less impressive calibre variation in the main pancreatic duct and its branches. The earliest changes ('minimal pancreatitis') are seen in the branch ducts alone. The clinical significance of minor branch duct changes remains controversial, but there are correlations with functional abnormalities and clinical follow-up. However, similar abnormalities in the branch ducts can occur with advancing age, and should be interpreted with caution.

The ERCP report should be the combined opinion of endoscopist and radiologist, given in the full knowledge of the clinical context and other imaging studies.

Specimen collection

Collection of pure bile and pancreatic juice

Pure bile can be collected by simple (gentle) aspiration after deep cannulation. Aspiration in the narrower pancreatic duct is rarely effective. Pure pancreatic juice is best collected with a catheter tip about 2 cm into the duct, using simple siphonage with the proximal end of the catheter near the floor, especially after an injection of secretin. For biochemical studies, the catheters should be primed with saline, and contrast materials should be avoided.

Duct cytology

Juice for cytology should also be free of contrast, but contamination is often inevitable, since it is the radiographs that provide the indication. If cancer is suspected and the duct cannot be cannulated, some juice may be aspirated from the orifice after injection of secretin. Specimens should be processed immediately using standard

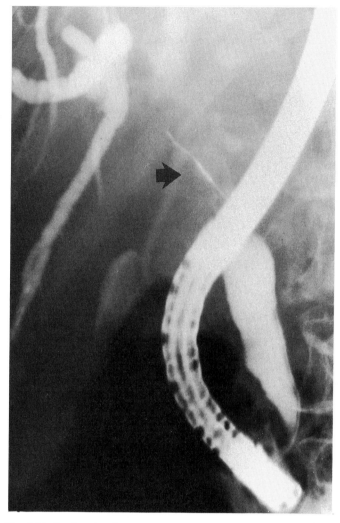

Fig. 6.56 Cytology brush (arrowed) passed deep into the common hepatic duct.

Fig. 6.57 Cytology brush with guidewire leader for use in ducts.

cytological techniques. The results of pancreatic juice cytology have been rather disappointing, although the sensitivity may reach 70% in lesions of the pancreatic head. Cell and diagnostic yields are higher with direct brushing techniques. Sleeved brushes can be passed deep into the biliary system (Fig. 6.56), but not far into the pancreatic duct because of its tortuosity. A brush with a guidewire leader is particularly useful since specimens can be taken without losing deep cannulation (Fig. 6.57).

Biopsies at ERCP

Tumours of the papilla, and those of the pancreas ulcerating into the duodenum, can be sampled by standard biopsy techniques,

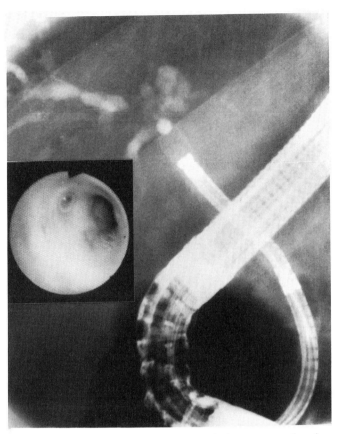

Fig. 6.58 Radiograph showing the baby choledochoscope passed up the bile duct through the 'mother' instrument.

including snare specimens where appropriate. Some tumours confined within the papilla are detected only after sphincterotomy has been performed for apparently benign papillary stenosis.

Biopsies can be taken from within the bile duct (less commonly the pancreatic duct) under fluoroscopic guidance with standard forceps. Biopsies can also be taken under direct vision within the duct systems using 'mother and baby choledochoscopes' (Fig. 6.58).

Attempts have been made to take aspiration cytology samples of the pancreatic parenchyma, using a fine needle passed via the duodenoscope through the wall of the stomach or duodenum. The safety and value of this technique has not yet been established.

Motivation to develop ERCP-related techniques for taking biopsy specimens was reduced by the widespread introduction of percutaneous aspiration cytology techniques. However, these do not give ideal results, and more emphasis should be placed on tissue diagnosis at ERCP, especially with the increased use of non-operative stenting.

Complications

ERCP carries the same potential rare risks of all endoscopic procedures, including medication reactions, cardiopulmonary accidents and perforation. The task of the nurse assistant in monitoring the patient may be made more difficult in a semi-darkened room. When working outside the confines of the usual endoscopy unit, it is essential to ensure ready access to all necessary equipment for resuscitation.

The act of duct cannulation carries risks specific to ERCP—pancreatitis and sepsis.

Post-ERCP pancreatitis

The incidence of pancreatitis after ERCP is around 3%, but this figure depends upon definition as much as technique. The serum amylase is almost always elevated for 4–48 hours after ERCP. Pancreatitis is defined as a consistent clinical picture with pain and raised amylase (without other cause) lasting for more than a few hours, and requiring in-hospital care. Most attacks are mild, settling in a few days with conservative management, but they can be complicated and life-threatening.

Pancreatitis is most likely to occur after repeated injections of contrast under undue pressure, usually in the context of a difficult bile duct cannulation. It is wise to limit the number of pancreatic injections to three—but pancreatitis can occur after the simplest ERCP and a single injection. Non-ionic contrast agents may reduce the risk, but there is not yet sufficient evidence to justify the cost of their routine use.

Sepsis after ERCP

Clinically apparent sepsis (cholangitis and septicaemia) can result from cholangiography in the presence of *infected bile*. The risk can be minimized by the prior use of antibiotics and avoiding increased bile-duct pressure (exchanging bile for contrast), and almost eliminated by providing effective drainage at the end of the procedure by endoscopic stone extraction, nasobiliary drainage or stent—or, when necessary, by percutaneous or surgical intervention.

Serious and avoidable sepsis can occur as a result of *introducing* infection with contaminated equipment. Several *Pseudomonas* outbreaks have been traced to contaminated endoscopes and ancillary equipment (particularly the water bottle). The development of sepsis due to *Pseudomonas* (or other hospital opportunist organisms) after ERCP strongly suggests contamination, and should result in immediate review of disinfection procedures.

Sepsis of this type is most likely to occur in the presence of duct strictures (or pseudocysts), but deaths have occurred after a normal-appearing ERCP. The presence of a pseudocyst has been considered to be a relative contraindication for ERCP, for fear of infection. However, the risk is minimal if proper disinfection is employed, and ERCP should be used when information about the duct systems will affect management decisions.

Sphincter of Oddi manometry

Dysfunction of the sphincter of Oddi can cause biliary pain (especially post-cholecystectomy), and recurrent pancreatitis. ERCP has brought the problem of 'papillary stenosis' into closer focus by ruling out other causes, such as stones and tumours. Pressures can be measured in the ducts and sphincter zones by standard manometric techniques, using a triple lumen perfused catheter system at the time of ERCP (Fig. 6.59). Endoscopic manometry is often difficult for the endoscopist and the patient, since no analgesic or duodenal relaxant can be used. Interpretation of the tracings is often subjective (Fig. 6.60). Furthermore, the addition of manometry appears to increase the risk of pancreatitis above that expected for standard ERCP. For these reasons, sphincter of Oddi manometry is restricted to a few special centres, and attempts are being made to obtain similar diagnostic information by less invasive methods.

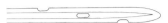

Fig. 6.59 Triple lumen catheter tip for manometry.

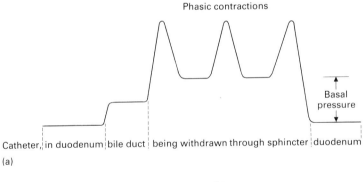

Phasic contractions

Basal pressure

Catheter, in duodenum | bile duct | being withdrawn through sphincter | duodenum

(a)

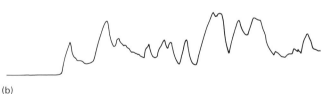

(b)

Fig. 6.60 (a) Stylized manometry trace. (b) Actual tracing from a patient showing potential difficulties in interpretation.

Indications for ERCP

The technique of ERCP was introduced in the early 1970s when ultrasound and computed tomographic (CT) techniques had not been developed, and before percutaneous transhepatic cholangiography (PTC) was widely available. The clinical role of ERCP has changed as these other techniques have developed, and changed again with the increasing dominance of ERCP therapeutic techniques.

Detailed discussion of the clinical role of ERCP is beyond the intended scope of this book. Its overall value depends much upon its quality, and its linkage to immediate therapy (e.g. for stones and strictures). ERCP, PTC and non-invasive imaging methods provide a spectrum of complementary approaches to patients with biliary and pancreatic disease, whose pattern of utilization will vary between different institutions.

Specific clinical contexts

Post-cholecystectomy pain

ERCP has a primary role in this common situation, allowing diagnosis (and treatment) of residual stones and post-surgical strictures, but also detection of other causes of pain including ulcer disease, pancreatitis, pancreas divisum, and sphincter of Oddi dysfunction (aided by manometry).

Unexplained pancreatitis

Any patient with unexplained (and especially recurrent) pancreatitis should undergo ERCP to detect or exclude abnormalities of the papilla and ductal systems. These examinations are traditionally delayed for a few weeks after the last attack of pancreatitis, but the risk of exacerbation appears minimal, even when performed earlier. Endoscopic techniques are also being used increasingly for the treatment of pancreatitis (Chapter 7).

Obscure abdominal pain

The diagnostic yield of ERCP is small in patients with no abnormalities of abdominal imaging, liver function tests, or amylase. Chronic pancreatitis can be detected by duct abnormalities when other tests are negative, but the interpretation of minor abnormalities of the branches remains controversial. It is unusual to detect pancreatic cancer in the presence of a normal CT scan (or good quality ultrasound study). Even if such scans do not detect the mass lesion itself, they usually show pancreatic duct dilatation upstream, indicating the presence of a lesion. ERCP is of limited value in investigating patients with *known* pancreatic mass lesions, since the duct appearances (obstruction or stricture) may appear similar in patients with benign and malignant disease. ERCP may detect pancreas divisum or other rare anomalies which may have clinical significance. ERCP may occasionally show gallbladder stones which had previously escaped detection, and the procedure allows sampling of bile for crystals or more sophisticated biochemical analyses.

Diagnosis and management of jaundice

ERCP is generally preferred to PTC in the investigation of jaundiced patients, mainly because so many of the likely causes are best managed immediately by endoscopic techniques (see Chapter 7). The method is also better for ruling out obstruction (e.g. in the context of primary biliary cirrhosis), since PTC is more likely to fail with normal calibre or small ducts.

Further reading

Axon, A. T. R., Classen, M., Cotton, P. B., Cremer, M., Freeny, P. C. and Lees, W. R. (1984) 'Pancreatography and chronic pancreatitis. International definitions'. *Gut*, **25**, 1107.

Cotton, P. B. (1977) 'Progress Report ERCP'. *Gut*, **18**, 316.

Cotton, P. B. (1988) 'Problems in ERCP interpretation', in *Diagnostic Radiology* (ed. Margulis, A. R. and Gooding, C. A.). Radiology Research and Education Foundation, UCSF.

Endoscopy (1988) Supplement on 'Disorders of the major duodenal papilla and sphincter of Oddi'. *Endoscopy*, **20**, 165–236.

Ferguson, D. R. and Sivak, M. V. (1987) 'Contraindications and complications of ERCP', in *Gastroenterologic Endoscopy* (ed. Sivak, M. A.). W. B. Saunders, Philadelphia.

Fink, A. S., Valle, Perez de Ayala, Chapman, M. and Cotton, P. B. (1987) 'Radiological pitfalls in endoscopic retrograde pancreatography'. *Pancreas*, **1**, 180.

Lail, L. M. and Cotton, P. B. (1990) 'Risks of ERCP and therapeutic applications', in *Gastroenterology Nursing*. In press.

Ohto, M., Ono, T., Tsuchiya, Y. *et al.* (1978) *Cholangiography and Pancreatography*. Igaku Shoin, Tokyo.

Reuben, A., Johnson, A. L. and Cotton, P. B. (1978) 'Is pancreatogram interpretation reliable? A study of observer variation'. *British Journal of Radiology*, **51**, 956.

Schapiro, R. H. (1989) 'ERCP in the diagnosis of pancreatic and biliary disease', in *ERCP, Diagnostic and Therapeutic Applications* (ed. Jacobson, I. M.), pp. 9–40. Elsevier, Amsterdam.

Silverstein, G. E. and Tytgat, G. N. J. (1987) 'ERCP and sphincterotomy', in *Atlas of Gastrointestinal Endoscopy*. Gower Medical Publishing, London.

Stewart, E. T., Vennes, J. A. and Geenen, J. E. (1977) *Atlas of Endoscopic Retrograde Cholangiopancreatography*. Mosby, St. Louis.

Vennes, J. A. (1987) 'Techniques of ERCP', in *Gastroenterologic Endoscopy* (ed. Sivak, M. V.). W. B. Saunders, Philadelphia.

7 Therapeutic endoscopic retrograde cholangio-pancreatography (ERCP)

The first therapeutic application of ERCP—sphincterotomy for duct stones—was described in 1974, and is now a commonplace procedure throughout the world. Overall satisfaction with the results and familiarity with the techniques has led to an expansion of indications, and many new therapeutic developments, including balloon dilatation of strictures, placement of stents and nasobiliary drains, and increasing interest in the endoscopic management of patients with pancreatic as well as biliary problems.

These procedures are amongst the most worth while, but also the most difficult and hazardous that endoscopists attempt. It is essential to be properly trained and to have a volume of work sufficient to maintain and develop expertise. ERCP and its complex therapeutic applications are not techniques that every endoscopist should expect to master, or attempt to do so. Many of the procedures replace others previously performed by surgeons, but it is unwise to view endoscopy and surgery as competitors. Therapeutic ERCP techniques such as sphincterotomy are really surgical procedures performed by endoscopists. The therapeutic endoscopist must work in close association with surgical colleagues, forming a team approach which involves other specialists (including radiologists and pathologists). Complex procedures should be performed only in institutions with facilities adequate to deal rapidly with major complications, such as bleeding.

The importance of trained GI nurses/assistants cannot be overemphasized. A minimum of two are required; one to ensure the patient's comfort and safety during the procedure, the other to assist the endoscopist, manage the complex equipment, and maintain sterility. The quality of this assistance can make the difference between success and failure, triumph and disaster.

Biliary sphincterotomy

Sphincterotomy equipment

Sphincterotomy is performed with standard side-viewing duodenoscopes, appropriate sphincterotomes and an electrosurgical source. Electrosurgical units used for polypectomy are suitable; operating room electrosurgical units are unnecessarily powerful, and can be hazardous if used without expert knowledge. Familiarity with a single source is probably more important than the precise specification. Most experts prefer equipment which allows the application of blended coagulation and cutting current. Regular maintenance of electrosurgery equipment and attachments is essential.

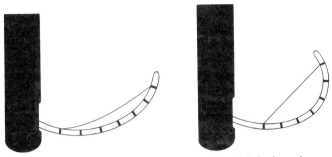

Fig. 7.1 Standard 'pull-type' sphincterotome: relaxed (left); bowed (right).

Sphincterotomes

A bewildering variety of sphincterotomes (papillotomes) are now available commercially. The original Demling–Classen design ('pull-type') is still the most popular (Fig. 7.1), but there are many variations. The main differences are the length of the exposed diathermy wire, and of the sphincterotome 'nose' (Fig. 7.2).

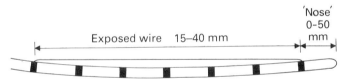

Fig. 7.2 Length variables of sphincterotomes.

A relatively short nose (5–8 mm) is convenient for cannulation. The tip can be engaged in the papilla without the wire interfering, and tension on the wire can be used to bow the tip into the correct axis (Fig. 7.3). This bowing facility is lost with a sphincterotome which has a long nose (2–5 cm beyond the wire), since the diathermy wire (tension on which causes the bow) inevitably remains inside the endoscope until deep cannulation has been achieved. The sole advantage of the long-nose sphincterotome is that cannulation is not lost as the wire is withdrawn during sphincterotomy. Sphincterotomes without any protruding nose are sometimes used for 'pre-cutting'; the diathermy wire extends into the tip of the catheter (Fig. 7.4).

The length of exposed wire in the original standard sphincterotomes was about 35 mm. Now versions are available ranging from 15 to 40 mm. Since most endoscopists perform sphincterotomy with only 5–8 mm of wire in contact with the mucosa, it seems illogical to have a much longer wire, especially since it is essential to avoid touching the endoscope tip with the proximal end of the wire during the application of diathermy current.

Unfortunately, attempts to make effective short-wire sphincterotomes have not been fully successful. Current models tend to

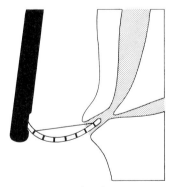

Fig. 7.3 Using the sphincterotome bow to obtain the correct axis for bile duct cannulation.

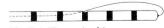

Fig. 7.4 'Pre-cut' sphincterotome.

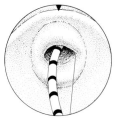

Fig. 7.5 Bad orientation, a common problem with short-wire sphincterotomes.

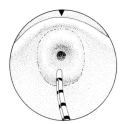

Fig. 7.6 Correct position of wire, which enters and leaves *left* side of catheter.

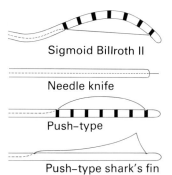

Sigmoid Billroth II

Needle knife

Push–type

Push–type shark's fin

Fig. 7.7 Specialized sphincterotomes.

flip sideways, especially towards 3 o'clock (Fig. 7.5), whereas the longer wire sphincterotomes (e.g. 35 mm) take the natural curve of the endoscope and elevator, and usually enter the papilla in the correct orientation (11 to 1 o'clock). All sphincterotomes are more likely to behave well if 'trained' before use. The tip should be curled so that the wire enters and leaves the catheter along its left side (Fig. 7.6). Assistants must appreciate that sphincterotomes with short wires require much shorter travel of the control handle to produce a bow; uninformed excessive 'tightening' will result in kinking.

All sphincterotome catheters should have a side port for injection of contrast.

Specialized sphincterotomes

Sphincterotomy (like cannulation itself) is more difficult in patients with Billroth II resections because of the reverse orientation. Sphincterotomes with a sigmoid shape (reversed bow) are available to facilitate correct placement (Fig. 7.7).

Larger diameter sphincterotomes which allow passage of a central guidewire can be very useful.

The 'needle knife' sphincterotome consists simply of a bare diathermy wire protruding about 3 mm from the end of a catheter (Fig. 7.7). A standard polyp snare can be used for the same purpose, with the tip just protruding from the sleeve or a standard sphincterotome cut down. The needle knife can be used exactly as a 'hot' knife, for pre-cutting, or for direct puncture of the bile duct above the papilla. 'Push-type' sphincterotomes (and a variant—the shark fin) are those in which the wire is pushed out to form a bow (Fig. 7.7). These types are rarely used, since the direction of protrusion is not predictable.

Preparation for sphincterotomy

Patient checks, preparation and sedation are broadly similar to those used for diagnostic ERCP. Detailed discussion of the aims, risks and alternatives must take place, for the patient's consent to be truly informed. An information leaflet helps this process (Fig. 7.8). Coagulation status is checked (prothrombin time, platelet count and partial thromboplastin time) and improved where necessary. The bleeding time should also be checked if there is a history of unusual bleeding, or if aspirin has been taken. Because of the serious potential risks, sphincterotomy is performed as an inpatient procedure—in an institution capable of dealing with any emergency.

Most experts use antibiotics routinely, starting 1 hour prior to any therapeutic ERCP procedure. Broad-spectrum antibiotic coverage is appropriate. We use gentamicin with ampicillin (with vancomycin as a substitute in patients who are penicillin sensitive).

We emphasize again the importance of quality assistants, and high-level disinfection of endoscopes and all ancillary devices.

THE BEST HOSPITAL ENDOSCOPY UNIT
ERCP/Sphincterotomy Information Sheet

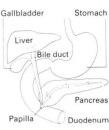

ERCP

ERCP (endoscopic retrograde cholangiopancreatography) is used in the diagnosis of disorders of the pancreas, bile duct, liver and gall-bladder. The doctor passes an endoscope (a thin, flexible telescope) through your mouth, to inspect your stomach and duodenum. The doctor then injects contrast dye into the drainage hole (papilla) from the bile ducts and pancreas, to take detailed X-rays (you should inform us if there is any possibility of pregnancy).

Preparation To allow a clear view, you should not eat or drink anything after midnight. If you must take prescription medicines, use only small sips of water. Do not take antacids.

What will happen? The doctor and nurse will explain the procedure, and answer your questions. Please tell them if you have had any other endoscopy examinations, or any allergies or bad reactions to medications or contrast dye. You will be asked to sign a consent form giving permission for the procedure, to put on a hospital gown, and remove eyeglasses, contact lenses, or dentures.

The examination is performed on an X-ray table. Local anaesthetic will be sprayed onto your throat to make it numb, and you will be given medication by injection through a vein to make you sleepy and relaxed. With you in a comfortable position on your left side, the doctor will pass the endoscope down your throat. A guard will be placed to protect your teeth. The endoscope will not interfere with your breathing and will not cause any pain. You may be asked to change positions during the examination, which takes 15–60 minutes.

Afterwards Your throat may feel numb and slightly sore. Because of the local anaesthetic and sedation you should not attempt to take anything by mouth for at least 1 hour. It is wise to keep to clear liquids for the remainder of the day. If you are an out-patient, you will remain in the clinic area for at least 1 hour. A companion *must* be able to drive you home as the sedation impairs your reflexes and judgments. For the remainder of the day you should not drive a car, operate machinery, or make any important decisions. We suggest that you rest quietly.

Risks? Endoscopy can result in complications, such as reactions to medication, perforation of the intestine, and bleeding. Injection of contrast dye through the endoscope can cause allergic reactions, inflammation of the pancreas (pancreatitis) and of the bile duct (cholangitis). These complications are rare, but may require urgent treatment, and even an operation. Be sure to inform us if you have any pain, fever or vomiting in the 24 hours after ERCP.

Questions or problems? Contact the nurse in charge, Endoscopy Unit (Tel: . . . .), 8 a.m. to 4.30 p.m. Monday to Friday. At other times, in case of emergency, call the Hospital Operator to contact the gastroenterologist on duty.

ERCP treatments

Sphincterotomy If the X-rays show a gallstone, or other blockage, the doctor can enlarge the opening of the bile duct. This is called 'sphincterotomy', and is done with an electrically heated wire, which you will not feel. Any stones will be collected into a tiny basket, or left to pass into the intestine.

Stenting A stent is a small plastic tube which is pushed through the endoscope and into a narrowed area in the bile duct. This relieves the jaundice, by allowing the bile to drain freely into the intestine. Stents are also sometimes placed in the pancreatic duct when it is narrow or blocked.

Naso-biliary tube Sometimes a small plastic tube is left in the bile duct, and brought out through the nose for a few days. This helps drainage of bile, and allows X-rays to check when the duct is clear. The tube may be slightly uncomfortable at first, but does not interfere with eating or drinking.

Risks? These treatments for stones and blockage have been developed and are recommended to you because they are simpler and safer than standard surgical operations. However, you should realize that they are not always successful, and problems can arise. Potential complications include perforation of the intestine, bleeding, inflammation of the pancreas (pancreatitis) and infection of the bile duct (cholangitis). These complications are rare, but may be serious enough to require urgent treatment, and even an operation. Death is a remote possibility.

It is very unusual for other biliary problems to develop in the months or years after sphincterotomy, but jaundice, fevers, and even new stones can rarely occur. Usually these can be dealt with by another endoscopic procedure.

Stents can become blocked with debris after some months. This will result in a recurrence of jaundice, usually associated with fevers and chills. If this happens, you should inform us or your local doctor quickly. You will need antibiotics, and consideration of a stent change.

Fig. 7.8 ERCP/sphincterotomy information leaflet.

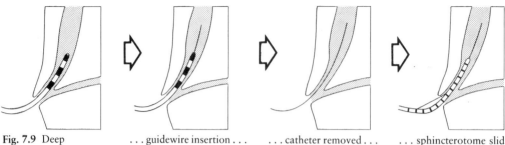

Fig. 7.9 Deep cannulation . . .

. . . guidewire insertion . . .

. . . catheter removed . . .

. . . sphincterotome slid over guidewire.

Technique of biliary sphincterotomy

Most endoscopists use a standard catheter to perform cholangiography before considering and initiating sphincterotomy. If deep cannulation has been achieved (especially when it has been difficult), there is merit in using the guidewire sphincterotome technique. An 0.035-in. guidewire is passed through the original diagnostic catheter; the catheter is then removed leaving the tip of the guidewire deep in the duct, and the sphincterotome is then slid over the wire (Fig. 7.9). Alternatively, the diagnostic catheter can be removed, a standard sphincterotome selected, and placed deep within the biliary system.

It is possible also to use a standard sphincterotome for the *initial* biliary cannulation and cholangiogram. This is an appropriate short-cut when the indication for sphincterotomy is strong (e.g. known duct stones). Deep cannulation can sometimes be easier to achieve with a sphincterotome than with a standard catheter as the tip is somewhat stiffer, and bowing the wire can be used to change the angle of approach. The sphincterotome tip is inserted into the roof of the orifice, angling and bowing up slightly. Deep cannulation is usually best achieved by lifting the sphincterotome tip up with the elevator, and *pulling back somewhat* on the endoscope, thus directing the tip into the duct axis (Fig. 7.10 a–d). Attempting to achieve deep cannulation by simply pushing the sphincterotome is usually unsuccessful (and counterproductive), since the tip is forced into the 'duodenal' wall of the bile duct, or between mucosal folds in the sphincter itself (Fig. 7.10 e). Confirmation that the sphincterotome is in the bile duct can be achieved by injecting

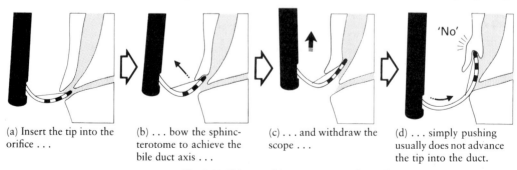

(a) Insert the tip into the orifice . . .

(b) . . . bow the sphincterotome to achieve the bile duct axis . . .

(c) . . . and withdraw the scope . . .

(d) . . . simply pushing usually does not advance the tip into the duct.

Fig. 7.10 Using a sphincterotome to achieve deep cannulation.

contrast. If pancreatography has been performed already, the position of the sphincterotome can be established by 'wiggling' it; the pancreatic duct will move if the tip is within it.

Once a sphincterotome is placed deeply in the bile duct and the indication for sphincterotomy is confirmed, it is time to check that the electrosurgical equipment is properly connected, and to assess the anatomical constraints on the procedure. The size of the papilla, and any stone, and the shape of the distal bile duct, can all determine the appropriate (and safe) length of incision (see below).

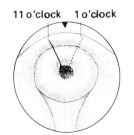

Fig. 7.11 Correct sphincterotomy sector.

The sphincterotome is withdrawn slowly under visual and fluoroscopic control until the proximal end of the wire is visible outside the papilla. The wire must be pointing between 11 and 1 o'clock, preferably at 12 o'clock (Fig. 7.11). Sphincterotomy should not be performed if the wire cannot be placed within these limits, since perforation is much more likely, especially beyond 3 o'clock. One way to swing the wire anticlockwise is to push the endoscope tip more deeply into the duodenum, whilst angling up. If good orientation cannot be achieved by manipulating the endoscope tip, it may be necessary to change to a different sphincterotome.

Experts use many different methods for the actual incision, but most use only slight bowing, and a short (5–8 mm) length of wire in contact with the mucosa (Fig. 7.12). The principle of incision should be 'hot and slow', achieved by lifting the sphincterotome upwards progressively to provide the necessary pressure. The principal aim is to use the sphincterotome as a short hot wire, which is 'walked up' from the tip of the papillary orifice (Fig. 7.12). The roof of the ampulla peels open to expose the distal bile duct mucosa.

Electrical settings vary with experts and machines. We use blended current, 2–3 on the Olympus PSD, and usually 4 cut, 7 coag on the Valley Lab. However, the effectiveness and safety of sphincterotomy depends much more on the *length of wire* in contact (and therefore the current density) than the precise settings. The commonest error is to have too much wire inside the papilla (partially for fear of falling out), and to apply too much bowing tension. Nothing will happen when current is applied—or only slow coagulation which increases the risk of subsequent pancreatitis.

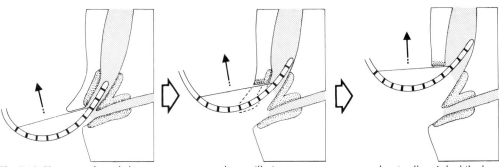

Fig. 7.12 Use up-angle and short wire contact . . .   . . . to cut the papilla in steps . . .   . . . and to 'walk up' the bile duct.

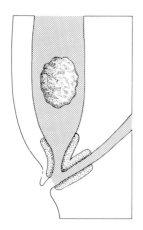

Fig. 7.13 Easy sphincterotomy: swollen papilla, big duct, 'square' termination.

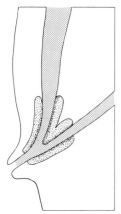

Fig. 7.14 More dangerous sphincterotomy: small papilla, small tapering duct.

There is then a temptation to increase the current settings, and pressure, which will eventually and suddenly cut through the coagulated area at alarming speed with a risk of significant bleeding (the 'zipper'). If nothing appears to be happening when current is applied, it is much better to reduce the length of wire in contact with the mucosa, which increases the local current density and should initiate the incision.

When to stop cutting?

The size of the sphincterotomy must be tailored to the size of the bile duct and stone, and will be influenced somewhat by the shape and direction of the terminal bile duct in relation to the duodenum. The simplest and probably safest sphincterotomies are those performed in patients who have (or have had) a stone impacted above the orifice; the papilla is large and oedematous, and cuts easily without bleeding, and the bile duct termination is somewhat 'square' (Fig. 7.13). Sphincterotomy is more hazardous in patients with a relatively small papilla and a duct which is either not dilated, or tapers distally (Fig. 7.14). Mainly for this reason, the risk of perforation is significantly greater when sphincterotomy is performed for 'papillary stenosis', when compared with sphincterotomy for ductal stones.

Judging when to stop cutting is obviously the crucial question—for which there is no easy answer. Some endoscopists rely on *external* landmarks, stating that it is safe to cut up to, but not beyond, the proximal hooding fold. Unfortunately, this fold varies in size and position, and bears little relationship to the underlying anatomy. More important is the size of the papilla itself, and whether or not any of the intramural bile duct can be seen from the duodenum. It is usually safe to cut down to the duodenal wall, but—although this may produce an impressive long cut on the surface—it may not reach the upper part of the biliary sphincter (Fig. 7.15). It is usually necessary to cut some more *inside*

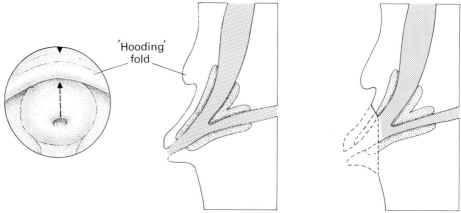

'Hooding' fold

Fig. 7.15 Probably safe to cut down to the estimated duodenal wall—but the upper sphincter is not necessarily divided.

(Fig. 7.16). Often the sphincterotome 'jumps' into the bile duct as the upper sphincter is broached, and bile flows out of the incision.

A useful sign of an adequate sphincterotomy is when the partially bowed sphincterotome slides easily to and fro through the orifice. The size of the orifice can also be measured using balloon-tipped catheters.

Difficult sphincterotomies

There are certain circumstances in which bile duct access and the resulting sphincterotomy is predictably more difficult than usual, and where additional skills and judgment may be required.

Peri-papillary diverticula

Many patients with bile duct stones have diverticula around the papilla. Cannulation and sphincterotomy may be extremely difficult when the papilla is inside the diverticulum. The site of the papilla is best identified by following the longitudinal fold upwards (Fig. 7.17). It is usually possible to bring the papilla out of the diverticulum by pressing firmly sideways (with a catheter or sphincterotome) on the duodenal folds which are flowing into the diverticulum (Fig. 7.18). There is no evidence that sphincterotomy is more dangerous in the presence of a diverticulum. The direction of the bile duct is somewhat unpredictable (unless it can be seen traversing the floor of the diverticulum) but the sphincterotome necessarily follows the bile duct direction.

Billroth II gastrectomy

The principles involved in performing a sphincterotomy are classical, the only problem being that the anatomy is 'upside down'. Standard sphincterotomes are designed to bring the wire out at 12 o'clock in the field of view. In the Billroth II situation, the wire needs to be pointing at 6 o'clock (using the standard side-viewing duodenoscope). It is probably easiest to use the specially-designed

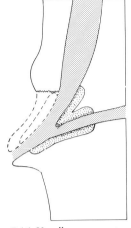

Fig. 7.16 Usually necessary to cut inside to ablate the biliary sphincter.

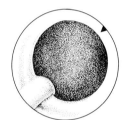

Fig. 7.17 Papilla within diverticulum—only the longitudinal fold shows.

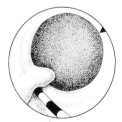

Fig. 7.18 Push with catheter or sphincterotome to evert papilla from diverticulum . . .

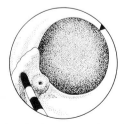

. . . then further pressure laterally brings orifice into view.

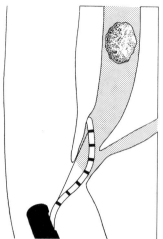

Fig. 7.19 A sigmoid loop sphincterotome is easiest in Billroth II patients.

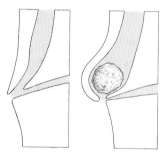

Fig. 7.20 Compared to the normal anatomy an impacted stone forces the orifice downwards.

sigmoid loop sphincterotome (Fig. 7.19). Sometimes a standard sphincterotome can be persuaded into the correct position by deft endoscopic manoeuvring.

An alternative method is to use a needle knife (see below), to make an incision above the papilla in the region of the bile duct termination, and then, either to complete the incision with the needle knife, or to insert a standard sphincterotome through this orifice, and guide the tip out of the main papillary orifice. The subsequent incision connects the two holes. Some experts first place a stent or naso-biliary drain and use this as a marker while cutting down with a needle knife.

Cannulation of the bile duct in patients with Billroth II gastrectomy may require the use of guidewire techniques (see Chapter 6). If cannulation has been achieved in this way, it is worth trying a long-nose sphincterotome designed to be passed over the guidewire.

Impacted stone

Stone impaction usually causes the papilla to bulge into the duodenum and forces the orifice downwards (Fig. 7.20). Cannulation can be achieved with a bowed sphincterotome, 'hooking' the tip into the orifice (Fig. 7.21 a). Alternatively, a needle knife (see below) can be used to incise the face of the papilla over the stone (Fig. 7.21 b).

Pre-cutting

Pre-cutting means starting an incision without having achieved deep biliary cannulation. It should not be used by inexperienced endoscopists. The procedure is uncontrolled. It may not be possible to complete the sphincterotomy, which can leave the patient worse off than before.

Some specialized types of sphincterotome may be used for pre-cutting. One is a variant of the standard sphincterotome, with the cutting wire extending to the tip (Fig. 7.4). This is placed in the common channel (as judged by injection of contrast) and electro-surgery is applied with firm upward pressure. This should permit

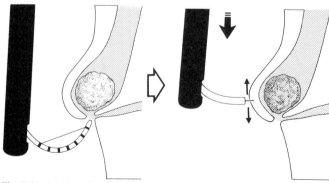

Fig. 7.21 (a) Use a bowed sphincterotome to cannulate . . . (b) . . . or a needle knife to incise over the stone.

deep biliary cannulation, but carries a risk of pancreatitis through coagulation of the pancreatic duct orifice. Another tool is the 'needle knife' (Fig. 7.7). The bare wire is inserted in the papillary orifice, and diathermy applied with pressure in the 12 o'clock direction (Fig. 7.22). The bile duct orifice can usually be identified in the floor of this incision, either immediately or on a subsequent day. Sometimes the needle knife can be used to make a direct 'drill' incision above the papilla into a dilated bile duct, or into the face of a markedly swollen papilla (as in the presence of an impacted stone, or choledochocele).

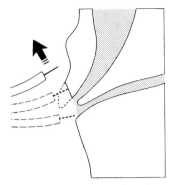

Fig. 7.22 Pre-cutting up from the orifice with a needle knife.

Pre-cutting is more dangerous than standard sphincterotomy. It should not be used as a substitute for proper training and experience in standard techniques, and should be reserved for use by experts in high-risk patients with a strong indication for sphincterotomy when other standard techniques and tricks have been exhausted. Pre-cutting cannot be recommended purely for diagnostic access to the bile duct.

The combined endoscopic–radiologic procedure. An alternative to pre-cutting when standard sphincterotomy fails is to work over a guidewire previously positioned through the papilla from above by an interventional radiologist. This procedure is more commonly employed for insertion of stents and it is described in more detail later (p. 145). Several related techniques have been described as aids to sphincterotomy. Probably the simplest is for the radiologist to position the guidewire (under endoscopic monitoring) about 1 cm outside the papilla. The endoscopist can then slide a 'guidewire' sphincterotome over the wire and into the duct (Fig. 7.23). Other variants have been described, including the use of percutaneous balloon dilatation of the papilla to facilitate deep endoscopic cannulation, the use of a basket (percutaneously) to grasp the sphincterotome and pull it into the duct, or the endoscopist pulling the guidewire all the way up the endoscope with a basket before sliding a sphincterotome over it.

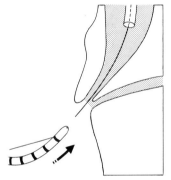

Fig. 7.23 'Combined procedure': a sphincterotome is slid over the percutaneously placed guidewire.

Results, problems and complications

Routine sphincterotomy (with stone extraction) should take less than an hour 'door-to-door'. Patients should be observed carefully overnight in hospital. They are usually given clear fluids the same evening, and are discharged on the following day if there are no adverse reactions, and after at least one full meal has been tolerated.

Success rates for sphincterotomy and for stent extraction vary between centres, with varying levels of expertise and different selection of patients. In the best hands, sphincterotomy can be achieved in > 95% of cases (without resorting to combined percutaneous–endoscopic approaches), and stone extraction in at least 90%, using standard methods.

Endoscopic sphincterotomy is the most risky of the therapeutic procedures currently performed by endoscopists. The usual quoted morbidity and mortality rates are approximately 10% and 1%, respectively. These figures vary somewhat with experience but are subject also to different definitions. We have recently proposed a definition of complications and their severity (see Cotton, 1990).

The big four complications are perforation, bleeding, pancreatitis and infection (mainly cholangitis). The risk of serious bleeding can be minimized by cutting 'hot and slow', avoiding the rapid 'zipper'. Bleeding that does not obscure endoscopic view can usually be controlled by injection of epinephrine (1 in 10 000) into the sides of the raw sphincterotomy, using a standard sclerotherapy needle. Bleeding sufficient to obscure the view within 1–2 min is unlikely to stop spontaneously. Skilled angiographic embolization may be effective. If surgery is necessary, it is wise to use non-absorbable sutures and to consider ligation of the major feeding vessel.

Perforation is more likely to occur with small common bile ducts and incisions off-centre (beyond 2 o'clock). If perforation is recognized whilst there are still stones in the duct, it is logical to proceed to surgery (unless the patient is a formidable surgical risk), in order to complete the procedure (by duct exploration and T-tube placement), and to drain the retroperitoneal space. When there are no stones present, many patients have been treated successfully by conservative means using a naso-biliary drainage catheter (on low-pressure suction), naso-gastric suction, 'nil by mouth' and anti-biotics. This course of action should be undertaken only after careful consideration and surgical advice, and continued only so long as the patient appears to be responding. Surgery (and/or percutaneous catheters) may be necessary to drain retroperitoneal collections and abscesses.

It is impossible to eliminate the risk of pancreatitis after sphincterotomy. It can probably be reduced by minimizing the number of pancreatic duct injections, and the amount of coagulation in the region of the pancreatic duct orifice. Some of the worst cases of pancreatitis have resulted from the use of contaminated equipment (particularly with *Pseudomonas*). Pancreatitis is managed by standard methods.

Cholangitis should not occur if drainage is instituted either by removal of the stones or placement of a naso-biliary catheter. Infection should be treated by appropriate antibiotics and drainage (percutaneous or surgical).

Other risks of sphincterotomy include all those of endoscopy and ERCP—and there are potential long-term problems.

Delayed complications

Most complications are obvious within 24 hours. Patients and their referring physicians should be given advice about potential delayed problems.

Complications which can occur in the early post-hospitalization phase include delayed bleeding (which is rarely severe), gallstone ileus, acute cholecystitis (if the patient still has a gallbladder), and cholangitis/pancreatitis (if stones have been left in the duct).

Late complications (up to 10 years) have been described in about

10% of patients after sphincterotomy, including stenosis of the orifice, new stone formation and recurrent attacks of cholangitis despite apparent adequate drainage. Gallbladder symptoms sufficient to warrant cholecystectomy occur in 10–20% of patients in whom the gallbladder is left in place in follow-up periods of 5–10 years.

Indications for biliary sphincterotomy

Detailed reviews of the clinical role of endoscopic sphincterotomy are published elsewhere. In general, sphincterotomy is performed for two main purposes—to relieve stenosis and to provide access to the duct. Organic papillary stenosis is well treated by careful sphincterotomy if correctly diagnosed. Sphincter of Oddi dysfunction is more difficult to define, and the results of sphincterotomy are predictably poorer in the absence of objective signs. It is wise to remember that the risks of sphincterotomy are higher in papillary stenosis than in patients with stones.

Sphincterotomy for bile duct access is performed mainly for extraction of stones, but also to facilitate insertion of some large stents, and (more rarely) for direct per-oral choledochoscopy.

Sphincterotomy is now the primary treatment for bile duct stones in most clinical contexts, whether emergency or elective. A radiological percutaneous approach may be preferred in patients with retained stones post-cholecystectomy and a suitable T-tube in place, but sphincterotomy provides an effective and safe alternative when the conditions are unfavourable for a percutaneous approach or when this fails. Surgical treatment for bile duct stones can now be restricted to those patients who need a cholecystectomy and any patients in whom endoscopic treatment fails or results in certain complications.

Sphincterotomy can also be used in highly-selected patients with biliary obstruction due to tumours of the papilla. This can be done to relieve jaundice as a preoperative measure, or as 'permanent' palliation in patients who are unfit for surgery or have established metastatic disease. Sphincterotomy for tumour carries a somewhat increased risk of bleeding (rarely severe), and may need to be repeated as the tumour grows.

Stone extraction

Techniques for extracting stones

Although most stones (at least those < 1 cm in diameter) will pass spontaneously in the days or weeks after an adequate sphincterotomy, most experts prefer to extract them directly. This immediately clarifies the situation, and reduces the risk of impaction, cholangitis and/or pancreatitis.

Stones can be removed using balloon-tipped catheters or baskets. Balloon catheters are useful for extracting large numbers of relatively small stones, and for sweeping the duct after extracting

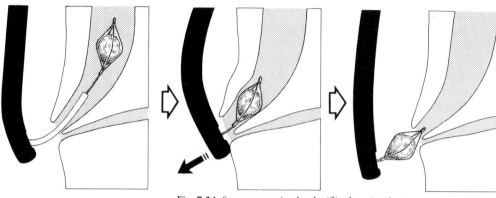

Fig. 7.24 Stone extraction by the 'flip down' technique.

stones to demonstrate that it is clear. The catheter is advanced to the hilum of the liver and contrast injected to fill the duct. The balloon is then inflated to the diameter of the duct, and pulled back slowly under fluoroscopic control. It is important to check the location of the catheter tip before inflating the balloon since damage can be caused if it is inflated in a narrow duct (e.g. pancreatic duct, cystic duct, or intrahepatic biliary tree). A major advantage of balloons over baskets is that they cannot become impacted. Unfortunately, balloons are not so effective for extracting larger stones (say > 10 mm in diameter), probably because the force is applied tangentially; the balloon may slip past the stone, or simply force it sideways against the duct wall. They are also fragile and expensive.

It is reasonable to start extraction attempts with a balloon, and turn to a basket if this fails. The basket is fully opened above the stone, taking care not to push the stone into the intrahepatic ducts. It may be necessary to 'jiggle' the basket to trap a stone within it. The basket is then trawled down the duct in the fully open position. Closing the basket may pop out the stone, and can impact the wires within a soft stone, so that it cannot be released. Usually there is resistance when the basket and stone reach the sphincterotomy orifice, so that pulling back further simply drags the endoscope tip onto the papilla. The final stage of extraction is then done under fluoroscopic control. Holding the basket position steady, the endoscope tip is angled sharply down, and rotated to the right; this applies force in the correct biliary axis, and is usually successful (Fig. 7.24).

There are several options when initial attempts at stone extraction fail. The stone can be released from the basket and the sphincterotomy enlarged. Releasing the stone can sometimes be embarrassingly difficult. It is best achieved by pushing the basket high in the common hepatic duct, and attempting to loop it (Fig. 7.25). Sometimes stones are easier to remove a few days after a sphincterotomy when the initial oedema has subsided. If this course is taken, it is essential to provide interim drainage (see below).

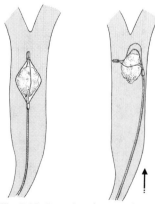

Fig. 7.25 Dropping the stone by advancing and distorting the basket.

An alternative approach when stone basket extraction fails is to use a 'mechanical lithotripter'—which is merely a stronger basket with a metal spiral sheath against which the stone is crushed.

Stone and basket impaction

Impaction should be avoidable if the sphincterotomy size is tailored to the stone, and appropriate trawling methods are used. However, if it occurs, it is essential somehow to provide the patient with biliary drainage to prevent life-threatening cholangitis. Cut off the basket handle (with pliers) and remove the endoscope, if possible leaving the plastic sleeve over the wires for protection. Replace the endoscope and try to enlarge the sphincterotomy, either with a standard sphincterotome, or by cutting down onto the stone with a needle knife. If this is not effective in releasing the stone up into the duct or down into the duodenum, try to pass a guidewire alongside the stone for placement of a naso-biliary drain. If this can be achieved, the situation is stable, and the stone (and basket) often fall out spontaneously in 1 or 2 days. Another method is to use a 'crushing sleeve' (Soehendra lithotripter, Wilson Cook Co.). This flexible spiral metal sleeve is advanced over the basket wires to the papilla under fluoroscopic control, by pulling on the basket wires. The wire is then pulled firmly by a type of reel mechanism (Fig. 7.26). Usually the stone will crush; alternatively the basket wires will break, which releases it from the stone.

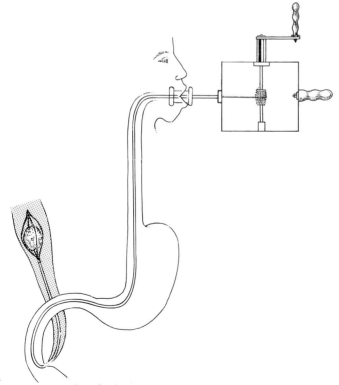

Fig. 7.26 Reel mechanism.

One of these methods usually will be effective. If they fail, the patient should undergo urgent percutaneous decompression or surgery. Do not be tempted to leave a patient overnight without drainage; serious cholangitis can result.

Specialized shock-wave lithotripsy devices are available for large stones (see below).

Naso-biliary catheter drainage

Leaving a naso-biliary drainage catheter in the duct is an essential part of safe, therapeutic ERCP, and should be within the armamentarium of every biliary endoscopist.

Naso-biliary catheters are simply long polyethylene tubes (5 or 7 French gauge), at least twice the length of the standard endoscope. The tip or distal part of the catheter is moulded to prevent it falling out. Several designs are available (Fig. 7.21) including catheters with terminal pigtails, terminal right-angle bends, mid-duct pigtails, and a variety with a pre-formed loop in the duodenum (Fig. 7.27). The advantage of the three latter designs is that the tip is straight, and that the tubes can therefore be inserted in the bile duct without the need for a guidewire. If a standard catheter is already in the bile duct when the decision is made to leave a naso-biliary drain, it is easiest to place a guidewire through the catheter, and then exchange the catheter for a drain. All of these models have multiple-site holes close to the distal tip.

Once the distal tip is in the correct position high in the biliary tree (and above any retained stone), the endoscope must be gradually removed without dislodging the catheter. It is easiest for an assistant to withdraw the endoscope slowly, while the endoscopist pushes the catheter and monitors the position by fluoroscopy (Fig. 7.28).

After the endoscope has been removed, the proximal end of the

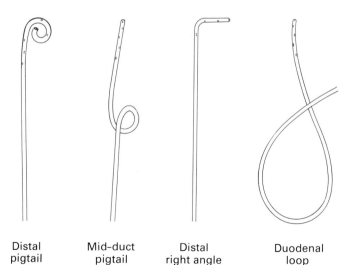

Distal pigtail   Mid–duct pigtail   Distal right angle   Duodenal loop

Fig. 7.27 Designs of naso-biliary catheters.

drain must be re-routed from the mouth to the nose. A short plastic tube is passed through a nostril into the pharynx, grabbed by surgical forceps (or fingers) and brought out through the mouth. The top of the biliary drain is then fed back through it; both are withdrawn at the nose until the drain lies straight in the pharynx. The drain should be strapped to the patient's face and connected to a bag with an injection/aspiration sideport.

Naso-biliary drains are usually well tolerated for several days, and have been left in place even for weeks. Their essential role is to provide effective drainage; therefore, the output should be monitored and the catheter flushed (and the position checked by fluoroscopy) if there is any question of dislodgement. The drain can be used for check cholangiography, infusion of saline to wash out biliary debris, or of solvents to attempt stone dissolution.

In patients with life-threatening suppurative cholangitis, it may be wise simply to place a naso-biliary drain tube quickly and not to attempt sphincterotomy and stone extraction (especially if coagulation is disturbed). This can be done under fluoroscopic control in an intensive care area.

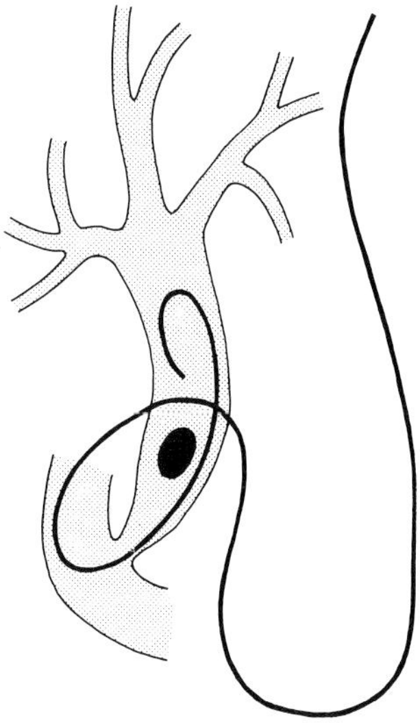

Fig. 7.28 Naso-biliary drainage.

Difficult and big stones

Many factors (not least the experience of the endoscopist) determine the success of stone extraction. Amongst the most important is stone size. A useful guideline is the size of the endoscope, approximately 15 mm on the radiographic film (because of magnification). Increasing difficulty must be expected with stones larger than the endoscope. Stones of up to 25 mm in diameter can be extracted (or even pass spontaneously) after endoscopic sphincterotomy, but the risks of bleeding and perforation presumably increase with sphincterotomy size. Stones > 25 mm have caused gallstone ileus when released into the duodenum.

The importance of the shape of the distal bile duct has already been emphasized in relation to the safety of sphincterotomy. It is much easier to remove a large stone when the lower end of the bile duct is 'square', and foolish to attempt it when there is a long distal taper (Fig. 7.13).

The site and shape of stones also affects success. Stones may be difficult to access in the cystic duct or intrahepatic ducts, and it is usually necessary to use guidewires (often best a guidewire with a J-tip) to guide a balloon-tipped catheter beyond a stone. Stones above strictures can be removed only if the stricture is first dilated satisfactorily.

Flat (coin-shaped) stones may be difficult to trap in a basket (or trawl in front of a balloon), and angulated stones may resist transit through the sphincterotomy. Stones which are 'sausage-shaped' are the easiest to remove, partly because they are usually relatively soft, brown pigment stones. The most difficult are the large square stones which fill the bile duct lumen like a piston (Fig. 7.29). Baskets usually deform around such stones, and fail to grasp them—which is sometimes just as well since their size and shape

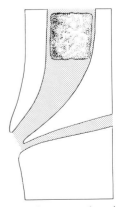

Fig. 7.29 The 'piston'-shaped stone. Difficult to grasp and extract.

make them difficult to extract through the sphincterotomy. Some of these large stones can be crushed with mechanical lithotripters (see above discussion on impacted stones). When these fail, a naso-biliary drain or stent should be placed and other options reviewed. A naso-biliary drain is preferred in this context if the patient is septic and when further intervention (endoscopic or surgical) is likely to take place within a few days. A stent is placed instead of a naso-biliary drain when the patient's condition is stable, and when there may be a significant delay before further attempts are made by specialist techniques (see below), particularly if these are to be at another institution. In some elderly and frail patients, stents provide adequate long-term treatment.

Options for the patient with a difficult big stone include surgical intervention, which may well be appropriate in younger and fitter patients (and certainly those with the gallbladder still in place). Infusion of solvents through naso-biliary drains has proved disappointing, largely because most of these big stones are not rich in cholesterol. In addition, solvent techniques (using mono-octanoin or methyl tert-butyl ether) are time consuming and not without serious hazard.

Large stones can be fragmented within the bile duct using endoscopically directed shock wave probes (pulsed lasers and electrohydraulic probes). Another alternative is the use of extra-corporeal shock-wave lithotripsy, focusing the stone radiologically using the naso-biliary drain for contrast injection.

Developments in sphincterotomy and stone disease

Most of the serious complications of endoscopic stone extraction are those of the sphincterotomy itself (particularly bleeding and perforation). The development of effective techniques for fragmenting (or dissolving) stones in the future should make it possible to clear the ducts in some patients without having to perform a sphincterotomy. Endoscopists have made sporadic forays through the cystic duct into the gallbladder over the last decade. The increasing interest in non-surgical treatment for gallbladder stone disease (extracorporeal lithotripsy, percutaneous dissolution, etc.) has focused attention again on the cystic duct approach. Methyl tertbutyl ether has been infused into the gallbladder via a tube placed through the cystic duct at duodenoscopy, but this and related techniques remain experimental.

Endoscopists are also teaming up with their interventional radiology colleagues to approach the bile duct and the gallbladder under direct vision through tracks made by percutaneous puncture techniques.

Balloon dilatation of biliary strictures

It is now relatively simple to dilate bile duct strictures with balloons at ERCP. The techniques were developed from those used for angioplasty. Sausage-shaped balloon catheters can be slid over standard guidewires. Balloon sizes vary in diameter from 4 to 10 mm (fully inflated) and in length from 2 to 5 cm. They are mounted on catheters of 5 or 7 French gauge. The 7 French gauge balloon catheters are preferred since they are sturdier, but must be used with a large endoscope channel (> 3.8 mm). For most purposes it is convenient to use a 2-cm long balloon of 8-mm diameter. Metal markers are incorporated to improve radiographic visualization (Fig. 7.30). The balloons are inflated to a predetermined pressure, and the procedure monitored under fluoroscopy for disappearance of the 'waist' (Fig. 7.31). Dilatation is often quite painful, and usually cannot be maintained for > 10–20 seconds. Smaller balloons are used to dilate tighter strictures and lesions of intrahepatic ducts.

Dilatation of strictures which are so tight that they will not accept a balloon catheter can be achieved using 'stepped' dilators

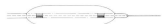

Fig. 7.30 Dilating balloon placed over guidewire; radio-opaque metal markers show up.

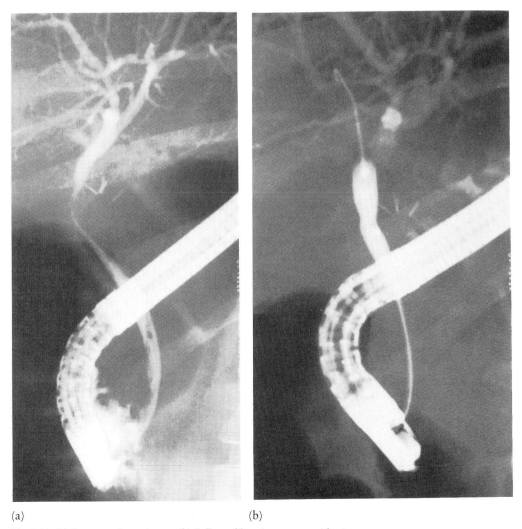

(a)   (b)

Fig. 7.31 (a) Postoperative stricture. (b) Balloon dilatation over a guidewire.

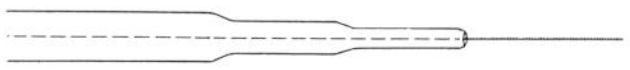

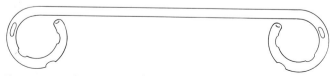

Fig. 7.32 Tapered 'stepped' dilator for use in the bile (or pancreatic) duct over a guidewire.

over a guidewire (Fig. 7.32). Various sizes are available; the commonest have three steps at 5, 7 and 9 French gauge. These dilators are most commonly used in patients with malignant strictures, prior to stenting (see below).

Most strictures recur quickly after simple dilatation; it is therefore customary to leave a stent in place for several months.

Balloon dilatation can be used at the main papilla, and has been proposed as a method of removing stones without sphincterotomy. However, there is a significant risk of developing pancreatitis (and cholangitis). Balloon dilatation (usually with subsequent stenting) is sometimes employed in the management of a stenosed choledochoduodenostomy stoma.

Indications for biliary balloon dilatation

Biliary strictures are most commonly due to operative accidents and sclerosing cholangitis. Whilst most can be managed by endoscopic dilatation, the long-term results are by no means clear. However, the techniques appear to be safe, and it thus seems reasonable to continue using them until further objective long-term data are available. For postoperative strictures, it is customary to perform up to three dilatations (with stenting) during a period of 1 year, and then to assess the outcome. Surgery should be considered at all stages, and certainly if there is an early recurrence.

Endoscopic biliary stenting

The techniques of endoscopic biliary stent placement are now well established, and the procedure has found an important clinical role in the palliation of elderly high-risk patients with biliary obstruction due to unresectable malignancy. The role in other contexts is more controversial, and will be discussed briefly later (p. 150).

Initially stents of 7 French gauge were used, since these were the largest which could be passed through a standard duodenoscope. Early stents had pigtails at both ends to prevent dislocation (Fig. 7.33) but these are now obsolete. These stents occlude (by bacterial and biliary debris) within a few months. This led to the development of larger channel (therapeutic) duodenoscopes (channels of 3.8–4.2 mm) to allow passage of stents of up to 11.5 French gauge. There are experimental instruments with even larger channels for insertion of up to 14 French gauge stents. Larger stents (and

Fig. 7.33 Pigtail stent—now obsolete.

endoscopes) are more difficult to manipulate, but the time to clogging is substantially prolonged. We strongly recommend using stents of at least 10 French gauge (in the biliary tree). Smaller stents must sometimes be used in very tight and tortuous strictures.

Equipment and preparation

Much of the preparation is similar to that for sphincterotomy techniques. The indication for the procedure is reviewed in detail with the patient, and appropriate informed consent is obtained. We check for coagulopathy and start prophylactic broad-spectrum antibiotics about 1 hour before the procedure.

The endoscopes should be completely disinfected by standard techniques and all the accessory materials gas sterilized or auto-claved. Great care should be taken during manipulation of catheters and guidewires to minimize contamination. The design of guide-wires is such that they cannot be adequately cleaned and disin-fected; they should therefore be discarded and not re-used. Stent placement requires high-quality fluoroscopy so that the movement of the guidewire can be followed, and it is essential to have two properly trained GI nurse assistants.

Stent 'sets' are produced by several manufacturers. Stents of 10 and 11.5 French gauge are inserted using a three-layer technique (Fig. 7.34). The stent is slid (with a pusher) over an inner guiding catheter, which itself lies over a standard guidewire (0.035-in. diameter). The guidewire should have a short, floppy tip and a length of at least 350 cm. The inner polyethylene guiding catheter is 5–6.5 French gauge, and 280 cm long. It has a removable adapter for injection of contrast.

Stents have a slightly tapered tip, flaps near each end to prevent migration upwards or downwards, and a curve at the lower end to correspond to the bile duct anatomy (Fig. 7.35). One or more side

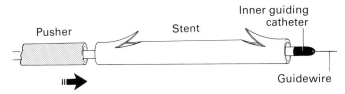

Fig. 7.34 Standard three-layer system for stent insertion.

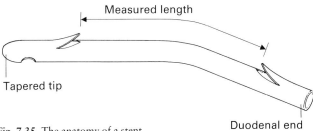

Fig. 7.35 The anatomy of a stent.

holes may be added close to the upper tip of the stent. Stent length is measured between the flaps (Fig. 7.35).

Techniques of stent insertion

Some endoscopists perform the initial cannulation and ERCP radiographs with a standard duodenoscope (which is slightly easier to manipulate than the larger stenting instrument). Once the anatomy has been demonstrated and the appropriateness of stent insertion confirmed, a small sphincterotomy is performed to facilitate subsequent re-cannulation and the passage of larger catheters; the endoscope is removed and replaced with the larger 'stenting' instrument.

Most experts have learned to short-cut this process and start the procedure (whenever there is a potential for stenting) with the larger channel endoscope (channel size 4–4.2 mm). Later versions are easier to manipulate than earlier ones, but it can still prove difficult sometimes to perform the initial deep cannulation; standard size catheters have a tendency to flip-flop in the larger channel and, also, it may be difficult to get the tip of the endoscope beyond the papilla to permit a good angle for biliary cannulation. (Equipment and manoeuvres to conquer these problems are described below.)

Cannulation is initially performed with a catheter (preferably with a metal radio-opaque 'ball' tip) large enough to accept a standard guidewire. The catheter (primed with contrast) is inserted into the bile duct orifice and radiographs are obtained. If possible, the catheter is passed directly through the stricture and into the dilated biliary system above. If this can be achieved, bile should be aspirated (as much as possible) to prevent over-distension of the biliary tree (and possible septicaemia) whilst injecting contrast. Bile specimens should be kept for culture and cytology.

If the catheter cannot be passed through the stricture, a guidewire must be inserted. Guidewire passage through the catheter is easier if a small quantity (1–2 ml) of saline is injected through it to flush out the viscous contrast. The guidewire is advanced (by the nurse/assistant) until the tip protrudes about 2 cm from the end of the catheter (Fig. 7.36). The endoscopist then advances both together to engage and pass through the stricture. Various manipulations of the catheter and guidewire independently may be necessary (Figs 7.37 and 7.38). Once the guidewire has passed through the stricture, the catheter can be slid over it. The guidewire is removed, bile is aspirated, and contrast injected. This contrast should be fairly dilute (15–20%) so as not to obscure the guidewire during subsequent manipulations.

Time should now be taken to examine the radiographs, which should define precisely the length and position of stricture, and the degree to which the whole biliary tree has been opacified. To get adequate radiographs, it is sometimes necessary to posture the patient or to aspirate more bile to be able to inject more contrast.

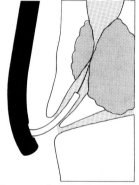

Fig. 7.36 The assistant protrudes the guidewire 2 cm beyond the catheter . . .

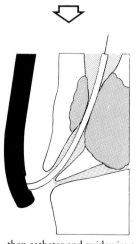

. . . then catheter and guidewire are advanced together to engage and pass the stricture.

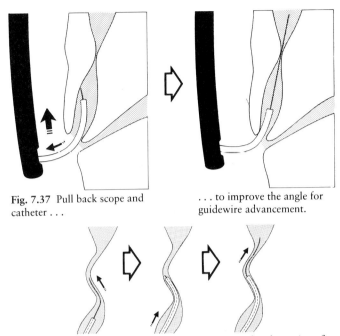

Fig. 7.37 Pull back scope and catheter . . .

. . . to improve the angle for guidewire advancement.

Fig. 7.38 Advancing through tortuous strictures one bend at a time, first guidewire, then catheter.

Selecting a stent, and passing through the endoscope

The aim is to place a stent so that its top flap is above the stricture and the bottom flap is just outside the papilla, usually leaving a margin of about 1 cm for movement and tumour growth. There is normally a 30% magnification factor on ERCP radiographs. A stricture whose upper margin is 8 cm above the papillary orifice requires a stent measuring 7 cm between the flaps (8 cm minus 30% = 6 cm, add 1 cm for safety). Likewise, a measured length of 15 cm would require a stent of 11–12 cm.

The guidewire and covering inner 'guiding' catheter should be lying well above the stricture, preferably in a major intrahepatic duct. The stent is passed over the inner catheter, down and into the biopsy port. The proximal flap of the stent is flattened into the biopsy channel. This can usually be done with the finger, but a short sleeve introducer is provided in some sets. The 'pusher tube' is then advanced over the inner catheter up to the stent, and is then used to push the stent down through the endoscope. There is considerable friction in this system, so that movement of the pusher will tend also to advance the inner catheter (and its contained guidewire). This risk can be minimized by lubricating the outside of the inner catheter (sterile saline seems to work as well as silicone fluid), and by attempting to 'hold' the inner catheter in position with the endoscope elevator in the fully 'up' position. Maintenance of the correct position of guidewire and catheter in the liver should be monitored repeatedly by fluoroscopy. The assistant informs the endoscopist as soon as the inner catheter

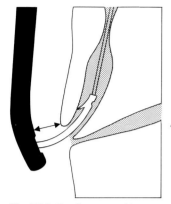

Fig. 7.39 Good scope position, close to papilla.

appears out of the top end of the pusher. The assistant can then help stent passage by pulling back on the inner catheter, against the pusher tube (Fig. 7.38). In fact, this merely maintains the inner catheter and guidewire in the same position in the liver as the stent advances. This collaboration between endoscopist and assistant is essential to success.

Inserting the stent.   The endoscopist can feel when the tip of the stent reaches the endoscope elevator. The crucial part is then about to begin. It is important to work carefully and deliberately, and to maintain the tip of the endoscope *close to the papilla*, without allowing any bow in the catheter (worse still the stent) between them (Fig. 7.39). Once everything and everyone is prepared the endoscope elevator is lowered, and the tip of the stent pushed 1–2 cm into the duodenum, into endoscopic view. The stent is then advanced into the papilla by lifting the elevator and angling up the tip of the endoscope in repeated small moves: elevator down, stent pushed out 1cm; elevator up, tip up, to insert stent; elevator down, etc. (Fig. 7.40). During this process, to reduce friction, the assistant (whilst watching the fluoroscopy screen) maintains traction on the inner catheter against the pusher tube. Resistance will be felt as the stent enters the stricture. Now movements must be even more deliberate; there is no way to withdraw a stent once it has passed too far out of the endoscope. Once the bottom flap is seen in the duodenum and pushed against the papilla, the insertion process is complete. If further injection of contrast is needed, the guidewire can be removed and contrast injected through the inner catheter. If not, the inner catheter and guidewire are removed together (by the assistant) whilst the endoscopist holds the pusher tube against the stent. It is gratifying to see a rush of bile into the duodenum as stent and pusher separate.

Straightening out a loop. Always try to prevent a loop developing. If this happens, it may be necessary to remove the endoscope completely (grasping the stent in the elevator), and to start the procedure over again. However, sometimes it is possible to escape from this predicament by pushing the endoscope tip further into

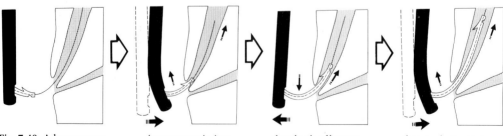

Fig. 7.40 Advance stent tip until just visible . . .

. . . insert stent tip into bile duct by angling scope tip up and lifting elevator . . .

. . . then back off scope slightly (angle down), drop elevator, and advance stent slightly . . .

. . . then push stent into bile duct by angling scope tip up and lifting elevator.

the duodenum so as to straighten the stent (Fig. 7.41b). The tip of the endoscope is then angled up, and the whole instrument 'jerked back'. This can produce enough force in the correct axis to advance the stent through the stricture.

Sphincterotomy for stents?

Many endoscopists routinely perform a small sphincterotomy as part of the stent insertion process. The risks of so doing are small, but we have found it to be unnecessary in most cases, even with stents of 11.5 French gauge. However, it is sometimes necessary to use the 'jerk back' manoeuvre (Fig. 7.41c) to get the stent tip through the sphincter. Sphincterotomy should be done if it is hoped to place more than one stent (as in some hilar lesions). Some endoscopists also recommend sphincterotomy to facilitate subsequent stent replacement.

If sphincterotomy is performed prior to stent placement, it is most convenient to use a 'guidewire sphincterotome', so as not to lose the initial cannulation. A guidewire is passed through the standard catheter deep into the bile duct, the catheter is removed and replaced with the sphincterotome. This is removed in turn after the sphincterotomy and replaced over the guidewire with the inner catheter of the stent set.

Routine dilatation of malignant strictures prior to stent insertion?

It is usually possible to pass a 10 or 11.5 French gauge stent through malignant strictures without prior dilatation. However,

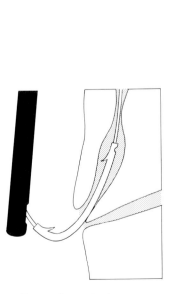 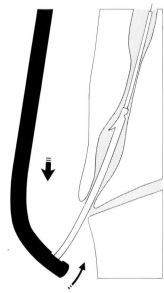 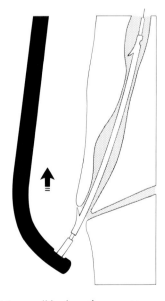

(a) Too much stent in the duodenum . . .

(b) . . . advance the scope and angle up to get the stent straight . . .

(c) . . . pull back on the scope to force the stent inwards.

Fig. 7.41 Getting out of loop trouble.

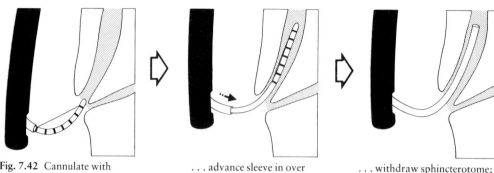

Fig. 7.42 Cannulate with sphincterotome and sleeve in position . . .

. . . advance sleeve in over sphincterotome . . .

. . . withdraw sphincterotome; sleeve allows catheter placement.

some strictures especially at the hilum are particularly sclerotic, and are also more difficult to pass because less force can be applied at a distance. Therefore, it may be wise to pass a dilating catheter through high lesions prior to stent insertion. This can be a 10 French gauge sleeve (Cunningham–Cotton sleeve, Wilson Cook Co.), passed over the inner guiding catheter, or a stepped dilator (5, 7 and 9 French gauge) over the guidewire alone.

Difficulties with initial deep cannulation

There are two useful techniques for facilitating deep cannulation when in difficulties using a standard catheter—which may occur especially when using large-channel endoscopes, with which it may be difficult to obtain a good position for biliary access. The first adjuvant method is to cannulate the papilla with a standard 5 French gauge sphincterotome protruding from a 10 French gauge sleeve (Fig. 7.42). The sleeve stabilizes the sphincterotome, the tip of which can be bowed to optimize the direction for cannulation. Once the sphincterotome has been placed deeply in the bile duct (as judged by contrast injection), a small sphincterotomy is performed. Then, without removing the sphincterotome, the sleeve is slid over it, into the distal bile duct. The sphincterotome is then removed completely, and the standard inner guiding catheter and guidewire are passed through the sleeve up to and through the stricture. Whilst there the sleeve can be used to dilate the stricture. The sleeve is then removed completely and the stent is placed by the standard technique.

An alternative method for cannulation is to use the tip of a guidewire protruding from the 'guidewire sphincterotome'. The sphincterotome can be bowed within the duodenum so as to produce an optimal cannulation angle (Fig. 7.43). Once the guidewire is deep in the bile duct, the sphincterotome is advanced over it, the guidewire is removed and contrast is injected. If this confirms a correct bile duct position, a small sphincterotomy is performed. The guidewire is re-inserted; then the sphincterotome is removed and replaced with the inner guiding catheter.

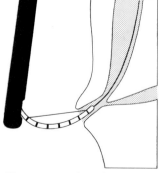

Fig. 7.43 Use a bowed sphincterotome to pass a guidewire, then follow with the sphincterotome—and remove the guidewire.

Smaller stents

Small stents are useful in the pancreatic duct, and may sometimes be used in the bile duct when it is impossible to pass a stent of standard size (10–11.5 French gauge); 7 French gauge stents can be passed through a standard-sized duodenoscope, using a 'two-layer' system. The stent is pushed directly over the guidewire (with a pusher), without any intervening inner catheter.

The procedure for inserting 7 French gauge stents is very simple. Sphincterotomy is unnecessary. Once deep biliary cannulation has been achieved, a guidewire is passed through the initial cannula, and worked through the stricture into an intrahepatic duct. The catheter is removed, and the stent simply advanced over it using a 7 or 8 French gauge pusher. Stents of 7 French gauge are unlikely to stay patent for more than 3 months, so that plans must be made for early exchange (hopefully for a larger stent) or for an alternative drainage method.

Hilar lesions

The technique for stent insertion is similar at all levels of the biliary tree up to the common hepatic duct. Type 1 hilar strictures (not involving the bifurcation) can be managed with a single stent. Stenting of hilar lesions of Types 2 and 3 (involving the bifurcation, or higher branches) is more difficult, less satisfactory, and more likely to result in complications. The strictures are often more tortuous and sclerotic—and they are further away from the power source (the duodenoscope tip). The main problem is the risk of sepsis developing in undrained segments of the liver. Whether or not it is necessary to attempt drainage of all obstructed ducts in every case remains controversial; in fact, this is often impossible. We have found that a correctly placed single stent will provide good palliation of jaundice in most hilar lesions, with an acceptably low risk of sepsis. Using disinfected equipment and prophylactic antibiotics, the early cholangitis rate is $< 10\%$. When sepsis does develop, it is essential to provide drainage to the obstructed duct system(s). Experts may try to place two or more stents endoscopically, but the success rate is low; the presence of the first stent may prevent cannulation of other ducts. There are some manoeuvres for steering into the required duct.

Steering into the intrahepatic ducts

Catheters preferentially enter the right intrahepatic ductal system, because of their natural curl (Fig. 7.44). There are several methods for attempting to steer into the left system. If the catheter is brought low into the bile duct the guidewire (which always goes straight) may be aimed appropriately (Fig. 7.45). A second method is to use a guidewire with a long flexible tip (or movable core). The tip is placed in a right intrahepatic duct: then, as the guidewire is

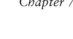

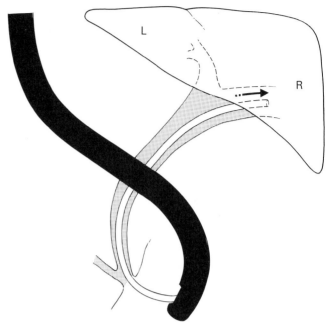

Fig. 7.44 (Patient prone) The natural curve of the catheter takes it into the right intrahepatic duct preferentially.

advanced, a knee develops into the left system (Fig. 7.46). The catheter is then advanced over the guidewire into the left duct (and the guidewire is withdrawn). Radiologists working percutaneously through the liver can employ torque stable and malleable tip wires. Unfortunately, similar wires do not work well over the long distances employed in the endoscopic approach. Another method for steering involves the use of a catheter with a preformed bend near the tip, which aims the guidewire in the correct direction (Fig. 7.47).

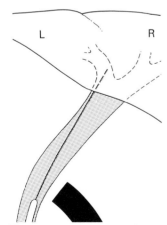

Fig. 7.45 (Patient prone) Pulling the inner 'guiding' catheter down the duct directs the straight guidewire into the left intrahepatic duct.

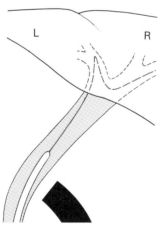

Fig. 7.46 (Patient prone) Gaining access to the left duct by making a 'knee' in a long floppy-tip guidewire.

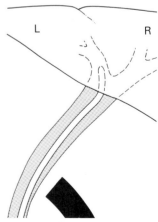

Fig. 7.47 (Patient prone) Using a preformed catheter for selective entry into the left duct.

When multiple stents are required it is often necessary to seek radiological assistance—either to place a drain followed by a stent percutaneously, or for a 'combined procedure' (see below).

Combined procedures (endoscopic–radiological techniques)

The use of a percutaneously placed guidewire has already been mentioned as a method for achieving bile duct access for sphincterotomy. 'Combined procedures' are more commonly used for insertion of stents, especially when initial cannulation fails. In experienced hands, failure is almost entirely restricted to tumours extending down to involve the papilla so that no normal orifice can be identified. Combined procedures are also used in patients with hilar lesions, when it proves necessary to drain more than one segment.

The principle behind the combined procedure is that it should be safer than pushing a stent through the liver; the liver puncture has to accommodate a catheter of only 5 or 6 French gauge. However, the superiority of the combined procedure over the primary percutaneous approach has not been proven in randomized studies.

In units with combined endoscopic–radiological facilities and excellent collaboration, the combined procedure can be performed immediately the indication arises (provided the patient's consent has been obtained beforehand). However, in most centres, the combined procedure is done in stages.

The first stage (after endoscopic access failure) is to perform a standard percutaneous drainage procedure, leaving the catheter through the stricture if possible. Radiologists usually prefer to do such procedures in their own specialized rooms.

Once the patient is stable (and whilst continuing antibiotics) the patient is brought back to the ERCP room. The radiologist places a standard 0.035-in. diameter guidewire through his catheter into the duodenum and the endoscopist places the therapeutic duodenoscope opposite the papilla. The radiologist pulls back his catheter until it is only just protruding from the papilla, and the guidewire 1–2 cm from it. The endoscopist places a snare loop (or basket) over the tip of the wire, and draws it back slowly through the endoscope channel (Fig. 7.48). The radiologist holds the catheter in place, and helps by pushing the guidewire at the skin surface. It is important to maintain the catheter in position, to prevent the wire traumatizing the liver. The guidewire is pulled at least 200 cm out of the endoscope (so a wire of about 400 cm should be used initially). This wire is then used in the standard way to insert the stent, using the three-layer system already described. As the endoscopist's inner catheter advances through the papilla, it pushes the radiologist's catheter back to a position above the stricture.

A significant danger with the combined procedure is advancing the stent too far, so that the tip is impacted in liver tissue, and no longer draining a duct (Fig. 7.49). One way to prevent this happening (after the radiologist has inserted a second wire) is for the

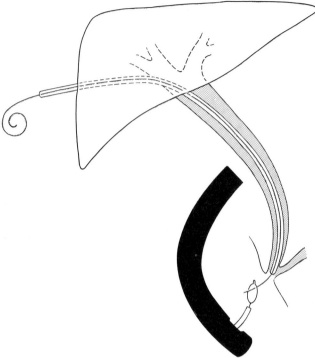

Fig. 7.48 'Combined procedure'—the endoscopist catches the radiologically-placed guidewire and pulls it back through the scope.

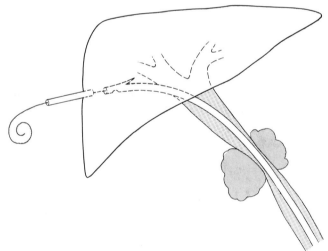

Fig. 7.49 A danger is to advance the stent too far, so that it no longer drains . . .

endoscopist to pull the original guidewire back until its tip is just above the stricture, then advancing it into an appropriate large duct (Fig. 7.50).

Once the stent is in place, it is customary to leave the percutaneous drainage catheter in for at least one night, and to do a

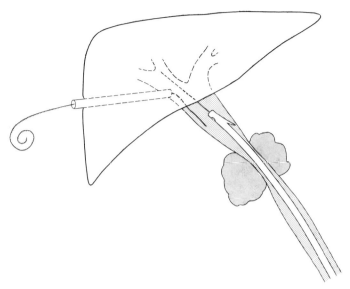

Fig. 7.50 . . . to avoid this the endoscopist can pull the guidewire back and then place it in a large duct.

check cholangiogram on the following day. The catheter can then be removed if the stent is functioning. Sometimes, with high lesions, there may be little room for the percutaneous catheter above the stent. This is another advantage of placing two guide-wires percutaneously (through a common sleeve). One is used by the endoscopist for the stent insertion, the other subsequently by the radiologist to place a temporary external drainage tube.

A variant of the combined procedure utilizes a forward-viewing endoscope to retrieve the guidewire from the duodenum. The stent is then inserted over this wire either under direct vision using the endoscope as the pusher, or under purely radiological control using a pusher tube alone. With this latter method it is sometimes difficult to judge when the stent is in the optimal position at the papilla.

Post-stenting care

Most stent procedures are straightforward and well tolerated. Patients are given fluids soon after the procedure. Antibiotics are continued overnight, and the patient is discharged on a normal diet the next day if there are no adverse developments. Provided everything has gone well it is usually not necessary to make any early check of stent function. The patient should usually be reviewed within a week, by which time stool and urine colour should be normal, and the bilirubin substantially lower. The patient should be told to return earlier if pain or fever develop.

Pain and fever usually signal inadequate stent function. This can be checked with serial liver function tests, and a plain abdominal radiograph; this should show air in the biliary tree if the stent is patent. Some recommend a 'Coca-Colagram' to accentuate this. Dynamic isotope scans have been used to check stent patency, but do not usually give definitive advice at an early stage. The only certain way to clarify the position is to repeat the ERCP procedure, and inject contrast into the stent itself (using a tapered-tip catheter and being careful not to push the stent further in). Often the stent is found to be patent and correctly placed, the slow response reflecting prolonged obstruction and poor liver function. Rarely the stent is blocked with blood clot, which can usually be flushed out. Sometimes the stent is found to have been placed in an inappropriate position (such as the cystic duct), and must be removed and replaced.

Early complications

The main complication of stent insertion is sepsis, which occurs only when drainage is inadequate. Treatment involves continuing full antibiotic coverage and institution of drainage by further endoscopic, percutaneous or surgical intervention. The small sphincterotomy sometimes performed to facilitate stent insertion carries virtually no risk of bleeding or perforation. It is, however, possible to perforate bile duct tumours with the guidewire, but this occurrence appears to be benign (provided adequate biliary drainage is achieved). There was concern that stents protruding from the bile duct might obstruct the pancreatic duct orifice and cause pancreatitis; this was one of the reasons for doing a small sphincterotomy. However, this fear has not been realized.

Late complications

Eventual stent occlusion is the significant long-term problem with stents. Those of 10–11.5 French gauge remain patent for a median period of about 6 months (range 3–9 months), whereas smaller stents rarely stay patent for < 3 months. Stent failure may also occur (rarely) from upward or downward migration.

Failure of stent function is announced by a return of jaundice and spiking fevers. The alkaline phosphatase rises somewhat before this if measured sequentially. Patients can become seriously ill very quickly with suppurative cholangitis. They should be warned about the early symptoms and the need to return to specialist care immediately when they develop. Because of the potential severity of this complication, consideration should be given to changing stents electively at about 4 months. This should always be done in patients with benign strictures, and should be discussed with any patient with malignant disease who is still in reasonable general condition at that stage. This will apply to approximately one-quarter of all patients with pancreatic and bile duct malignancy.

It is usually straightforward to remove a blocked (or migrated) stent, and to replace it. The stent tip in the duodenum is grasped with a snare loop or basket and simply pulled out through the

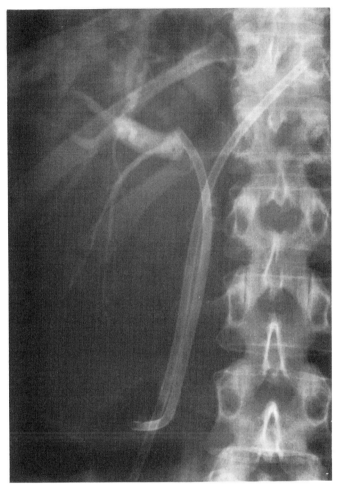

Fig. 7.51 Pull the stent down by inflating a balloon above its upper tip.

mouth. A new stent is placed by the standard technique. It is wise to make a visual note of the endoscopic appearances of the papilla before withdrawing the stent (or to take an instant photograph or videotape), since removal may cause some trauma and bleeding, making it more difficult to find the orifice for re-insertion. Should re-insertion fail, an alternative drainage procedure must be arranged immediately.

Stents which have migrated upwards are more difficult to extract since the tip is no longer within the duodenum. However, it is usually possible to 'lasso' the tip with a basket, or to pull the stent down again by inflating a balloon above its upper tip (Fig. 7.51). If these techniques fail, it is usually satisfactory to place another stent alongside the old one.

The lower end of the stent has occasionally damaged the duodenal wall and caused bleeding, or even perforation, but these events are extremely rare with appropriate techniques.

Indications for endoscopic biliary stents

Malignant obstruction

The success rate for stent insertion (excluding hilar lesions) exceeds 90%, and severe procedure-related complications occur in less than 1% of patients. The technique provides an ideal method of palliation for elderly high-risk patients with mid and distal bile-duct obstruction due to tumours which are not operable or resectable (Fig. 7.52). Recent randomized studies indicate that the short-term results are as good as—or better than—standard surgical bypass, at lower cost and patient discomfort. These advantages are somewhat eroded (but not eradicated) by the need for subsequent stent changes, and for surgery if duodenal obstruction develops (< 10% of cases). Patients with potentially resectable malignant lesions should undergo surgery. This raises the complex issue of the assessment of resectability—which is outside the scope of this chapter.

Another issue is that of histological (or cytological) confirmation of the diagnosis. It is important not to miss rarer lesions such as lymphoma and islet cell tumours. Good tissue cores can be obtained by the Trucut 'Biopty' gun technique under ultrasound or computed tomographic control.

The role of stenting for tumours at, and above, the liver hilum is more controversial. The results are less satisfactory at this level, but such lesions also pose major problems for surgical and percutaneous radiological intervention. Further objective studies are required.

Stents for preoperative drainage?

We place stents in all patients with malignant biliary obstruction documented at the time of ERCP, even if resection may be attempted later. This provides preoperative drainage, eliminates the risk of obstructive cholangitis, and starts the treatment should the patient prove not to be a surgical candidate.

Stents in benign disease

Biliary stents are placed after stricture dilatation in patients with benign disease (postoperative strictures and sclerosing cholangitis), but their contribution is still speculative. Stents can also be used in the acute management of patients with acute suppurative cholangitis due to stones; an advantage over the nasobiliary drain is that the patient cannot dislodge them. Endoscopic stents are also used temporarily in the management of patients with postoperative biliary leaks (e.g. a 'blown' cystic duct stump), and for patients with large bile duct stones which cannot be extracted by standard techniques—whilst reviewing other therapeutic options (Fig. 7.53).

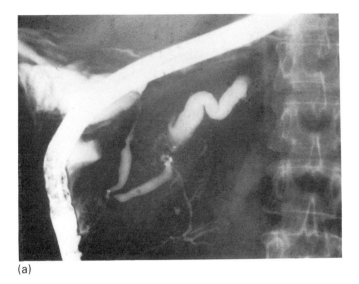

(a)

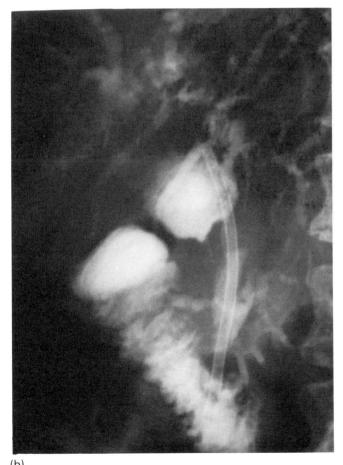

(b)

Fig. 7.52 Palliation for elderly, high-risk patients with mid and distal
bile duct obstruction due to tumours.

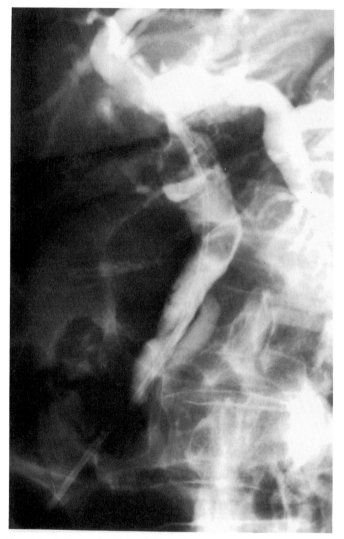

Fig. 7.53 Endoscopic stents can be used in some patients with large bile duct stones which cannot be extracted by standard techniques.

Possible developments in stricture management

Current attempts to overcome the stent occlusion problem (or to delay its development) include evaluation of new stent materials and their chemical impregnation, and the use of wire mesh stents which expand *in situ* up to about 10 mm diameter. Attempts are being made to core out malignant strictures with multi-polar thermal probes and laser balloons. Iridium wires can be placed within the bile duct via a naso-biliary catheter, for internal ir-radiation, but the contribution of this technique cannot be estab-lished without randomized studies.

Some golden rules for stenting

1 Make sure everyone understands what is being attempted before the procedure, including the patient, GI and radiology assistants.
2 Maintain sterility as much as possible.
3 Do not hurry. This can lead to inadvertent withdrawal of the guidewire or to the development of loops in the duodenum—both of which often mean that the procedure has to be re-started.
4 Make certain that the patient has adequate drainage at the end of the procedure.

Failure of drainage, either initially or after stent occlusion, places the patient at grave risk of serious sepsis. It is essential to quickly place the patient on parenteral antibiotics and to provide adequate drainage—by further stent insertion, naso-biliary catheterization, or percutaneous or surgical techniques.

Endoscopic management of pancreatitis

The success of endoscopic treatment for bile duct stones and biliary strictures has encouraged endoscopists to explore their potential in patients with pancreatitis. Several techniques are available, but the indications require clarification.

Gallstone pancreatitis

Many anecdotal reports indicate that ERCP and sphincterotomy can be performed in the acute phase of gallstone pancreatitis with remarkable safety, and that it is usually easy to remove small impacted stones—with impressive clinical recovery. The problem in defining the role for urgent endoscopy is that most patients settle spontaneously within 48 hours; they are well managed by standard conservative measures, usually leading to elective cholecystectomy. A recent randomized study indicates that urgent ERCP and sphincterotomy are preferable to a standard conservative and surgical approach in patients who had admission characteristics predicting a severe outcome. A reasonable approach is to recommend the ERCP/sphincterotomy if the patient is not improving after 48 hours, and especially if there is evidence of increasing biliary obstruction and sepsis.

Standard techniques are employed, although it is usual to avoid injecting the pancreatic duct if possible. Pancreatography should be performed if no stone is found within the bile duct, since (occasionally) gallstones cause problems by migrating into the pancreatic duct—and can be removed from it with appropriate techniques.

Pancreatic duct sphincterotomy for stones and stenosis

Solitary stones in the main duct in the pancreatic head can often be removed endoscopically by performing a small pancreatic orifice sphincterotomy, and using baskets and balloon catheters for extraction. We usually perform a biliary sphincterotomy initially, and then use a short-wire sphincterotome to incise the pancreatic orifice upwards to a length of 5–8 mm.

Sphincterotomy is also sometimes performed in patients with idiopathic recurrent pancreatitis judged to be due to sphincter stenosis or dysfunction—but this entity is difficult to define, and the results even more difficult to evaluate.

Pancreatic duct strictures

Symptoms in some patients with chronic pancreatitis may be related to single dominant strictures—although this judgment is difficult to make. Such strictures can be dilated (using a balloon or graduated stepped dilators over a guidewire) and it is probably wise to leave a stent in place to splint the stricture for a few months (Fig. 7.54). Pancreatic duct stents can induce duct abnormalities, and the indications for their use remain to be clarified. When pancreatic stents are inserted, it is wise to have additional flaps outside the papilla, since stents are very difficult to remove if they migrate into the duct.

Pseudocysts

ERCP may be useful in patients with pseudocysts to define the integrity of the duct system, and whether or not the cyst is

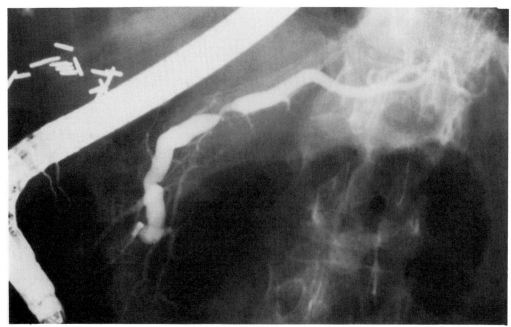

Fig. 7.54 A solitary stricture which may be managed by endoscopic dilatation/stenting.

communicating. The risk of introducing infection is minimal if properly disinfected equipment (and antibiotics) are used.

If the pseudocyst communicates with an intact duct system, the endoscopist may consider placing a naso-pancreatic drain (on continuous low-pressure suction), with subsequent temporary stenting once the cyst has collapsed.

Pseudocysts adjacent to, and compressing, the wall of the duodenum or stomach can be managed by direct endoscopic cyst puncture. A needle knife (or the tip of a polyp snare) is used to drill a hole into the cyst. This hole is then enlarged with a standard sphincterotome. It is customary to leave a naso-pancreatic drain in place for a few days to monitor progress. This method should not be employed unless it is clear that the cyst and gastric or duodenal wall are in intimate contact, as judged by CT scanning or endoscopic ultrasound. Short-term results appear good in selected cases, but there is a significant risk of haemorrhage, and these techniques should be used only by experts.

Pancreas divisum

The clinical relevance of the congenital anomaly 'pancreas divisum' remains a subject of controversy. The hypothesis that the anomaly can result in obstructive pancreatic pain and pancreatitis rests on the assumption that the accessory papilla orifice may be insufficient to allow the full flow of pancreatic juice. This belief has led some endoscopists to attempt treatment by improving drainage at the accessory papilla. Initial attempts at accessory sphincterotomy resulted in an unacceptably high rate of re-stenosis. Currently, selected patients with undoubted pancreatic pathology are being managed by the insertion of a stent through the accessory papilla after initial catheter dilatation. Short stents of 5 or 7 French gauge are used, with additional external flaps to prevent inward migration. The stents are changed at 3–6 month intervals, and are usually left in place for about 1 year, in the hope that this results in significant long-term dilatation. An alternative approach is to place a stent, and then to do a sphincterotomy onto it with a needle knife, leaving the stent to prevent early re-stenosis. The efficacy of these techniques is still being assessed.

Further reading

Berkelhammer, C., Kortan, P. and Haber, G. B. (1989) 'Endoscopic biliary prostheses as treatment for benign post-operative bile duct strictures'. *Gastrointestinal Endoscopy*, 35, 95–101.

Carr-Locke, D. L. (1988) 'Endoscopic management of gallstone disease', in *Annual of Gastrointestinal Endoscopy* (ed. Cotton, P. B., Tytgat, G. N. J. and Williams, C. B.). Gower Scientific Publications, London.

Carr-Locke, D. L. (1989) 'Endoscopy and pancreatic disease', in *Annual of Gastrointestinal Endoscopy* (ed. Cotton, P. B., Tytgat, G. N. J. and Williams, C. B.). Current Science, London.

Cotton, P. B. (1984) 'Endoscopic management of bile duct stones (apples and oranges)'. *Gut*, 25, 587–597.

Cotton, P. B. (1985) 'Pancreas divisum—culprit or curiosity?' *Gastro-enterology*, **89**, 1431–1435.

Cotton, P. B. (1988) 'Endoscopic management of biliary obstruction due to pancreatic cancer', in *Surgical Clinics in North America* (ed. Reber, H.). W. B. Saunders, London.

Cotton, P. B. (1989a) 'Complications of ERCP and therapeutic procedures', in *Gastrointestinal Emergencies* (ed. Taylor *et al.*). Williams & Wilkins, Baltimore.

Cotton, P. B. (1989b) 'Endoscopic management of biliary strictures', in *Annual of Gastrointestinal Endoscopy* (ed. Cotton, P. B., Tytgat, G. N. J. and Williams, C. B.). Current Science, London.

Cotton, P. B. (1990) 'Complications, comparisons and confusion', in *Annual of Gastrointestinal Endoscopy* (ed. Cotton, P. B., Tytgat, G. N. J. and Williams, C. B.). Current Science, London.

Cotton, P. B., Forbes, A., Leung, J. W. C. and Dineen, L. (1987) 'Endoscopic stenting for long-term treatment of large bile duct stones; a 2–5 year follow-up'. *Gastrointestinal Endoscopy*, **33**, 401–412.

Cremer, M. and Deviere, J. (1986) 'Endoscopic management of pancreatic cysts and pseudocysts'. *Gastrointestinal Endoscopy*, **32**, 367–368.

Deviere, J., Baize, M., DeToeuf, J. and Cremer, M. (1988) 'Long-term follow-up for patients with hilar malignant strictures treated by endoscopic internal biliary drainage'. *Gastrointestinal Endoscopy*, **34**, 95–101.

Dowsett, J. F., Russell, R. C. G., Hatfield, A. R. W. *et al.* (1989) 'Malignant obstructive jaundice, a prospective randomized trial of bypass surgery *vs.* endoscopic stenting'. *Gastroenterology*, **96**, A128.

Dowsett, J. F., Vaira, D., Hatfield, A. R. W. *et al.* (1989) 'Endoscopic biliary therapy using the combined percutaneous and endoscopic technique.' *Gastroenterology*, **96**, 1180–1186.

Dowsett, J. F., Vaira, D., Polydoron, A. *et al.* (1988) 'Interventional endoscopy in the pancreatico-biliary tree'. *American Journal of Gastroenterology*, **83**, 1328–1336.

Grimm, H., Huibregtse, K. and Tytgat, G. N. J. (1989) 'New modalities for treatment of chronic pancreatitis'. *Endoscopy*, **21**, 70–74.

Huibregtse, K. (1988) *Endoscopic Biliary and Pancreatic Drainage*. George Thieme Verlag, Stuttgart, New York.

Huibregtse, K., Katon, R. M., Coene, P. P. and Tytgat, G. N. J. (1986) 'Endoscopic palliative treatment in pancreatic cancer'. *Gastrointestinal Endoscopy*, **32**, 334–338.

Leung, J. W. C. (1989) 'Endoscopic management of gallstone disease', in *Annual of Gastrointestinal Endoscopy* (ed. Cotton, P. B., Tytgat, G. N. J. and Williams, C. B.). Current Science, London.

Miller, B. M., Kozarek, R. A., Ryan, J. A. *et al.* (1988) 'Surgical versus endoscopic management of comon bile duct stones'. *Annals of Surgery*, **207**, 135–141.

Neoptolemos, J. P. and Carr-Locke, D. L. (1989) 'ERCP in acute cholangitis and pancreatitis', in *ERCP, Diagnostic and Therapeutic Applications* (ed. Jacobson, I. M.). Elsevier, Amsterdam.

Satterfield, S. T., McCarthy, J. H., Greenen, J. E. *et al.* (1988) 'Clinical experience in 82 patients with pancreas divisum'. *Pancreas*, **3**, 248–253.

Silvis, S. E. (1984) *Therapeutic Gastrointestinal Endoscopy*. Igaku-Shoin, New York.

Speer, A. G. (1988) 'Endoscopic management of biliary strictures', in *Annual of Gastrointestinal Endoscopy* (ed. Cotton, P. B., Tytgat, G. N. J. and Williams, C. B.). Gower Scientific Publications, London.

Speer, A. G., Cotton, P. B., Russell, R. C. G. *et al.* (1987) 'Randomized trial of endoscopic versus percutaneous stent insertion in malignant obstructive jaundice'. *Lancet*, **2**, 57–61.

Small Intestinal Endoscopy

It is fortunate for the endoscopist that small intestinal disease is so relatively rare, since instrumental access is restricted; 5–50 cm of the terminal ileum can be examined by passing a colonoscope through the ileo-caecal valve (Chapter 9) and standard upper GI endoscopes can be passed into the third part of the duodenum; sometimes these, or paediatric colonoscopes, can be guided past the ligament of Treitz into the proximal jejunum, but only with difficulty and considerable patient discomfort.

Malabsorption biopsies

The mucosal lesions of sprue or coeliac disease are as prominent in the second part of the duodenum as they are in the jejunum. The coeliac lesion can be recognized macroscopically with high-resolution instruments, especially after dye-spray; the mucosa appears pale and oedematous, without normal villous structures. Biopsies taken at endoscopy are smaller than those obtained by a standard capsule, but they are adequate for histological diagnosis, and can also be used for biochemical studies. At least four specimens should be taken from beyond the papilla of Vater, preferably with a large-channel therapeutic endoscope.

Dye-spraying gives dramatic accentuation of abnormalities of mucosal architecture (and excellent photographs). A dilute coloured dye (washable blue ink, methylene blue, indocyanine green or indigo-carmine) is sprayed over the mucosa via a Teflon tube and enters the interstices between villous structures. A similar effect is sometimes inadvertent, and less obvious, when blood spills across the mucosa from a biopsy site. Dye-spraying can be used throughout the GI tract and provides particularly good documentation of ulcer scars and the extent of small tumours.

Enteroscopy

Examination of the small intestine beyond the ligament of Treitz is difficult. Suitably sterilized colonoscopes, adult or preferably paediatric, are suitable for jejunoscopy since they are significantly more flexible than gastroscopes. This extra flexibility, together with longer shaft length, is the main characteristic of purpose-built 'enteroscopes' (both fibreoptic and video-based) which are available from some manufacturers. A 'sonde-type' small intestinal endoscope can be used (Fig. 8.1). Essentially this is a very long and passive fibreoptic bundle without biopsy capability, with a distensible balloon at the tip to let intestinal peristaltic movements carry it down towards the ileum (in 4–8 hours). The partial views obtained and lack of biopsies makes this a 'heavy' and rarely used

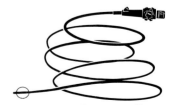

Fig. 8.1 A 'sonde-type' small intestinal endoscope, with a terminal weighted balloon.

157

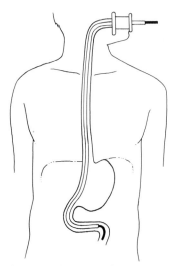

Fig. 8.2 A long overtube may facilitate jejunoscopy.

approach, not least because of its demands on the patient. The 'best buy' for limited small intestinal endoscopy is likely to be the use of a floppy or extra flexible paediatric colonoscope used in conjunction with a special soft-teflon (Gortex) 60-cm-long overtube, passed with the instrument into the duodenum (Fig. 8.2). This overtube has low-friction characteristics which allow the endoscope to pass down without the intragastric looping which normally limits attempted jejunoscopy. Another experimental approach is to use a variable stiffening device inside the proximal 70 cm of the instrument channel, also to prevent looping in the stomach.

Total enteroscopy has been achieved with the use of a weighted Teflon string, which the patient swallows and eventually passes (after a few days). The string at the patient's mouth is threaded back up the channel of an extra long double-channelled instrument. The endoscope is then advanced over the string, the two ends being pulled apart to straighten it. The whole of the small intestine and colon can be intubated by this means, from mouth to anus, with examination on withdrawal. This technique has not proved worth its expense, discomfort and occasional hazard.

Intra-operative enteroscopy

Until new methods are developed, the whole small intestine can be accurately examined only at laparotomy; the surgeon guides the endoscope through the small bowel with the abdomen open. A long colonoscope is the preferred instrument because of its flexibility. There are three possible modes of access:

1 *Via the mouth.* While the surgeon makes the skin incision, the endoscopist passes the endoscope as far as comfortably possible into the duodenum. Intubation of the duodenum is easier if done before the abdomen is opened and the tamponade effect of the abdominal wall lost.

2 *Via a surgical enterotomy.* Opening the bowel for intra-operative endoscopy has historical precedent but should rarely be required and in general is to be avoided. The infection risk will be increased.

3 *Via the anus.* The colonoscopy takes up about 70 cm of instrument, leaving less for examination of the small bowel.

The endoscope used for enteroscopy should be of the immersible type, and fully disinfected before the procedure. The patient's bowel is prepared by standard techniques. Intra-operative enteroscopy must be managed carefully and methodically, with special care taken to avoid overinsufflation and rough handling of the intestine. Counter pressure is applied by the surgeon to straighten out acute angles, and particularly (whilst working through the mouth) to prevent large loops from forming in the stomach and duodenum (Fig. 8.3)—or in the colon during a transanal approach.

The instrument tip is advanced slowly by the surgeon, under endoscopic vision, keeping air insufflation to a minimum. A kocher manoeuvre is usually not necessary.

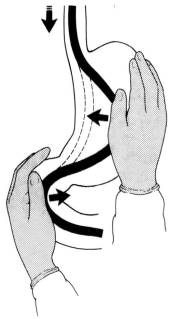

Fig. 8.3 Per-operative straightening of the stomach and duodenum.

During the withdrawal phase, placing fingers at appropriate positions across the bowel can help to localize distension to the part being examined—this 'sausage' of air being moved backwards as examination proceeds. If enteroscopy is being performed to look for a site of bleeding, it is important to view during advancement, so as not to be confused by haematomas caused by rough handling of the instrument against the mucosa. Angiomas are often best seen by transillumination, performed simply by switching off the operating room lights. Sometimes, reverse transillumination is also helpful; the bowel is viewed endoscopically, using only the operating room lights for illumination.

Noted lesions should be marked by the surgeon with a suture, and a decision is made regarding simple oversewing or resection only after the examination is completed.

Intra-operative endoscopy appears to be a remarkably safe procedure when performed by an expert—but indications are few, so that experts are rare. The most important things for the beginner to appreciate and avoid are:

1 Review the technique with the surgeon preoperatively. Co-operation is necessary.

2 Position the anaesthesiologist and his equipment to the patient's right. Position the patient supine in stirrups.

3 Place a naso-gastric tube before passing the endoscope. This will avoid over-distending the stomach during the procedure.

4 Be patient. Passage of the endoscope through the small bowel may at first appear to be difficult, but it is not.

5 Always advance under direct vision. This requires constant dialogue with the surgeon.

6 Use minimal amounts of air.

7 Examine the mesentery frequently. Do not allow tension on it to become excessive.

8 Do not worry if the entire small bowel cannot be examined from above. The distal ileum can be intubated after passage of the endoscope through the colon.

9 Decompress the bowel completely after each segment is examined.

Direct complications have been rare. Postoperative ileus may be somewhat prolonged, and both mucosal and serosal tears have been described.

Further reading

Axon, A. T. R. (1989) 'Endoscopy of the duodenum and small bowel' in *Annual of Gastrointestinal Endoscopy* (ed. Cotton, P. B., Tytgat, G. N. J. and Williams, C. B.) Current Science, London.

Bowden, T. A. (1985) 'Intraoperative endoscopy of the gastrointestinal tract', in *Surgical Endoscopy* (ed. Dent, T. L., Strodel, W. E. and Turcotte, J. G.), pp. 167–188. Year Book, Chicago.

9 Colonoscopy

Indications

The place of colonoscopy in clinical practice is outside the scope of this book and depends in any case on local circumstances and available endoscopic or radiological expertise. In large centres where both techniques are equally available, colonoscopy and barium enemas are performed in approximately equal numbers. Double-contrast barium enema (DCBE) is a safe way (one perforation per 25 000 examinations) of showing the configuration of the colon, the presence of diverticular disease and the absence of strictures or large lesions in patients with pain, altered bowel habit or constipation; it also shows extramural leaks or fistulae which are invisible to the endoscopist. Colonoscopy has a higher complication rate (around one perforation per 1700 examinations in series overall) but achieves more, partly in greater accuracy and also through its biopsy and therapeutic capabilities. Where rigid proctosigmoidoscopy, rectal biopsy and barium enema have made a diagnosis of inflammatory bowel disease, colonoscopy may have little to add in a patient who responds to treatment. However, in many circumstances it is simply easier to go for the golfer's 'hole in one' by performing colonoscopy straight off; this policy is particularly relevant to patients with bleeding, anaemia, prolonged bowel frequency or diarrhoea, and to any patient at risk for cancer—in whom detection and removal of any adenomas is important for the patient's future. Colonoscopy is thus the method of choice for cancer surveillance examinations and follow-up, the only proviso being that a few patients who are very difficult to colonoscope for anatomical reasons may be best examined by combining limited left-sided colonoscopy (much more accurate than DCBE in the sigmoid colon) with barium enema to demonstrate the proximal colon. If carbon dioxide insufflation is used during the endoscopy, the colon will be absolutely deflated within 10–15 min and DCBE can follow immediately, whereas after air insufflation the enlarged colon presents difficulties to the radiologist. In a very few high-risk patients, such as those with numerous adenomas, it may be justified to combine a check DCBE with colonoscopy for extra accuracy. Much more often the endoscopist is required to check uncertain radiological findings, and this adds to the tendency to go for colonoscopy as the first procedure. The notion of having a prior barium enema 'to show the shape of the colon' is largely irrelevant to the endoscopist, since short colons with short mesenteries can be difficult to endoscope, whereas some very long colons prove to be painless and easy.

If colonoscopy was technically easier and more predictable, the 'direct look' would be preferable to the indirect X-ray image in all cases, but some examinations in inexpert hands prove to be difficult, painful and even dangerous. Limited examination by flexible sigmoidoscopy may therefore have a major role in patients with minor symptoms such as left iliac fossa pain or altered bowel habit, and DCBE alone is safer and adequately effective in patients with constipation or others with minor functional symptoms where the result is expected to be normal or to show minor diverticular disease.

Contraindications and hazards

Against this clinical background, there are few patients in whom colonoscopy is contraindicated. Any patient who might otherwise come to diagnostic laparotomy because of colonic disease is fit for colonoscopy, and colonoscopy is often undertaken in very poor-risk cases in the hope of avoiding surgery. For a 3-week period after myocardial infarction, it is unwise to perform colonoscopy due to the risk of arrhythmias. If fluoroscopic control is to be used during the examination of young women, a menstrual history should be taken as for any other radiological procedure. In any acute and severe inflammatory process, such as ulcerative, Crohn's or ischaemic colitis, where abdominal tenderness suggests increased risk of perforation, colonoscopy should only be undertaken with good reason and extreme care. If large and deep ulcers are seen, the bowel wall may be weakened and it can be safest to limit or abandon the examination. In the chronic stage of irradiation colitis, a year or more after exposure, the bowel can be perforated even without excessive force; if the diagnosis has been made, and insertion proves difficult, it may be wiser to withdraw.

Colonoscopy is absolutely contraindicated in 'acute diverticulitis' which is due to local sepsis and threatened perforation. It should not be performed in any patient with marked abdominal tenderness, peritonism or peritonitis from whatever cause because of the high risk of causing perforation.

Passage of the colonoscope, and indeed any other instrumentation including air or barium insufflation, causes transient release of bowel organisms into the bloodstream and peritoneal cavity. This constitutes a relative contraindication to endoscopy of patients with known ascites or on peritoneal dialysis. They, and patients with known heart valve replacement, and also marasmic infants or immunosuppressed or immunodepressed adults, should be protected by prior administration of antibiotics (see the section on medication below). There is no contraindication to examination of infected patients (viz. infectious diarrhoea, hepatitis) since *all* normal organisms and viruses will be inactivated by routine cleaning and disinfection procedures including 4-min soak/channel perfusion with 2% glutaraldehyde. Mycobacterial spores, however, require a much longer period, and therefore after examination of suspected tuberculosis patients, and before and after examination of AIDS patients who are susceptible to, and possible carriers of, *Mycobacteria*, a 60-min soak of the instrument in glutaraldehyde is recommended (see Chapter 12).

Patient preparation: out-patient, day-case or in-patient?

Most patients can organize their bowel preparation at home, present themselves for examination and walk out shortly afterwards. Routines depend on national, organizational and individual factors. In some countries (USA, France, Italy, West Germany) patients are prepared to administer their own cleansing enemas; in others this has to be done by the endoscopy nursing staff. Some nationalities (Dutch, German, Japanese) do not expect sedation whereas others (British, American) frequently insist on it. Whether a doctor recommends admission for endoscopy is influenced, amongst other things, by cost, the type of bowel preparation and sedation used, the potential for therapeutic procedures and the availability of adequate facilities and nursing staff for day-care and recovery. Colonoscopists in private practice are motivated to organize stream-lined day-case routines. These variables result in an extraordinary spectrum of routines from the many skilled colonoscopists who require the patient for less than an hour in an office or day-care unit, to others with less experience and a traditional hospital background who feel that hours, even days, in hospital are essential.

Colonoscopy should be made as quick and easy as possible; this requires both a reasonably planned day-care facility and an endoscopist with the confidence and skill to work gently and fast. Some patients must be admitted before or after the procedure; the very old, sick and very constipated may need professional supervision during bowel preparation, and frail patients often merit overnight observation. Some endoscopists feel that all patients undergoing polypectomy (Chapter 10) should be in hospital afterwards; for the endoscopist's first few polypectomies this may be correct, but we admit only a few patients with polyps ≥ 2 cm, when the lesion is broad-stalked or sessile and has a greater likelihood of complications.

Bowel preparation

Patients and colons vary. No single preparation regime suits every patient and it is often necessary to adapt to individual needs. The doctor, or his nurse or secretary, should *talk to* the patient to find out about his normal bowel habit (loose or constipated, laxative requirements, results of previous purgatives, etc.) and explain the need for special diets and purgation. Minutes spent in explanation and motivation may prevent a prolonged, unpleasant and inaccurate examination due to bad preparation. A preparation which has made the patient vomit or has failed on one occasion is unlikely to be a success on another.

Limited preparation

Diverticular disease or stricturing makes preparation more difficult and phosphate enemas are unlikely to work for mechanical reasons. For limited colonoscopy in the 'normal' colon, limited preparation should be enough. The patient need not diet and is simply given one or two disposable phosphate enemas (Fleet's, Fletcher's) 20–30 min before colonoscopy; early examination is performed so that there is no time for proximal bowel contents to descend. The colon is often perfectly prepared to the transverse or hepatic flexure, especially in young patients. Note that patients with any tendency to faint or with functional bowel symptoms (pain, flatulence, etc.) are more likely to have severe vaso-vagal problems after phosphate enemas; make sure they are supervised or have a call button and that lavatory doors open from and to the outside in case the patient faints against the door.

If there is a serious possibility of obstruction, per-oral preparation is dangerous, even potentially fatal, and in ileus or pseudo-obstruction normal preparation simply does not work; one or more large-volume enemas are administered in such circumstances (up to a litre or more can be held by most colons). A contact laxative such as oxyphenisatin or bisacodyl can be added to the enema to improve evacuation (see below).

Full preparation

Diet

Iron preparations should be stopped 3–4 days before, since organic iron tannates produce an inky black stool which interferes with inspection and can make the stool viscous and difficult to clear. Constipating agents should also be stopped 1–2 days before, but other medication is continued as usual. The patient should have no indigestible or high-residue food for 24 hours before colonoscopy; if he can be persuaded to stay for 24 hours on clear fluids so much the better. Written instructions are well worth while.

Purgation and enemas

To be effective, sufficient contact laxative or purgative must be taken to produce fluid diarrhoea, which shows that unaltered small intestinal contents are emerging and the colonic residue has been cleared. Any agent producing this result may also cause nausea or abdominal cramps in some patients. It takes only about 8 hours for colonic water absorption to reform ileal effluent into solid stool so it is best if diarrhoea stops only shortly before examination. However, since some people respond to laxatives in 1–2 hours and others take as much as 8 hours, exact timing is difficult. If the patient is to get some sleep and then be able to travel without risk of accident, the best compromise is for the laxative to be taken at 3–4 p.m. on the previous afternoon. For a mid-afternoon colonoscopy the purge can be taken early the same morning.

The most widely used purge was castor oil (30–40 ml) which acts on both small and large intestine, but is disliked by most patients. Its after-taste and oily texture can be masked by mixing with orange juice or an effervescent drink immediately before taking it, and following with a 'chaser' of orange juice. Senna preparations work equally well providing a large dose is given (140 mg of sennosides) either as syrup or tablets. Osmotic purges such as the magnesium salts (citrate tastes better than sulphate or hydroxide) can also be effective with repeated 2-hourly doses and high fluid intake until there is clear diarrhoea.

A proprietary combination (Picolax), which tastes acceptable and works well in most patients, produces both magnesium citrate (from magnesium oxide and citric acid) and bisacodyl (from bacterial action on sodium picosulphate). Providing enough fluid is drunk, no enema is needed. Failures occur mainly in older patients with diverticular disease and colons damaged by colitis.

Constipated patients should be primed with senna at bedtime on the nights preceding normal preparation. Really stubborn constipation, as in cases of megacolon or cystic fibrosis, can be cleared by hourly doses of magnesium sulphate crystals (Epsom salts, 15–30 g) with large volumes of clear fluid, but since this and the subsequent colonoscopy are likely to be unpleasant, the experience should be avoided if at all possible.

Tap-water, isotonic saline or purgative (bisacodyl or oxyphenisatin) enemas are self- or nurse-administered 1–2 hours before examination until the returns are clear. Two or three enemas each of 1–3 litres may be needed. The fluid should reach the caecum; lavage or 'washouts' of the social variety, where small volumes of water are run in and out of the distal colon, are useless. Having got the fluid in it must also be got out, which entails the patient being able to sit relaxed on the lavatory for 15–20 min initially and then to revisit and evacuate at will afterwards. The returns are inspected and, if any solid matter remains, the enema is repeated.

Patients with diverticular disease or painful spasm obstructing enema inflow are given an intramuscular antispasmodic injection (hyoscine *N*-butylbromide, 40 mg i.m.; glucagon, 0.5 mg i.m.).

Oral lavage regimes

Oral lavage regimes are supplanting purge plus enema in many practices because they are quicker, more effective and cause no pain. On the other hand, some patients will not or cannot drink the 3–6-litre volumes of fluid required, experience uncomfortable distension, become nauseated or vomit, or simply dislike the taste of the chosen solution. Further work is needed to provide the ideal compromise—a powder which can be sent through the mail, dissolved to produce perhaps 2–3 litres maximum of a pleasant-tasting combination of non-absorbed solutes and electrolytes, with a physiological gut-activator or prokinetic agent to speed transit.

Saline

Saline 0.9% alone is effective and used successfully by a number of centres. Not surprisingly it tastes salty, especially at first, but over the 3–4 litres usually needed, the saltiness is less and less apparent.

Balanced electrolyte solution

This solution, including the requisite amount of KCl and bicarbonate to avoid body losses, is physiologically correct, but for one-off preparation it is debatable whether the loss is significant, whereas the taste of the additives (especially KCl) may be unpleasant.

Balanced electrolyte solution with PEG (Golytely)

Polyethylene glycol (PEG)/electrolyte mixture is widely used, primarily because it has formal (FDA) approval allowing commercial packaging (Golytely) and easy prescription by doctors. Even chilled, its taste is more unpleasant than either saline or balanced electrolyte solution, due to the addition of $NaSO_4$ (as well as bicarbonate and KCl) to minimize body fluxes. However, modification of the original formula, lowering the sodium content by omitting $NaSO_4$ and reducing KCl, much improves the taste; the necessary increase in PEG makes the solutes bulky for postage but this is still feasible.

Patient acceptance of electrolyte/PEG oral preparation is enhanced, without impairing results from the endoscopist's point of view, by the simple expedient of administering it in two half doses (2 litres evening before and 2 litres morning of examination).

Mannitol

Mannitol (and similarly sorbitol or lactulose) is a sugar for which the body has no absorptive enzymes. In solution it presents an iso-osmotic fluid load at 5% (2–3 litres) or a hypertonic purge at 10% (1 litre) with corresponding loss of electrolyte and body fluid during the resulting diarrhoea, although this is only of concern in the elderly and normally can be rapidly reversed by drinking. The solution tastes very sweet and can be nauseous to those without a sweet tooth. Unfortunately colonic bacteria possess the necessary enzymes to metabolize mannitol and other carbohydrates to form explosive quantities of hydrogen, so that any electrosurgical or laser procedure is hazardous unless CO_2 insufflation has been used, or all colonic gas several times exchanged by aspiration and air re-insufflation.

Administration of oral lavage

The night before oral lavage some patients are best given a dose of senna or bisacodyl. Half an hour before starting to drink, a prokinetic metoclopramide or domperidone tablet (10 mg) reduces the chance of duodenal dilatation and vomiting. Using a barrier cream, petroleum jelly or other ointment will avoid perianal soreness. Electrolyte solutions should be drunk steadily at a rate around 1.5 litres per hour (250 ml per 10 min initially) and mannitol chilled and drunk more slowly still. The patient walks around to encourage transit, but should stop drinking temporarily if nausea or uncomfortable distension occur.

Bowel actions should start within about an hour, returns are often clear by 2–3 hours and colonoscopy can be started 1–2 hours later. The endoscopist may have to aspirate large quantities of fluid during the examination but the patient is spared the dietary changes, cramps and enemas of a purge regime and the result is usually excellent.

Special circumstances

Children

Children accept pleasant-tasting oral preparations such as senna syrup or magnesium citrate very well. Drinking large volumes is less well accepted and mannitol may cause nausea or vomiting. The childhood colon normally evacuates easily except, paradoxically, in some cases with colitis which prove perversely difficult to prepare properly. Small babies in particular may be almost completely prepared with half a phosphate enema (see also paediatric colonoscopy, p. 217).

Colitics

Relapses of inflammatory bowel disease are said occasionally to occur after over-vigorous bowel preparation, although they can also be provoked by simple distension during an unprepared barium enema, which suggests that the cause may be mechanical rather than chemical. Magnesium citrate, senna preparations, mannitol, saline or balanced electrolyte/PEG solutions are all generally well tolerated and the latter preparations are favoured in patients with diarrhoea from active colitis. A simple tap-water enema will clear the distal colon sufficiently for limited colonoscopy. Patients with severe colitis are unlikely to need colonoscopy at all, since plain abdominal X-ray or unprepared barium enema will usually give enough information; for severely ill patients even barium enema is risky and colonoscopy positively contraindicated due to the potential for perforation. If colonoscopy is advised to exclude cancer or to reach the terminal ileum to help in differential diagnosis, full and vigorous preparation is necessary. If a patient is fit for total colonoscopy, he is fit for full bowel preparation, which is needed because inflammatory change often makes the proximal colon difficult to prepare properly.

Constipated patients

Having elicited a story of long-standing constipation (or having seen evidence of it on previous barium enema), extra bowel preparation is needed. This is very difficult to achieve in patients with megacolon, Hirschsprung's disease, cystic fibrosis, etc., in whom colonoscopy should be avoided if at all possible. Constipated patients should continue any habitually-taken purgatives in addition to the colonoscopy preparation, and preferably in large doses for several days beforehand. The principle is to achieve regular soft bowel actions during the days before taking the main purge, if necessary using additional doses of paraffin emulsion, magnesium citrate/sulphate, etc. Larger-than-standard doses of senna or other purgatives are unlikely to produce any extra effect, but frequent doses of magnesium salts and large volumes of fluid are guaranteed to move mountains (see above), providing there is no obstruction.

Colostomy patients

The colons of colostomy patients are as difficult to prepare as normal colons (and often more so). The preparation regime should not be reduced just because the colon is shorter, if anything increased, with a prior 'pump-priming' dose of senna on the night before. Oral preparation with one of the lavage regimes described above is well tolerated, whereas enemas/colostomy washouts are tedious and difficult to perform satisfactorily unless the patient is accustomed to this and used to performing it personally.

Stomas and pouches

Ileostomies are self-emptying and normally need no preparation. Kock or ileo-anal pelvic pouches can either be managed by saline enema or by oral lavage.

Ileo-rectal anastomosis

The small intestine can adapt and enlarge to an amazing degree within some months of surgery, so that if the object of the examination is to examine the small intestine, full oral preparation should be given. For a limited look, a saline or tap-water enema is usually enough.

Defunctioned bowel

Defunctioned bowel, for instance the distal loop of a 'double-barrelled' colostomy, will contain a considerable amount of viscid mucus and some inspissated residue which will block the colonoscope. Conventional tap-water/saline enemas or tube lavage through the colostomy are needed before examining defunctioned bowel.

Active colonic bleeding

Blood is a good purgative and some patients need no other preparation providing examination is started *during* the phase of active bright-red bleeding. Posturing the patient during insertion of the instrument will shift the blood and create an air interface through which the instrument can be passed; changing to the right lateral position clears the proximal sigmoid and descending colon, which is otherwise a blood-filled sump. Bleeding patients requiring preparation for total colonoscopy are best managed by nasal tube or oral electrolyte/mannitol lavage. This allows examination within an hour or two and ensures that blood is washed out distal to the bleeding point, rather than carried proximally with enemas. Blood can be refluxed to the terminal ileum from a left colon source, which makes localization difficult, unless it is being constantly washed downwards by per-oral high-volume preparation. Massively bleeding patients may best be examined per-operatively with on-table colon lavage combining a caecostomy tube with a large-bore rectal suction tube.

Medication

Sedation/analgesia?

When the examination is arranged, the patient should be given verbal and written explanation both of bowel preparation and of the procedure. On arrival for colonoscopy, a few minutes of further explanation will reassure and calm most patients and allow the endoscopist to judge whether the particular individual is likely to require sedation. Most people tolerate some discomfort without resentment if they understand the reason for it. Few people expect to be semi-anaesthetized for a visit to the dentist, but on the other hand they expect the intensity and duration of any pain to be within 'acceptable' limits—a threshold not always easy to predict before colonoscopy, because both individual anatomy and tolerance to the unpleasant quality of visceral pain vary so much. It is sensible to warn the patient that there can be some stomach ache or air distension during the procedure, but to ask him to complain at once rather than to suffer in silence, and also to ask for analgesia if he wants it. It is worth pointing out that pain is a useful warning to the endoscopist, is not dangerous, and can usually be terminated in a short time (by straightening out the responsible loop).

The use of sedation has advantages and disadvantages. Without it, the bowel is more tonic, shorter and possibly easier to examine; the patient can co-operate with any changes of position, needs no recovery period and can travel home unaided immediately. The colonoscopist is also forced to develop good technique. With sedation the patient is more likely to find the examination tolerable even if it is prolonged, and the endoscopist can be more thorough and is more likely to achieve total colonoscopy in a shorter time. However, with heavy sedation endoscopists can get away with ham-handed technique, which is a bad investment in the long term, perhaps more likely to result in complications and certainly more expensive in instrument repair bills. It is often said that it is dangerous to sedate because the safety factor of pain is removed, but this is not strictly true providing that the endoscopist raises his own threshold of awareness as the patient's pain threshold is raised, responding to restlessness or changes of facial expression as a warning that the tissues are being overstretched.

General anaesthesia in particular is hazardous when used by inexperienced endoscopists, but may be needed occasionally in special circumstances. The endoscopist must take care not to use brutal technique when the patient cannot protest.

Using moderate or no sedation, employing the skills, changes of position and other 'tricks of the trade' described hereafter, the only pain experienced by the patient during a correctly-performed colonoscopy in a 'normal' colon should be for 20–30 seconds in the sigmoid, with only a feeling of distension or apparent desire to pass flatus at other times. Total colonoscopy should be absolutely safe and achievable in > 95% of patients; some endoscopists employing no sedation admit to only 70–80% success in performing total colonoscopy. With the heavy sedation employed by other endoscopists (e.g. diazepam, 10 mg i.v., especially if combined with pethidine, 75–100 mg i.v.) the drowsy patient cannot either co-operate or complain effectively, the possible subtleties of colonoscopic technique may be ignored and there is no 'negative feedback' when loops form; the end result is that colonoscopy risks becoming a 'heavy' procedure with a significant complication rate due to air distension and excessive force, but the total colonoscopy rate may be disappointing because of loops formed but not removed.

Most endoscopists use a balanced approach to sedation which will be affected by many factors including personal experience and the patient's attitude. A relaxed patient with a short colon having a limited examination rarely needs sedation, but a tense sick patient with a tortuous colon or severe diverticular disease requiring total colonoscopy needs some protection. Exceptional patients have such a morbid fear of colonoscopy, or such a low pain threshold that it is justified to resort to general anaesthesia if colonoscopy, rather than barium enema, is particularly indicated.

The ideal sedative for colonoscopy would last 5–10 min with strong analgesic action but no respiratory depression or after-effects. The nearest approach to the ideal at present is given by the combination of a benzodiazepine hypnotic such as diazepam (Valium) (5–10 mg) or midazolam (Versed) (2.5–5 mg) with an opiate such as pethidine (Demerol) (25–75 mg) given slowly over a period of 1–2 min whilst observing the patient's conscious state and ability to talk coherently. The benzodiazepine contributes anxiolytic, sedational and amnesic effects (midazolam often causes complete amnesia, including unfortunately any explanation given after the examination is over). The opiate contributes analgesia and, in the case of pethidine (Demerol), a useful sense of euphoria. In general only a small dose of benzodiazepine should be given unless the patient is very anxious; for pathologically anxious or neurotic patients, premedication may be helpful, e.g. a beta-blocker (propranolol, 40 mg or equivalent orally) or an opiate, pethidine (Demerol, 75 mg i.m.). If increments of medication are needed during insertion use extra opiate, rather than extra benzo-diazepine which makes some patients even more restless and has no useful pain-killing properties.

Diazepam (Valium) is poorly soluble in water and the injectable form is therefore carried in a glycol solution which can be painful and cause thrombophlebitis, especially if administered into small veins. If a hand vein is to be used, and also for paediatric practice, it is better either to use diazepam in lipid emulsion (Diazemuls, where available) or water-soluble midazolam (Versed), both of which are less irritant. Pethidine (Demerol) may cause pain when administered through small veins, particularly in children, but this can be avoided by diluting the injection 1:10 in water. Some endoscopists prefer to give pethidine (Demerol) i.m. an hour beforehand, which we do not favour. Others have used the neurolept-analgesic combination of haloperidol and droperidol, which is effective but has the disadvantage of prolonged after-effects. Pentazocine (Fortral) is a weaker analgesic, more hallucinogenic and seems to have little to recommend it. Inhalational analgesics such as nitrous oxide alone are not enough to relieve the visceral pain of colonoscopy. Benzodiazepines and opiates potentiate each other in effectiveness and also in side-effects such as depression of respiration and blood pressure, which can be sudden or gradual, and potentially serious. Pulse oximetry should be available to monitor elderly or heavily sedated patients and if in doubt oxygen should be administered.

Availability of antagonists to benzodiazepines (adnexate) and opiates (naloxone) is an invaluable safety measure; some endoscopists routinely give them (i.v. and/or i.m.) to speed the recovery period.

Antispasmodics

Either hyoscine *N*-butylbromide (Buscopan, 20–40 mg) or glucagon (0.5–1 mg) i.v. give good colonic relaxation for 5–10 min and are helpful during examination of the over-active bowel for polyps or other lesions. The ocular side-effects of hyoscine may continue for several hours and the patient should not drive if vision is impaired, although cholinesterase inhibitor eye drops will restore normality. Fears about anticholinergics initiating glaucoma are misplaced since patients previously diagnosed are completely protected by their eye drops, and those with undiagnosed chronic glaucoma are best served by precipitating an acute attack, which will cause the diagnosis to be made. Glucagon is more expensive, but has no ocular or prostatic side-effects.

The short duration of action of intravenous antispasmodics means that it is often best to give them when the colonoscope is fully inserted, making inspection on withdrawal more complete. Experienced endoscopists sure of a rapid procedure may give them at the start, although there is some suspicion that a redundant and a tonic bowel is more difficult to examine. In the unsedated patient (flexible sigmoidoscopy, etc.) and in diverticular disease, antispasmodics may make insertion easier. Diazepam alone has an antispasmodic effect which will relax most colons except for those which are 'irritable' or spastic. Patients with functional bowel disorder or diverticular disease may suffer from increased air retention after using antispasmodics, with sudden onset of colic an hour or more after the procedure when the pharmacological effects wear off (see section on carbon dioxide, p. 173).

Antibiotics

It is well proven from studies in which multiple blood cultures are taken during colonoscopy, that transient bacteraemia occurs while the instrument is being inserted. Both aerobic and anaerobic organisms can be released into the bloodstream at this time. Patients with ascites or on peritoneal dialysis have been reported to develop peritonitis following colonic instrumentation, presumably by transmural passage of bacteria as a result of local trauma. At-risk patients (such as those with heart valve disease or replacement) and immunosuppressed or severely ill patients (especially immuno-compromised infants) should have a suitable antibiotic combination administered beforehand so as to give therapeutic blood levels at the time of the procedure. Ampicillin orally at 2 hours with gentamicin i.m. 1 hour beforehand would be a possible regime, dosage depending on size. Alternatively, a single i.v. dose of gentamicin (80 mg) and ampicillin (500 mg) before premedication has been advised. Vancomycin can be substituted for ampicillin in patients with a history of penicillin sensitivity. In high-risk subjects it may be wise to continue antibiotics for up to 48 hours.

Equipment

Where to do colonoscopy

The only special requisite for a colonoscopy room is good ventilation to overcome the evidence of occasional poor bowel preparation. In a few patients with particularly difficult and looping colons, it can be helpful to have access to X-ray facilities, which also make the learning process quicker. Most units perform colonoscopies in the ordinary endoscopy area, but arrange to have access to a mobile image-intensifier or to an X-ray screening room on the rare occasions that this is necessary.

Which colonoscope?

Colonoscopes are, regrettably, engineered similarly to upper gastrointestinal endoscopes, except in having a more flexible shaft and provision of carbon dioxide insufflation and syringe lens-washing facilities. The bending section at the tip is also more gently curved, to avoid impaction in acute bends such as the splenic flexure. The ideal colonoscope would be modified so that one-handed steering in all directions was easily possible at the same time as activation of other control buttons, thus leaving the right hand free to manage the precise shaft movements needed to manoeuvre through the tortuous bends of the colon.

Ignoring the slight differences between different makes of colonoscope, there are significant advantages in choosing the 'right colonoscope for the job' both at the stage of purchase and for the particular patients. Long colonoscopes (165–180 cm) are able to reach the caecum even in redundant colons, but their longer control wires may be more easily damaged, and their longer accessories are slightly more awkward to handle and clean; they are also more expensive. Medium- or intermediate-length instruments (130–140 cm) are a good compromise and, with the occasional use of a stiffening overtube, can almost always reach the caecum. The shortest instruments (70–110 cm) used for flexible sigmoidoscopy or limited colonoscopy have the advantage that the endoscopist knows from the onset that he is doing a quick procedure and is not tempted to go further and prolong it; they have the disadvantage of tending to result in 'cheek-to-cheek colonoscopy'. Video-colonoscopes, since they do not need to be held near the endoscopist's face, have both positional and hygienic advantages and intermediate-length video-colonoscopes seem likely to become the routine 'work horse' instruments for busy units. Since flexible sigmoidoscopy can be performed with a longer instrument, there is little need for a flexible sigmoidoscope in an endoscopy unit, although it has an essential role in the office of a primary care physician or a general clinic facility.

Apart from length, the other current variable is in the size of the suction/instrumentation channel; a larger channel usually results in marginally greater shaft diameter and consequent slight stiffness and clumsier handling characteristics. Doubtless, engineering skills will in future allow increased channel size without this penalty, for a larger channel has every advantage. It permits aspiration of fibrous food residues or polyp fragments which would otherwise cause blockage and allows fluid aspiration whilst standard accessories (snare, biopsy forceps, etc.) are in place, and the use of larger 'jumbo' forceps to obtain substantial biopsies for more certain diagnosis of malignancy or Crohn's disease.

Paediatric colonoscopes, of intermediate length and smaller diameter (9–10 mm) with either standard or 'floppy' shaft characteristics are also available. They are invaluable for examination of babies and children up to 2–3 years of age (see Chapter 10). They also have a role to play in adult endoscopy. As well as allowing examination of strictures, anastomoses or stomas impassable with the full-sized colonoscope, they are often much easier to pass through areas of tethered postoperative adhesions or severe diverticular disease. Floppy paediatric instruments are particularly comfortable and easy to insert to the splenic flexure, tending to conform to the loops of the colon and form a spontaneous alpha loop which avoids difficulty in passing to the descending colon. The smaller diameter of the shaft is, however, less easy to torque or twist and is more easily damaged if used routinely for more extensive examination.

Few endoscopists have the luxury of having a variety of instruments available. It is therefore important when buying a colonoscope to consider its likely major use, and in the individual patient to select one with regard to the clinical situation, the distance to be examined (and the tortuosity of the colon if a previous barium enema is available). The most experienced endoscopists are the least worried by changing instruments, but vary amazingly in their opinions as to what is the ideal—longer/shorter, more or less stiff—which suggests that there will never be such a thing as a single 'ideal colonoscope'. A physician who will want to be sure of being able to examine the proximal colon must either have a long instrument or have an intermediate length instrument with a split overtube and/or fluoroscopy available. A busy unit needs at least two functional colonoscopes used alternately to permit adequate disinfection during a routine list, a third instrument being available as back-up during any period of breakdown. A surgeon who is only interested in occasional and left-sided examinations or per-operative procedures will be satisfied with a single instrument of intermediate length. Ideally any endoscopist should also have access to a paediatric endoscope for special cases.

Which accessories?

All usual accessories such as biopsy forceps, snares, retrieval forceps, sclerotherapy needles, laser light-guides, cytology brushes, washing catheters, etc. are used down the colonoscope. Long- and intermediate-length accessories work equally well down shorter instruments, so it is sensible to order all accessories to suit the longest instrument in routine use. Other manufacturers' accessories also work down any particular instrument and, since some are better than others, it is worth taking advice when buying replacements.

The only specialized accessory in colonoscopy is the 'stiffening tube', 'stiffener' or 'split overtube', the use of which is described later (pp. 202–203). This is occasionally invaluable in avoiding recurrent loop formation after straightening of the sigmoid colon, for exchange of instruments or for retrieving multiple polyps.

Carbon dioxide?

All colonoscopes have carbon dioxide (CO_2) buttons, but few colonoscopists use CO_2 insufflation. This is because—with the exception of bowel preparation using mannitol (and other similar agents such as sorbitol, lactulose or lactitol)—colonoscopic bowel preparation has been shown to leave no residual explosive gas in the colon as a polypectomy hazard. However, for certain routine examinations, the use of CO_2 offers the striking advantage that it clears (through the circulation, to the lungs and breathed out) 100 times faster than air. This means that after CO_2 insufflation the colon and small intestine are free of any gas in 15–20 min, whereas air distension can remain and cause discomfort for many hours. Colonoscopy with CO_2 insufflation can therefore be followed immediately by double-contrast barium enema (DCBE) whereas air distension increases the amount of barium needed to fill and then coat the colon, with a likelihood of a resulting substandard procedure. Additionally, patients with ileus, pseudo-obstruction, stricturing, severe colitis, diverticular disease or functional bowel disorder with pain should all benefit from the added safety and comfort of using CO_2 rather than air distension. In some instruments it is now possible to fit a CO_2 insufflation button as a replacement for the usual air button and cheaper low pressure metered-flow CO_2 delivery systems are also available, which removes the previously valid objection that CO_2 was cumbersome to use and expensive to install.

Instrumental technique

General principles

The occasional severe difficulties of colonoscopy come as a surprise to those with experience only in gastroscopy or rigid procto-sigmoidoscopy. The bends of the colon resemble those of the duodenum, where subtlety and instrumental rotation are more likely to allow advance than any amount of pushing, but colonic bends are numerous, unpredictable and frequently mobile as well—compared to only two fixed anatomic bends in the duodenum. The proctosigmoidoscopist is additionally not used to the close-up view of the colonoscope, nor to its perverse habit of flexing when he wants to advance; he therefore tends to lose patience, use force and then be surprised that insertion becomes difficult and painful.

The colon is an elastic tube (Fig. 9.1). Inflated, it becomes long and tortuous; deflated, it is significantly shorter, as after-evacuation X-ray pictures show convincingly. Stretched by a colonoscope the bowel forms loops and acute bends (Fig. 9.2) but shortened down by the colonoscope it can be telescoped into a few centimetres on convoluted length (Fig. 9.3).

The fundamentals in colonoscopy are therefore:
1 To inflate as little as possible consistent with vision, aspirating excess air at every opportunity.
2 To be gentle and avoid forming unnecessary loops—by pushing as little as possible.
3 To pull back and shorten the colon at every opportunity.
4 To look at the distance of colonoscope inserted, keeping it appropriate to the anatomic location (viz. 50 cm at splenic flexure).
5 To pay attention to patient discomfort, which indicates excessive looping or insufflation.
It is also necessary to appreciate and use the normal functional anatomy of the colon, and to be aware of possible anatomical variants.

Endoscopic anatomy of the colon

The endoscopist is not concerned with many of the normal anatomical considerations, such as the blood and nerve supply and lymphatic drainage. Visually he is aware of the fixed infoldings of

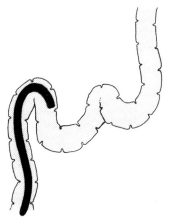

Fig. 9.1 The sigmoid colon is an elastic tube . . .

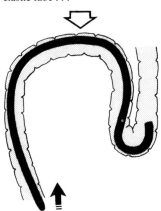

Fig. 9.2 . . . pushing loops it . . .

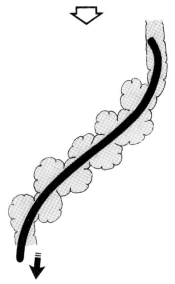

Fig. 9.3 . . . but pulling back shortens and straightens the colon.

the circular muscle haustrations which, when pronounced, can interfere with complete mucosal visualization. In the sigmoid and descending colon the haustra and the colonic outline are generally circular (Fig. 9.4). The longitudinal muscles fused into three straps or 'taeniae coli' are responsible for the characteristic triangular cross-section often seen in the transverse colon (but which can be present in the descending colon) (Fig. 9.5). Only in certain places, notably at the hepatic flexure (but sometimes also in the mid-transverse colon if there is a deep transverse loop), are the haustra seen face on as thin knife-like folds (Fig. 9.6). As well as these structural circular folds, there can be variable active contractions of the bowel circular muscle, narrowing it like a row of clenched fingers, but opening up with time or after administration of antispasmodics.

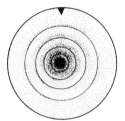

Fig. 9.4 The descending colon is usually circular.

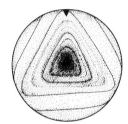

Fig. 9.5 The transverse colon is usually triangular.

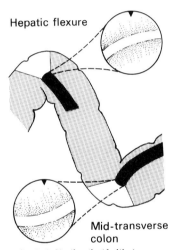

Fig. 9.6 Similar 'knife-like' haustral folds at the mid-transverse colon and hepatic flexure.

Visible evidence of extra-colonic viscera normally occurs at the hepatic flexure where there is seen to be a bluish indentation from the liver; a similar appearance may however sometimes occur at the splenic flexure or elsewhere. The combination of an acute bend with sharp haustra and blue coloration is thus characteristic of the hepatic flexure and a useful, but not infallible, endoscopic landmark.

In the more thin-walled proximal colon the longitudinal muscle bands of the taeniae coli may be visible endoscopically as a longitudinal fold running in the direction of the lumen, sometimes a useful guideline. At the pole of the caecum the taeniae fuse down into the appendix (Fig. 9.7); between the taeniae and the marked caecal haustra there can be cavernous outpouchings which are difficult to examine. The appendix orifice is normally an unimpressive slit, which is often crescentic since the appendix lies tangentially. Sometimes the opening resembles a solitary caecal diverticulum; only rarely is it tubular, and it may not be obvious in a local whirl of mucosal folds. The operated appendix usually looks no different unless it has been invaginated into a stump, when it can sometimes resemble a polyp (*take care*—biopsy but no polypectomy).

The ileo-caecal valve is situated on the medial part of the prominent ileo-caecal fold which encircles the caecum about 5 cm from its pole (see p. 209). Unfortunately for the endoscopist, the

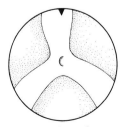

Fig. 9.7 Appendix orifice.

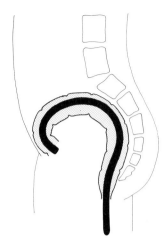

Fig. 9.8 Sigmoid colon—lateral view.

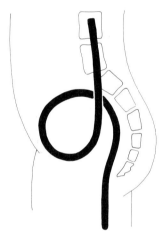

Fig. 9.9 Sigmoid loop—lateral view.

orifice of the valve is often a slit on the invisible 'caecal' aspect of the ileo-caecal fold. The most the endoscopist normally sees is the slight bulge of the upper lip—much as the mouth would look if seen by an endoscope emerging from the nose. It is therefore rare to see the orifice directly without specific close-up manoeuvres (p. 209).

Normal mesenteric anatomy, colonic attachments and their effect on colonoscopy

The anatomy and variations of the attachments of the colon are well known to surgeons but they are given little coverage in textbooks and are invisible on X-ray. Most inexperienced colonoscopists have difficulty in understanding the anatomical explanations for the weird loops and configurations of the colonoscope as seen on fluoroscopy and why the 'rules' of colonoscopy do not always work—usually due to mobility of the colon and its attachments.

The inserted colonoscope may stretch the bowel to the limits of its attachments or the confines of the abdominal cavity. The shape of the pelvis, with curved sacral hollow and the forward-projecting sacral promontory, cause the colonoscope to pass up anteriorly (Fig. 9.8) from the pelvis and the shaft can often be felt looped onto the anterior abdominal wall before it passes posteriorly again to the descending colon in the left paravertebral gutter (Fig. 9.9). The result is that an antero-posterior loop forms during passage of the sigmoid colon and, since the descending colon is usually laterally placed, it forms a clockwise spiral loop (Fig. 9.10); the importance of this will be discussed later. Because the sigmoid loop runs anteriorly against the abdominal wall it is possible partially to reduce or modify the sigmoid looping of the colonoscope by pressing against the left lower abdomen with the hand (Fig. 9.11).

The descending colon, after running up the paravertebral gutter, then bends medially and anteriorly into the transverse colon,

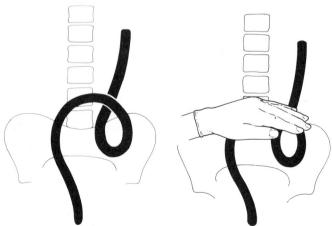

Fig. 9.10 Sigmoid loop—anterior view (clockwise spiral).

Fig. 9.11 Hand pressure restricts the sigmoid loop.

which also lies just beneath the abdominal wall, held forward by the vertebral bodies, the duodenum, pancreas and other viscera (Fig. 9.12). The hepatic flexure loops backwards into the right paravertebral gutter and the ascending colon—a further clockwise spiral. The caecum rises anteriorly against the anterior abdominal wall, permitting transillumination and explaining why changes of position (front or back) can help reach the pole.

The bowel is normally fixed at the rectum, descending and ascending colon (Fig. 9.12), leaving the sigmoid and transverse parts free on mesenteries or 'mesocolons' (Fig. 9.13). The rectum is bound down onto the sacral hollow by the peritoneum.

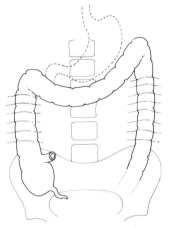

Fig. 9.12 The transverse colon is anterior; the descending and ascending colon are fixed retroperitoneally.

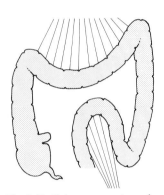

Fig. 9.13 Colon mesenteries—the transverse and sigmoid 'mesocolons'.

Mesentery

The longer the sigmoid colon, the longer its mesocolon; thus it is unusual to cause pain in a patient with a redundant sigmoid unless there are surgical adhesions. Patients with short colons and mesenteries may conversely be easily hurt by colonoscopic loops and manoeuvres.

The descending colon is normally bound down retroperitoneally and forms a fixed straight which is easy to pass with the colonoscope, but which also results in a fixed 'hairpin' bend at the junction with the sigmoid colon (Fig. 9.14). This junction is only a theoretical landmark to the radiologist, but a real and often difficult one for the endoscopist to pass. The acuteness of the sigmoid-descending angle depends not only on several anatomical factors, including how far down in the pelvis the descending colon is fixed, but also on colonoscopic technique—since it is only the forced upwards bowing of the sigmoid colon by the colonoscope which creates the bend at all. A really acute hairpin bend results when the sigmoid colon is long or elastic enough to make a large loop and the

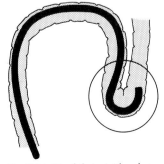

Fig. 9.14 Fixed 'hairpin' bend at the sigmoid-descending junction.

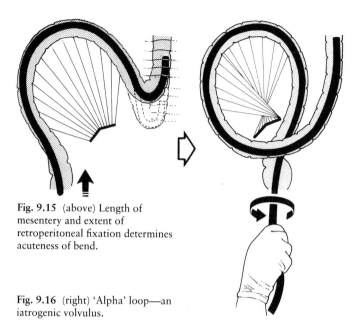

Fig. 9.15 (above) Length of mesentery and extent of retroperitoneal fixation determines acuteness of bend.

Fig. 9.16 (right) 'Alpha' loop—an iatrogenic volvulus.

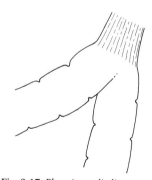

Fig. 9.17 Phrenico-colic ligament.

retroperitoneal fixation of the descending colon happens also to be low in the pelvis (Fig. 9.15). Fortunately it is when the sigmoid colon is long that the alpha loop occurs and avoids any angulation at the sigmoid-descending juntion, the 'alpha' being the fluoroscopic description of the loop of sigmoid colon twisted around on its mesentery or sigmoid mesocolon in what is, in effect, a partial iatrogenic volvulus (Fig. 9.16). Formation of the loop depends on the anatomical fact that the base of the sigmoid mesocolon is a short inverted 'V' at the pelvic brim, which allows easy rotation (Fig. 9.16).

The splenic flexure is partially tethered by a fold of peritoneum, the 'phrenico-colic ligament' (Fig. 9.17). The laxity of this ligament determines to what extent the splenic flexure can be pulled down and rounded off during passage of the colonoscope (see p. 202 for effect of positional changes). A lax phrenico-colic ligament can also make control of the transverse colon difficult (see p. 206). The configuration and behaviour of the transverse colon (like the sigmoid) varies according to its length, elasticity and the supporting transverse mesocolon (a double fold of peritoneum investing the transverse colon and attaching it to the posterior abdominal wall over the pancreas). The depth of the looped transverse colon also affects the angle at which the endoscope approaches the hepatic flexure, in the same way that the size of the sigmoid colon loop causes an acute sigmoid-descending bend. Because the transverse mesocolon (Fig. 9.18a) is broad-based it does not usually allow a gamma loop to form (Fig. 9.18b). The colonoscope tends to push a downward loop in the transverse colon which can, if necessary, be resisted (making use of its anterior position against the abdominal wall) by pressing upwards with a hand under the left costal margin or in the epigastrium according to results. From an anatomical and

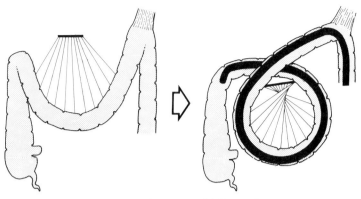

Fig. 9.18 (a) Transverse mesocolon. (b) Gamma loop.

endoscopic viewpoint, the hepatic flexure is a nearly 180° hairpin bend, similar in many respects to the bend at the sigmoid-descending junction but more constant in its fixation and more voluminous.

Anatomical variations and 'mobile colons'

Any endoscopist who has done 50–100 examinations, especially if he has used fluoroscopy in the more difficult ones, will know that the classical technical manoeuvres do not work in every case and that some strange colonoscopic configurations occur which do not fit the 'normal' textbook anatomy of the colon and its attachments. For instance:

1 When the looped instrument is in the descending colon, a counter-clockwise twist, rather than the usual clockwise rotation, is sometimes helpful in straightening it, because an anti-clockwise 'reversed-alpha' sigmoid loop has formed. Equally, fluoroscopy may show the tip of the instrument, although in the descending colon, to be in the centre of the abdomen (Fig. 9.19).

2 When straightened out the instrument may run centrally and pass into a 'reversed splenic flexure' (Fig. 9.20).

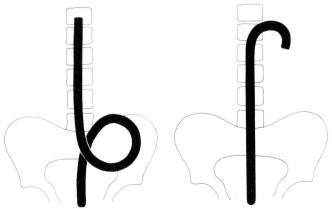

Fig. 9.19 Reversed alpha loop (X-ray appearance).

Fig. 9.20 Reversed splenic flexure.

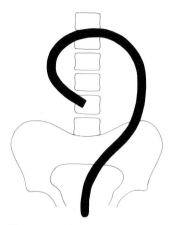

Fig. 9.21 Mobile caecum.

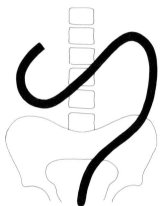

Fig. 9.22 Inverted caecum.

3 Sometimes when the tip of the instrument is in the caecum and visualizing the ileo-caecal valve, it can be seen on fluoroscopy to be in the centre of the abdomen (Fig. 9.21) or right hypochondrium (Fig. 9.22) rather than in its conventional position in the iliac fossa.

Surgeons are well aware that there is great patient-to-patient variation in how easily the colon can be mobilized and delivered outside the abdominal cavity; occasionally the whole colon can be lifted out without dissection. It is this mobility which results in the endoscopic confusion described above, because normal fixation has not occurred in fetal life. A mobile colon which is 'easy' for the surgeon is difficult for the endoscopist. The embryology of the colon is complex. The fetal intestine and its longitudinal mesentery elongate beyond the capacity of the abdominal cavity and herniate into the umbilical sac. When the intestine returns to the abdomen after the third month of intrauterine development, the colon is rotated around so that the caecum lies in the right hypochondrium and the descending colon on the left of the abdomen (Fig. 9.23). With further elongation of the colon the caecum normally 'migrates' down to the right iliac fossa. At this stage, the mesentery of the colon is free but then the mesenteries of the descending and ascending colon, pushed against the peritoneum of the posterior abdominal wall, fuse with it and are absorbed so that the ascending and descending colon become retroperitoneal (Fig. 9.24). In some cases incomplete fusion of mesocolon and posterior wall occurs and a variable amount of the original mesocolon remains, resulting in variable mobility of the right and left colon. How often this incomplete fusion occurs is not clear from the literature but a persistent descending mesocolon has been found in 36% and an ascending mesocolon in 10% of subjects. Occasionally the caecum fails to descend and becomes fixed in the right hypochondrium; in others where a free mesocolon persists, the caecum remains completely mobile. The persistence of a descending mesocolon

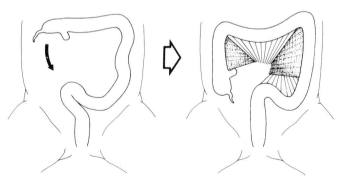

Fig. 9.23 The embryonic colon extends on its mesentery at 3 months' gestation . . .

Fig. 9.24 . . . then partial fusion of the mesentery and peritoneum occurs at 5 intrauterine months.

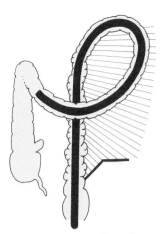

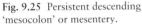

Fig. 9.25 Persistent descending 'mesocolon' or mesentery.

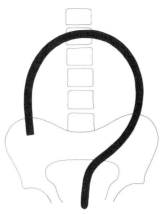

Fig. 9.26 The ideal 'question mark' shape at the caecum.

explains most of the strange configurations caused by the colonoscope in the left colon (Fig. 9.25). The presence of such a mesocolon does not however prevent the colon from being made to adopt its conventional position. This may occur when the endoscopist suddenly succeeds in straightening the grotesquely looped instrument (and colon) onto the walls of the abdominal cavity into the ideal 'question mark' shape (Fig. 9.26) which represents the 'normal' anatomical position.

Knowledge of functional colonic anatomy is the basis of colonoscopic technique and appreciation of the range of possible anatomical variations explains the frustrations which occur in 10–15% of colonoscopies due to a mobile colon.

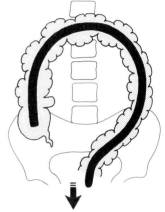

Fig. 9.27 Pulling back the scope shortens the colon.

Localization of the colonoscope tip

Inexperienced colonoscopists sometimes try to express the position of the instrument or of lesions in the colon in terms of length of instrument inserted ('the colonoscope was inserted to 90 cm', 'a polyp was seen at 30 cm', etc.). The elasticity of the colon makes this information meaningless; at 70 cm the instrument may be in the sigmoid colon or in the caecum. On withdrawal however, providing no adhesions are present, and the mesenteric fixations are normal, the colon will shorten and straighten predictably (Fig. 9.27) so that measurement gives approximate localization. On withdrawal the caecum should be at 80 cm, the transverse colon at 60 cm, the splenic flexure at 50 cm, the descending colon at 40 cm and the sigmoid at 30 cm (Fig. 9.28). The last two figures depend of course on the sigmoid colon being straightened. It is sometimes difficult to convince enthusiasts for rigid proctosigmoidoscopy that at 25 cm their instrument may still be in the rectum, whereas the flexible colonoscope (on withdrawal) may be in the proximal sigmoid colon. Equally, it is sometimes possible for

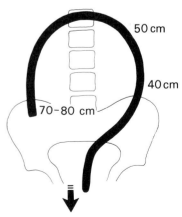

Fig. 9.28 If the scope is in the caecum at 70–80 cm, other anatomic sites are predictable by measurement.

a skilled endoscopist to pass a 60-cm flexible sigmoidoscope to the right colon, providing that he can shorten and deflate the bowel sufficiently.

One of the problems of flexible sigmoidoscopy or limited colonoscopy is the uncertainty of localization; anatomical location of the limit of insertion (when judged by withdrawal distance) in a personal series was wrong in almost half the cases when checked on fluoroscopy. In 25% a persistent loop ('alpha' or 'N') caused the endoscopist to judge tip location as 'splenic flexure' when actually at the sigmoid-descending colon junction (Fig. 9.29). In 20%, a mobile splenic flexure pulled down to 40 cm from the anus causing the endoscopist wrongly to judge the instrument to be at the sigmoid-descending colon junction (Fig. 9.30).

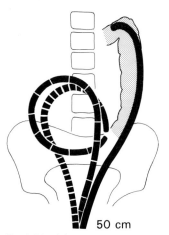

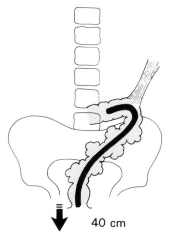

Fig. 9.29 If there is an 'N' or 'alpha' loop the sigmoid-descending junction may only pull back to 50 cm.

Fig. 9.30 The splenic flexure can pull back to 40 cm if there is a free phrenico-colic ligament.

The internal appearances of the colon have been described on p. 175, but they too can be misleading. The descending colon may look triangular or the transverse colon circular in outline, blue 'hepatic' coloration can be seen in the descending colon or the splenic flexure and the hepatic flexure can be mistaken for the caecal pole. The only definite landmark in the colon is the ileo-caecal valve, which is not always easy to find.

Transillumination of the abdominal wall by instruments with bright enough illumination (not all video-endoscopes) can be very helpful, but in obese patients may need a darkened room. It should be remembered that the descending colon is so far posterior that no light is usually visible and that the surface marking of the splenic and hepatic flexures is by transillumination through the rib cage posteriorly (Fig. 9.31). Light in the right iliac fossa is suggestive, but not conclusive, that the instrument is in the caecum; similar appearances can be produced if the tip stretches and transilluminates the sigmoid or mid-transverse colon.

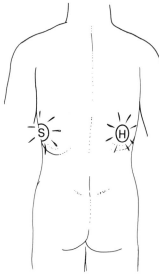

Fig. 9.31 The surface markings of splenic and hepatic flexures on transillumination.

Palpatation or balloting with the fingers can be effective, particularly in the ascending colon or caecum, where close apposition to the abdominal wall should make the impression of the palpating fingers easily visible to the endoscopist, unless the patient is fat.

Fluid levels can be surprisingly useful in localization, especially after oral lavage. Just as the radiologist rotates the patient into the right lateral or left lateral position to fill the dependent parts of the colon with barium (Fig. 9.32a,b), the endoscopist (with the patient in the usual left lateral position) knows that the instrument tip is in the descending colon when it enters fluid and in the transverse colon when it leaves fluid for the triangular and air-filled lumen of the transverse (Fig. 9.32c).

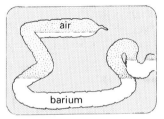 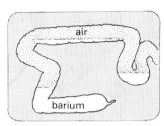 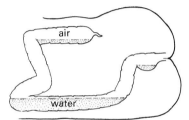

Fig. 9.32 (a) Ba enema—left lateral. (b) Ba enema—right lateral. (c) Colonoscopy—fluid levels in the left lateral position.

Localization of the instrument tip or lesions found in the colon should always be reported in broad anatomical terms (e.g. 'the polyp was seen on withdrawing the instrument 30 cm in the proximal sigmoid colon'), or even omit the measurement altogether so that there is no chance of confusion in the mind of someone unfamiliar with the shortening of the colon possible during flexible endoscopy. Inaccurate localization can occur even when fluoroscopy is employed and the endoscopist usually needs to rely on a combination of assessments—distance inserted, distance after withdrawal and straightening of the shaft, appearances and visualization of palpating fingers or transillumination. Knowing the pitfalls and being careful should make localization reasonably accurate, but even experienced endoscopists can mistake the sigmoid colon for the splenic flexure, or the splenic for the hepatic, which can be a serious error if localizing a lesion before surgery.

Handling the colonoscope

In upper gastrointestinal endoscopy the instrument runs a relatively short and fixed course in the body and, except perhaps during ERCP or 'push enteroscopy', looping and twisting of the shaft is of less importance than it is during colonoscopy. The mechanical construction of an endoscope, with its protective wire claddings and four pull-wires controlling tip movement, is such that each loop formed increases the resistance of the instrument to twisting/torqueing movements and decreases tip angulation due to friction in the control wires. This is as much true of the instrument *outside* the body as *inside* it. Excessive twisting stresses on the shaft can be reduced if the endoscopist turns the control body one way or the other to minimize rotational stresses; the shaft should also run in an easy curve to the anus, without unnecessary bends, and any loops forming outside the patient should be de-rotated and straightened (Fig. 9.33). Where possible the shaft of a long colonoscope lying outside the patient on the table is arranged so as to make it easy and comfortable to twist *clockwise*, since this is such a frequent action.

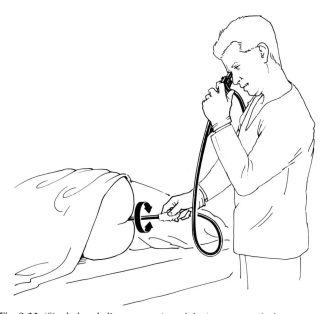

Fig. 9.33 'Single-handed' manoeuvring of the instrument shaft.

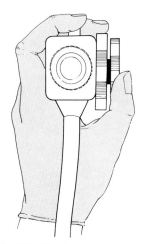

Fig. 9.34 The thumb can reach the lateral control knob if the hand is positioned appropriately.

The endoscopist should stand in a relaxed manner, comfortable for what can be a prolonged examination but in a neutral position so that he can manoeuvre the instrument in all directions. For the single-handed endoscopy that we recommend, each hand is disciplined to fulfil only its appropriate tasks; the left hand holds the instrument in balance, manages the air/water/suction buttons and up/down control knob (Fig. 9.33) with minor adjustments of left/right angling as well (Fig. 9.34), while the right hand controls the shaft of the instrument with only occasional major alterations to the lateral control knob. With so many different instruments, techniques, hand sizes and degrees of dexterity, it is pointless to suggest that there is only one method of handling an endoscope, although the single-handed method seems to us the most logical and is favoured by most skilled colonoscopists. Others prefer an assistant to advance and withdraw the instrument, especially during the learning phase and difficult phases of insertion. The exact handling technique is relatively unimportant if it is relaxed, gentle and effective. The colon is a continuous series of short bends requiring multiple combinations of tip and shaft movement as well as frequent air/water and suction button activations, so that small delays and inco-ordinated movements rapidly add up to prolong the procedure unnecessarily. Discipline the hands so that (as detailed above) only the left forefinger activates the air/water/suction buttons and only the left thumb (with help from the left middle finger; Fig. 9.33) controls the up/down knob; the right hand is then free for co-ordinated rotational/twisting/torqueing movements of the shaft and also feels whether the shaft moves easily (is straight) or there is resistance (due to looping). To feel and manipulate the shaft deftly, hold it in the fingers (Fig. 9.35) as you would any other delicate instrument (and not in the fist like a hammer or an offensive weapon). Rolling the shaft between fingers and thumb, like a cigar, allows major steering rotations with minimal effort. Quick, almost reflex, logical responses develop with practice and colonoscopy, from slow careful beginnings, can become a rapid and fluent procedure.

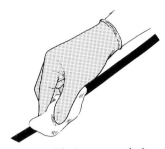

Fig. 9.35 The instrument shaft held delicately between thumb and finger.

Twisting and torqueing

With the single-handed method, twisting the shaft becomes second nature and a most essential part of the colonoscopist's range of tricks and manoeuvres. It should be appreciated, however, that there are three different twisting effects.

1 Twisting with the shaft and tip straight rolls the instrument around on its axis. This can be useful to re-orientate the biopsy forceps, injection needle or polypectomy snare into the ideal quadrant to target a particular lesion, or to place the suction channel precisely over a fluid pool to be aspirated (Fig. 9.36). When approaching a bend, twisting may adjust the axis of the instrument so that up/down angulation alone will steer around the bend. Appreciating the 'free-and-easy' feel and responsiveness of a really straight colonoscope to twist and to push/pull movements is an essential part of skilled colonoscopy.

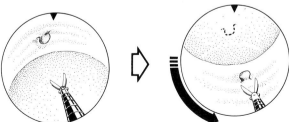

Fig. 9.36 (a) If a lesion is difficult to reach with the forceps . . .

(b) . . . 180° rotation of the straightened shaft makes it easy to reach without losing the view.

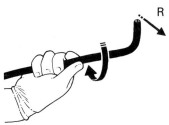

Fig. 9.37 With clockwise shaft twist: (a) up-angling moves tip to right;

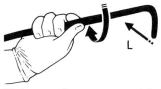

(b) down-angling moves tip to left.

2 Twisting with the shaft straight but tip angulated deviates the tip very rapidly according to the direction of twist and angulation. Thus with the tip angled *up*, twisting clockwise moves it *right* (Fig. 9.37); with the tip *down*, the same clockwise twist will move it *left* (droop or cock your wrist and then rotate the forearm one way or the other to simulate this). Such 'corkscrewing' movements are particularly effective when the colon is fixed, as by adhesions or diverticular disease, or when the tip is already acutely angulated in a sharp bend.

3 Twisting with a loop in the shaft will alter the position of the loop, and often its size and configuration as well. Because the course of most sigmoid colon loops is spiral—usually a clockwise spiral due to passage anteriorly from the pelvis and then curving laterally and posteriorly into the descending colon (Fig. 9.10)—twist is particularly effective in this region. Since the colonoscope is free to move within the colon, but the colon itself is fixed at the rectum and retroperitoneally in the descending region (as well as being constrained by the anterior and lateral abdominal wall), a clockwise twist will also usually shorten (pleat/concertina/accordion) the mobile sigmoid over the shaft, whilst the tip moves forward up the fixed descending colon. Other loops (large 'alpha', large 'N', reversed splenic or 'gamma') usually need to be first reduced in size by pulling back, before they can be successfully twisted about and straightened in the confined space of the abdominal cavity.

Torque is the application of continued twist whilst inserting or withdrawing the instrument. Clockwise torque is a major help in keeping the colonoscope shaft straight in the sigmoid colon whilst advancing up the descending colon, but also in controlling the sigmoid (and other potential loops) during the later phases of insertion. Whether to torque/twist clockwise or anticlockwise is an empirical decision according to results, but with conventional mesenteric anatomy clockwise is the more likely to help.

Insertion of the colonoscope

All functions of the colonoscope, light source and accessories should be thoroughly checked before insertion. In particular make sure that air insufflation is fully operational, briskly bubbling when the tip is held underwater (if in doubt wrap a rubber glove around the tip and watch it inflate). It is very easy during the examination to think the colon is hypercontractile and difficult to inflate when in fact one of the connections is loose, resulting in decreased pressure. Polishing the objective lens with a silicone stick or spectacle lens fluid helps to keep it clean during the examination.

The patient is placed in the left lateral position and made as comfortable as possible. A few moments of relaxed and friendly conversation at this stage often save much unnecessary sedation. The colonoscope tip and perianal region are liberally lubricated; most endoscopists use a clear water-soluble jelly (for instance

'K-Y' or local anaesthetic lubricating jelly). Further lubrication may be needed from time to time during the procedure. It is wise to do a digital examination before inserting the instrument, both to check for pathology in this 'blind' area and to pre-lubricate and relax the anal canal. The instrument tip is blunt and, unless digital examination is easy, it should not be inserted 'head on' (Fig. 9.38a) but pressed in sideways supported by the examiner's forefinger until the sphincter relaxes (Fig. 9.38b); alternatively the examiner can use his thumb to push the tip down his forefinger as it withdraws from the anal canal (Fig. 9.38c).

The squamous epithelium of the anus and the sensory mechanisms of the anal sphincters are the most pain-sensitive areas in the colorectum, and digital examination and insertion of the endoscope should be gentle. Particularly tight or tonic sphincters may take some time to relax; asking the patient to 'bear down' is said to help this. Inflating air down the endoscope whilst pressing the tip into the anal canal under direct vision also facilitates insertion.

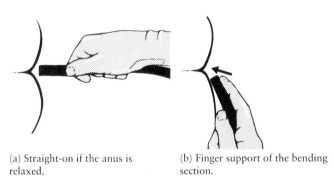

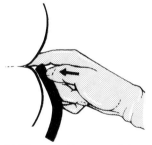

(a) Straight-on if the anus is relaxed.

(b) Finger support of the bending section.

(c) Tip pushed in as examining finger withdraws.

Fig. 9.38 Different methods of colonoscope insertion.

Flexible sigmoidoscopy and passing the sigmoid colon

On entering the rectum there is usually little to see except a 'red-out' because the rectal mucosa is pressed against the lens.

1 *Insufflate some air*.

2 *Pull back and angulate or rotate* slightly to find the lumen; this is the first of many times during the examination when withdrawal, inspection and thought bring success more quickly than following instinct and pushing blindly. Gentle air insufflation is needed throughout the examination, except when there is an excellent view; holding the forefinger close to and over (but not occluding) the orifice of the air button avoids excessive pressure but produces mild inflation. Throughout a colonoscopy, the policy is 'as much as necessary, as little as possible'; it is essential to see, but counter-productive and uncomfortable to overinflate. Whenever fully distended colon is seen or if the patient feels discomfort it takes only a second or two to suction off the excess until the colon outline starts to wrinkle and collapse.

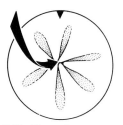

Fig. 9.39 Aim at the convergence of folds.

3 *Push in* once an adequate view has been obtained. A perfect luminal view is not needed for progress; the lumen of the colon when deflated or in spasm is at the centre of converging folds (Fig. 9.39). The object is to reach the caecum as fast (and as comfortably) as reasonably possible and full inspection should be on the return journey.

Keeping or regaining the view

In the rectum, and at any other point in the examination, if the view is lost, *keep the control knobs still or let them go entirely and gently withdraw the instrument* until the mucosa and its vascular pattern

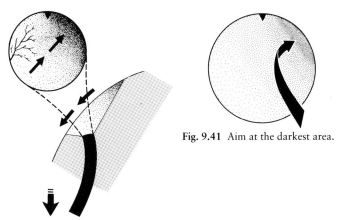

Fig. 9.41 Aim at the darkest area.

Fig. 9.40 Pull back when lost—the mucosa slides away into the direction of the lumen.

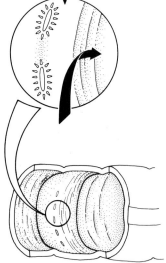

Fig. 9.42 Aim at the centre of the arc formed by folds, muscle fibres or reflected 'highlights'.

slides slowly past the lens proximally (Fig. 9.40). Then stop withdrawing and angle or rotate the tip to follow the vessel pattern proximally and the lumen of the colon will be found. Even with only a partial or close-up view of the mucosal surface, there are usually sufficient clues to detect the luminal direction. Always aim towards the darkest area, which is worst illuminated because it is furthest from the instrument and nearest the lumen (Fig. 9.41).

Acquiring the visual skill to detect the luminal axis, even in close-up, is of paramount importance. As well as light/dark (Fig. 9.41), the convex arcs formed by visible wrinkling of the circular muscles, the haustral folds, or the highlights reflected from the mucosa over them, all indicate the centre of the arc as the correct direction in which to angle (Fig. 9.42). The expert can make his steering decisions on evidence which would be inadequate for the beginner. On the other hand, each time the expert is 'lost' for more than 5–10 seconds he pulls back quickly to re-orientate, whereas the beginner can flounder around blindly for a minute or more in each difficult spot and is surprised that the overall examination takes so long.

When directing the tip towards the lumen, first angle up or down slightly (with the thumb); next—rather than using the right/left control knob—try rotating the instrument shaft clockwise or anticlockwise with the right hand. Because the tip is already slightly hooked this gentle rotation should corkscrew it around precisely and quickly. Each individual movement is slow and purposive. Every action during insertion should be thought out and executed in response to the view, or whatever visual clues there are to suggest the correct luminal direction; if there is no view, pull back at once and if the view is still lost, reverse the previous action(s) until the view is regained (i.e. de-angle or de-rotate back to the previous position) and then start again.

Suctioning

Residue in the rectum or low sigmoid colon is no reason to abandon the examination, because bowel contents naturally pass distally and the proximal colon may be clean. It is worth aspirating to evacuate the rectum completely and avoid explosive soiling during the rest of the procedure. Thereafter only aspirate during insertion when absolutely necessary to keep a view, so as to get the discomfort of insertion over as quickly as possible, suctioning any residue on the way back for a perfect view. Especially after oral preparation there may be numerous local 'sumps' or pools of residual fluid; aspirating each one wastes a lot of time and it is usually possible to inflate a little and steer in over the fluid level rather than plunging into it and having to suction. Even solid stool can often be successfully passed, deliberately angling the tip to slide along the mucosa for a few centimetres rather than impacting against a bolus (which often coats the lens irrevocably). Remember that bubbles are caused by insufflating under water, which can usually be avoided; if fluid preparation and bile salts do result in excessive bubbles, these can be instantly dispersed by injecting a solution containing simethicone (particulate silicone) down the instrument channel or through the lens-washing syringe attachment, as preferred.

Multiple bends

Single-handed manoeuvring is particularly useful in the multiple bends of the rectum and recto-sigmoid, where co-ordination with an assistant can be difficult. Each of the succession of serpentine bends requires a conscious steering decision. The quicker and more accurately each decision is made, the faster the whole examination will be. It is easier to judge direction around a bend from afar, so the tip should not be rushed into it. First observe the bend carefully from a distance; it will be seen as a bright semi-lunar fold of mocosa against the shadowed background (Fig. 9.43). Having decided on the direction to be taken, work out and pre-rehearse the correct combination of angling and rotation needed to steer around correctly when subsequently pushing through the bend close-up

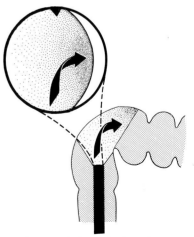

Fig. 9.43 Endoscopic view of an acute bend, with bright fold on the inner angle—and the 'aerial view'.

and relatively blind. There are a limited number of possible tip movements.

1 The easiest is thumb control up/down.

2 The next easiest is clockwise/anticlockwise twist.

3 *The least convenient is left/right angling* (by thumb on the lateral knob or taking the right hand off the shaft to activate the lateral control knob).

Start each steering movement *slowly* so that there is time to stop or reverse the action if it does not move the view in the required direction (or starts to lose it altogether). Avoid any superfluous movements during insertion such as swinging or scanning, which, being fast and not thought out, cannot be reversed to regain the view if the lumen is lost.

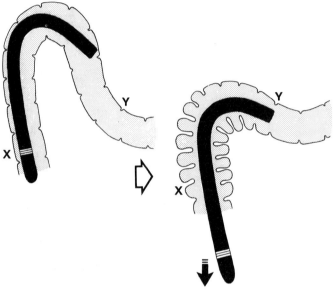

Fig. 9.44 (a) Poor view around a bend . . .   (b) . . . pulling back shortens the colon and improves the view.

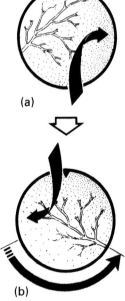

Fig. 9.45 Rotation of vessel pattern from (a) to (b) indicates rotation of the colon (requiring complete change of steering direction).

Having angled in the correct direction, if the view is poor (Fig. 9.44a) *gently pull back* the angled/hooked tip, which should both reduce the angle, shorten the bowel distally, straighten it out proximally and disimpact the tip to improve the view (Fig. 9.44b). If all fails, de-angle, pull back below the bend again and re-check its direction more carefully; the colon can flop around and the nature of bends may change during manoeuvring, any rotation being visible in close-up as a rotation of the visible vessel pattern (Fig. 9.45a,b); watching the direction towards which the vessels rotate indicates in which direction to follow a mobile bend. Occasionally altering the patient's position will alter the lie of the bowel and the air within it so as to improve the view. For instance, changing to right lateral will cause air to rise and distend the sigmoid-descending junction whereas the water within it and the colon itself will fall by gravity.

Push—but then withdraw

As an absolutely last resort, if it is quite clear that the instrument is pointing in the correct direction but attempts at angling and twisting and simultaneous gentle pull or push have not given a luminal view, it is permissible simply to push blind for a few centimetres; providing the tip is pointing correctly, it should slip gradually over the mucosa with the '*slide by*' appearance of the mucosal vascular pattern traversing the field of view. Continue to push if 'slide by' continues smoothly; *stop* if the mucosa blanches (indicating excessive local pressure) or if the patient experiences pain (indicating undue strain on bowel or mesentery).

As soon as a luminal view is achieved the instrument should be withdrawn again to shorten the loop that forceful insertion will inevitably have caused. Intermittent withdrawal is instinctively unnatural to most endoscopists, and yet one of the most important points of colonoscopic technique. However much of a struggle has been involved in rounding a bend, as soon as the tip is well past the instrument must be partially withdrawn until resistance is felt or the tip begins to slide back, indicating that the shaft is straight.

Expert versus learner

Much of colonoscopy is a matter of patience—'two steps forward and one step back'. Impatience or relentless pushing tend to result in loops, pain and a slower examination in the end. The more experienced colonoscopist, being more careful and rational, and using less air, ends up with fewer acutely angled bends. He also steers accurately in spite of the more restricted view of only partially inflated and shorter bowel. He is more fluent because he chooses the right combination of movements to move the tip in the desired direction, with simultaneous twist, push or pull as necessary to straighten the bowel or advance the tip, without losing control or sense of luminal direction. He slows down, or even pulls back, before an acute bend to maintain a view at all times. Whilst he does nothing different from the beginner, there are fewer mistakes, little waste of time and effort and the colonoscope seems magically to snake up the colon.

In the learning phase the two commonest reasons for becoming 'stuck', particularly in the sigmoid colon, are either that the instrument has become looped and jammed in a bend (it should be withdrawn as far as possible both to straighten it out and get a proper view) or simply that, having manoeuvred into the right position, the endoscopist has not the courage of experience to 'slide by' through the difficult area by pushing hard for a few seconds to get around the bend—before pulling back to straighten it out again.

Be prepared to abandon

A caveat is called for. Not every sigmoid colon can be safely intubated. Operative or peri-diverticular adhesions may fix the pelvic colon so as to make the attempt impossible or dangerous. If there is difficulty, if the instrument tip feels fixed and cannot be moved by angling or twisting, and the patient complains of pain during attempts at insertion, there is a danger of perforation and the attempt should be abandoned. Sometimes a different endoscope (e.g. paediatric) or endoscopist may succeed where another has failed, but only a very experienced colonoscopist with very good clinical reasons should risk patient and instrument under these circumstances; usually the most experienced are the most prepared to stop.

Adhesions and diverticular disease

Adhesions, as after hysterectomy, cause angulation and difficulty but rarely failure because of the ability of the colon to straighten over the instrument. Even in severe diverticular disease, where there are the difficulties of a narrowed lumen, peri-colic adhesions and the difficulty in choosing the correct direction (Fig. 9.46a), once the instrument has been laboriously inched through the area, the 'splinting' effect of the abnormally rigid sigmoid usually facilitates the rest of the examination. In the presence of diverticular disease the secret is extreme patience, with care in visualization and steering combined with greater than usual use of withdrawal, rotatory or corkscrewing movements. It helps to realize that a close-up view of a diverticulum means that the tip must be deflected 90° (by withdrawal and angulation or twist) to find the lumen (Fig. 9.46b). Using a thinner and more flexible paediatric colonoscope may make an apparently impassable narrow, fixed or angulated sigmoid colon relatively easy to examine—which sometimes also saves the patient from surgery.

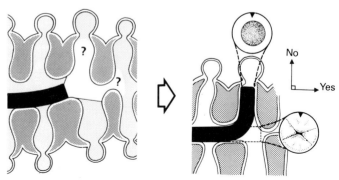

Fig. 9.46 (a) Choosing the correct path can be difficult in diverticular disease . . . (b) . . . a circular view is a diverticulum—the correct direction is at right angles.

Passing the sigmoid-descending junction

All colonoscopists occasionally—and the inexperienced frequently —have trouble in passing the junction of the sigmoid and descending colon. It will be clear from the preceding section and previous comments on anatomy that a colonoscopist who rounds the sigmoid with panache will probably have stretched up a sigmoid 'N' loop (Fig. 9.47) and created difficulty for himself, whereas one who has been more careful, using less air and frequent withdrawal should be rewarded by a straighter or even direct passage from sigmoid to descending colon (Fig. 9.48a,b); on the other hand an alpha loop may be formed—intentionally or unintentionally. So much depends on the anatomy of the particular patient that anything can happen and the colonoscopist may need all his skills and some luck to pass this region reasonably quickly and without undue pain. It is often the most difficult part of the colonoscopy and the greatest challenge to the endoscopist.

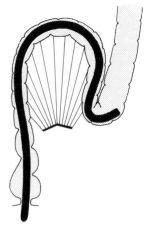

Fig. 9.47 'N' loop stretching up the sigmoid colon.

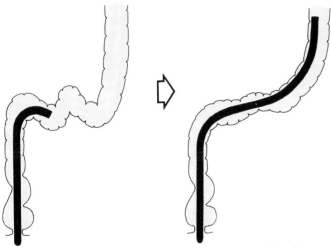

Fig. 9.48 (a) Pull back and using less air to keep the sigmoid short . . .

(b) . . . which may allow direct passage to the descending colon.

Direct approach to the descending colon

Although the endoscopist may not be certain when he has reached the proximal sigmoid, the appearance of an acute bend at approximately 40–70 cm is suggestive evidence, particularly (in the left lateral position) if it is water filled. The sigmoid-descending junction can be so acute as to appear at first to be a blind ending, especially if the bowel is over-inflated. Sometimes there is a longitudinal fold pointing towards the correct direction of the lumen, caused by the muscle bulk of a taenia coli (Fig. 9.49); follow the longitudinal fold closely to pass the bend.

It can prove difficult to wriggle the tip around the sigmoid-descending bend, particularly when acute because of a large 'N'

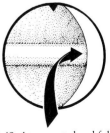

Fig. 9.49 At an acute bend follow the longitudinal fold (taenia coli).

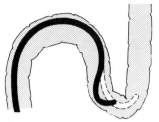

Fig. 9.50 In acute bends, pre-steer before pushing in.

loop. If during withdrawal while trying to reduce the size of this loop the instrument slips out, it can be helpful to deflate the colon, which may both shorten it and help to relax the flap-like inner angle of the bend. Alternatively, changing the patient to the right lateral position may both improve visualization (air rises) and cause the distal descending colon to fall into a more favourable position. The mechanical difficulty of flexing the instrument tip around the bend can also present difficulties; the technique of 'pre-steering' of the bend can be used, the tip being steered at the mucosa just before the inner angle (Fig. 9.50), so that on pushing in the 'pre-steering' causes the tip to slip past the angle and be pointing straight at the lumen of the descending colon.

Once hooked into the descending colon the sigmoid loop can be reduced by pulling back gently because the tip is now retroperitoneal and relatively fixed (Fig. 9.51a). One of the consequences of pulling back is, however, that the hooked tip will inevitably impact into the mucosa (Fig. 9.51b) and must be straightened carefully to pass further into the descending colon. A wrong move at this point will lose the critical retroperitoneal fixation and the instrument will fall back into the sigmoid. Careful interpretation of the close-up view, minimal insufflation, twist (usually clockwise), delicate steering movements and patience are all needed to pass in without re-looping (Fig. 9.51c) which results from excessive push or tip impaction. The importance of using clockwise torque rotation to prevent re-looping of the straightened instrument is such that this method of direct passage is sometimes called the 'right twist (clockwise)—withdrawal manoeuvre'. The 3-D looping of the sigmoid colon, with both left-right and antero-posterior components

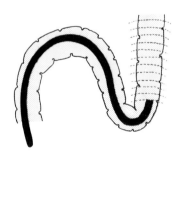

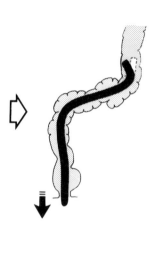

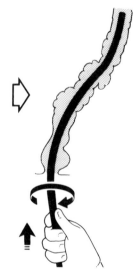

Fig. 9.51 (a) First the tip is hooked into the retroperitoneal part of the descending colon, then pulled back . . .

(b) . . . when fully straightened the hooked tip is re-directed . . .

(c) . . . and pushed in with clockwise twist to pass into the descending colon.

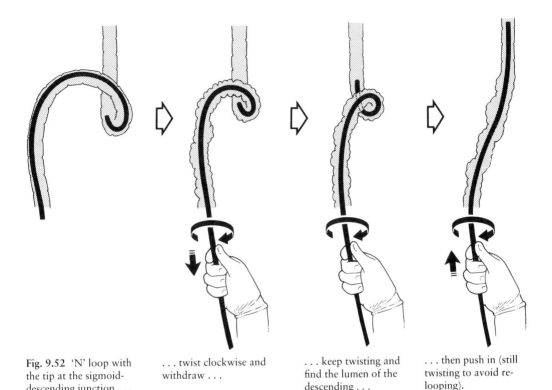

Fig. 9.52 'N' loop with the tip at the sigmoid-descending junction . . .

. . . twist clockwise and withdraw . . .

. . . keep twisting and find the lumen of the descending . . .

. . . then push in (still twisting to avoid re-looping).

creating a clockwise spiral is illustrated (Fig. 9.52) to show why twisting is so important at this stage.

The 'N' loop

The occurrence of a transient 'N' loop in the sigmoid colon has been described above (Fig. 9.47) and is the commonest loop to form during colonoscopy. Most of the difficulties experienced whilst passing the proximal colon (splenic flexure, transverse colon and hepatic flexure) also stem from recurrent 'N' looping in the sigmoid, which removes the motive power of the endoscopist's inward push unless this loop can be avoided, removed or minimized. 'N' looping is also the major cause of pain during colonoscopy.

An 'N' loop can be anything from a minor zig-zag—which may be fixed and not straightened following hysterectomy or previous diverticulitis—to a huge loop reaching towards the diaphragm in some patients with a redundant or megacolon. Most 'N' loops can eventually be straightened out completely, which is why it is worth attempting this *during* passage through the sigmoid colon, or certainly when the sigmoid-descending junction is reached, so as to attempt direct or straight scope passage to the descending colon, as described above. With a longer colon, complete removal of the 'N' loop may be difficult until the instrument tip has reached nearly to (or around) the splenic flexure, so as to give adequate purchase for forcible withdrawal. However, as for direct passage, manual pressure by the assistant in the left lower abdomen will often contribute by reducing or minimizing the size of the loop (Fig. 9.11), acting as a buffer to transmit of the inward push on the shaft laterally towards the descending colon. If the assistant can actually feel the loop, the objective is to reduce it back towards the pelvis (i.e. with downward, as well as inward, pressure). Although it is worth the endoscopist trying one or two withdrawal movements to shorten the 'N' loop, especially near the apex of the sigmoid colon but also at any obvious fold or bend which allows 'hooking', often there is little to be done until the sigmoid-descending junction is reached and an attempt can be made at the clockwise-twist-withdrawal manoeuvre, described above.

Again the final resort is to use force; having warned the patient to expect discomfort, a few seconds of careful 'persuasive pressure' may slide the instrument tip successfully around the bend.

Pain in the sigmoid

Remember that if the patient experiences excessive pain there is a potential danger of damage to the bowel or mesentery. In the longest colons, however, there may be sufficient length of sigmoid colon and mesentery to let the instrument loop below the sigmoid-descending junction and pass relatively easily into the descending colon without the acute hairpin bend usually formed when an 'N' loop is present (Fig. 9.53). Having to use force or cause pain is inelegant and to be avoided if possible; however, it may be preferable for the patient to suffer briefly and get the instrument into the descending colon quickly and successfully rather than to struggle on and on with repeated failed attempts at gentle passage, particularly as the analgesic effects of i.v. pethidine diminish considerably by about 5 min after administration. Before using force, and at any stage during colonoscopy when pushing in may cause pain due to looping, the patient is warned beforehand (e.g. 'this will hurt for a few seconds, but there is no danger'). Inward push should also be applied gradually, avoiding any sudden shove and, to keep faith with the patient, should be limited to a tolerable time—say 20–30 seconds. Looping pain stops at once when the instrument is withdrawn slightly.

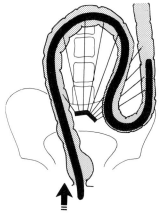

Fig. 9.53 A very long sigmoid may allow sufficient loop to avoid a hairpin bend.

The alpha loop and manoeuvre

When the colonoscope is passed through the sigmoid colon it can form spontaneously into the configuration known as an 'alpha' loop (Fig. 9.54). Even on barium enema the colon can sometimes be seen in this position. From the endoscopist's point of view, the formation of an alpha loop is a blessing, as there is no acute bend between the sigmoid and descending colon and the splenic flexure can always be reached. If no particularly acute flexure is encountered in the sigmoid colon and the instrument appears to be sliding in a long way without problems, it can be suspected that an alpha loop is being formed. If so (perhaps confirmed on fluoroscopy if this is

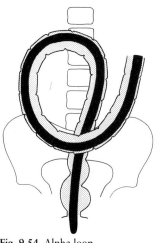

Fig. 9.54 Alpha loop.

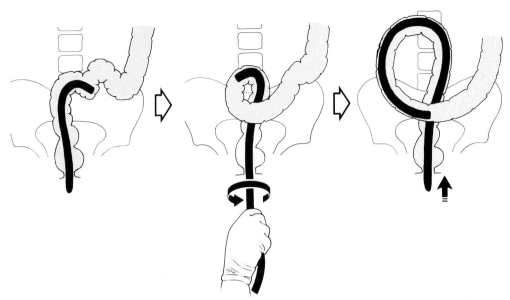

Fig. 9.55 (a) At the first sigmoid colon bend, 15–20 cm from the anus . . .

(b) . . . rotate the angled tip *counter*-clockwise . . .

(c) . . . and push in to make an 'alpha' loop.

available) it is better to spend a little time and care passing to the proximal descending colon or splenic flexure at 90 cm (sometimes even around the splenic flexure into the transverse colon) before trying any withdrawal/straightening manoeuvre, which can cause the alpha configuration to flop across and form the more difficult 'N' loop.

The 'alpha manoeuvre' is the intentional formation of an alpha loop. This was originally always performed with fluoroscopy, but if the colon is known to be long or feels long and mobile during normal insertion into the distal sigmoid colon, it is worth trying to make an alpha loop so as to avoid the greater problems of an 'N' loop. The principle is to twist the sigmoid colon around into a partial volvulus (see Fig. 9.16)—which is easy to demonstrate but difficult to explain. As soon as the instrument is felt to be angling upwards into the distal sigmoid colon at around 15–20 cm from the anus (Fig. 9.55a), start to rotate the shaft firmly *counter*-clockwise at every opportunity, so that the angled tip swings anteriorly across the pelvic brim to point towards the caecum, pulling the sigmoid colon across with it (Fig. 9.55b). Continue the insertion through the sigmoid with as much counter-clockwise twist as possible at all stages (Fig. 9.55c) and avoid clockwise twist (so that the loop does not swing back to the 'N' position). Equally do not withdraw or attempt to straighten the shaft (even if the patient has mild stretching pain) but push and steer carefully until the tip has passed through the fluid-filled descending colon to the splenic flexure, reached at 90 cm (Fig. 9.56).

It is not always possible to achieve the alpha manoeuvre. Endoscopists who claim 'always' to do so are shown, when they

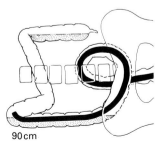

90 cm

Fig. 9.56 In an alpha loop the scope runs through fluid-filled descending colon to the splenic flexure at 90 cm.

demonstrate their techique under fluoroscopy, equally often to form an unrecognized 'N' loop, which they pass with élan (and extra sedation because of the pain). A short or fixed sigmoid mesocolon probably prevents formation of an alpha loop; thus patients with diverticular disease or any other cause of peri-colic adhesions are not suitable for the manoeuvre, and are most unlikely to form a spontaneous alpha loop.

Straightening an alpha loop

Any loop puts some stress and limitation on tip angulation due to friction in the control wires, as well as often being uncomfortable for the patient, so it is logical to remove the alpha loop at some stage. Opinions differ concerning the correct time to do so. With current very flexible and full-angling instruments, it is sometimes preferable to attempt to pass straight on into the proximal transverse colon with the alpha loop in position rather than to straighten it at the splenic flexure and then have difficulty keeping it straight.

Most colonoscopists prefer to straighten out the alpha loop as soon as the upper descending colon is safely reached and to pass the splenic flexure with a straightened instrument. However every colonoscopist has also experienced the chagrin of struggling to reach the descending colon and the frustration of seeing the tip slide back out of the descending colon when the instrument is withdrawn to straighten it. A reasonable compromise is to pass the tip up to, but not necessarily around, the splenic flexure at about 90 cm and then to take care that it does not slip back excessively during removal of the alpha loop. This can be checked by looking down the instrument during withdrawal to watch for mucosal slippage. If fluoroscopy is used the whole alpha loop cannot be seen in one fluoroscopic field and the best plan is to centre the view over the point where the looped shaft crosses itself (Fig. 9.57). The

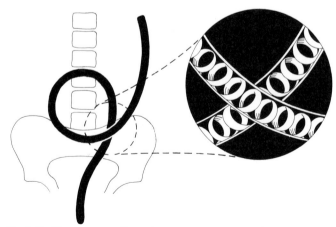

Fig. 9.57 Fluoroscopy will not show the whole alpha loop; watch the cross-over point.

metallic wrappings of the shaft are easily seen and any movement in the descending colon can be watched, as well as reduction of the loop itself. If the instrument is seen to be moving too far down the descending colon it is quickly advanced again and the tip hooked around the splenic flexure for extra support before repeating the straightening manoeuvre.

The alpha loop is straightened by combined withdrawal and clockwise de-rotation. Slightly withdrawing the shaft initially reduces the size of the loop and makes de-rotation easier, but the tip can start to slide down the descending colon; de-rotation alone will undo the 'alpha' volvulus of the sigmoid into the 'N' position, but does not reduce the size of the loop. The two actions must be combined by simultaneously pulling back and twisting the whole instrument (Fig. 9.58a,b,c). Strong clockwise twist during straightening will tend to push the tip up towards the splenic flexure and any tendency of the tip to slip back can usually be stopped by applying more twist and less pull. Twisting forces are not harmful to the colonoscope providing that they are not excessive. Having rotated the colonoscope 180° or more in the process of straightening an alpha loop it is often sensible to unplug the instrument from the light source and undo any twists in the umbilical; alternatively untwist the external shaft loop (*anti*-clockwise) whilst steering the tip into the lumen so that the colonoscope rotates on its axis within the colon.

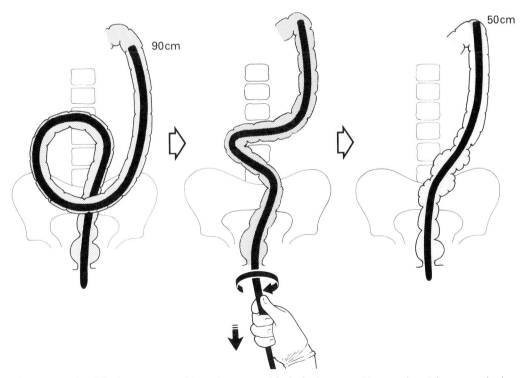

Fig. 9.58 (a) An alpha loop . . .   (b) . . . de rotates with clockwise twist and withdrawal . . .   (c) . . . and straightens completely.

Again a caveat. De-rotation should be easy and atraumatic; if straightening the loop proves difficult or the patient has more than the slightest discomfort the situation should be re-assessed. Adhesions make de-rotation difficult and occasionally impossible. Do not use force. The sigmoid loop that has formed may not be a true alpha loop but a 'reversed alpha', which can form when there is persistent descending mesocolon and freely mobile left colon (Fig. 9.19). This reversed loop may need *counter*-clockwise de-rotation during straightening.

Descending colon

The descending colon is, with the exception of a few individuals with unusually long and tortuous colons, normally traversed in a few seconds as a 20 cm long 'straight'. For the gravitational reasons described above when the patient is in the left lateral position (Fig. 9.32c), fluid residue can impede the endoscopist's view, and if this makes steering difficult, it may be quicker to turn the patient onto the right side to fill the descending colon with air, rather than to waste time suctioning and re-inflating.

Apart from this positional trick and the frequent use of clockwise twist and persistent hand pressure to minimize sigmoid colon looping, no particular skills or manoeuvres are needed in the descending colon.

Passing the splenic flexure

After fluid bowel preparation it is obvious when the instrument has passed around the apex of the splenic flexure, because it emerges from fluid into air-filled, and usually triangular, transverse colon. However, whilst the flexible and angled tip section of the colonoscope passes around without effort, the stiffer segment at 10–15 cm at the leading part of the shaft does not follow so easily. This problem is accentuated in the left lateral position, because drooping of the transverse colon causes the splenic flexure to be acutely angled (Fig. 9.59a) compared to its configuration when opened out by gravity in the right lateral position (Fig. 9.59b).

To pass the splenic flexure, follow these rules:

1 Ensure that the colonoscope is truly straight and therefore mechanically efficient. Pulling back with the tip hooked around the flexure until the instrument is 50 cm from the anus, both straightens any sigmoid loop and pulls down and rounds off the flexure. *Note:* splenic avulsions or capsular tears have been reported, *so be gentle*.

2 Avoid over-angling the tip. Full angulation of a colonoscope can result in the bending section effectively impacting in the splenic flexure preventing further insertion (the 'walking-stick handle' effect). Having obtained a view of the transverse colon and pulled back, consciously de-angulate a little so that the instrument runs

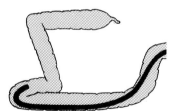

Fig. 9.59 (a) In the left lateral position the transverse can flop down making the splenic flexure acute . . .

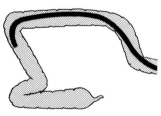

(b) . . . changing to right lateral causes gravity to round off the splenic flexure, making it easy to pass.

around the *outside* of the bend (Fig. 9.60) even if this means worsening the view somewhat—but avoid the tip impacting in haustral folds.

3 Continue assistant hand pressure over the sigmoid colon. Any resistance encountered at the splenic flexure is likely to result in stretching upwards of the sigmoid colon into an 'N' or alpha loop, which dissipates more and more of the inward force applied to the shaft as the loop increases (Fig. 9.61). It is immediately obvious to the single-handed endoscopist that such a loop is forming, because the 1:1 relationship between insertion and tip progress is lost—in other words, the shaft is being pushed in but the tip moves little or not at all. Pull back again to re-straighten the shaft if this occurs.

4 Use clockwise torque on the instrument shaft during inward push. As explained above, the clockwise spiral course of the sigmoid colon from the pelvis to its point of fixation in the descending colon means that applying clockwise torque to the colonoscope shaft whilst pushing in tends to counteract any looping tendency in the sigmoid colon (Fig. 9.62). Clockwise twist will only work if the colonoscope has previously been straightened, if the descending colon is normally fixed and any sigmoid loop is small. Obviously the instrument tip will not advance around the splenic flexure without inward push, so as well as clockwise twist, continued gentle inward push is needed (aggressive pushing only re-forms the sigmoid loop).

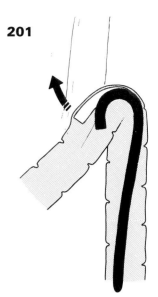

Fig. 9.60 De-angulate at the splenic flexure to avoid impaction (walking-stick handle effect).

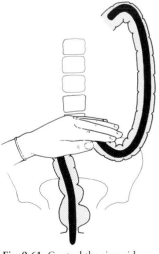

Fig. 9.61 Control the sigmoid colon looping with hand pressure whilst passing the splenic flexure.

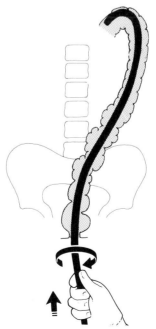

Fig. 9.62 Advance while twisting the shaft clockwise to hold the sigmoid colon straight.

5 Combine actions 1 to 4 with movements of the angling control knobs. A combination of these various manoeuvres, together or in sequence, whilst using the control knobs to 'squirm' the bending section, may help the tip and the stiffer shaft behind it to slide around the splenic flexure. Occasionally it is quickest to abandon these attempts and resort to change of position.

6 Change the patient's position to right lateral. As pointed out earlier, the left lateral position used by most endoscopists has the undesirable effect of causing the transverse colon to flop down (Fig. 9.59a) and make the splenic flexure acutely angled. Turning the patient to right lateral has the opposite effect, the transverse colon sagging to the right side and, together with gravity, pulling the splenic flexure into a smooth curve without any apparent 'flexure' at all (Fig. 9.59b). The first angulation encountered by the instrument on passing round after this change of position is usually at the mid-transverse colon, or even the dependent and fluid-filled hepatic flexure. Change to the right lateral position is almost invariably and immediately effective in passing the splenic flexure, but it does take 30–40 seconds to achieve, and the patient has to be returned to left lateral position to inflate and visualize the proximal colon properly and reach the caecum. It is also cumbersome if the patient is obese, disabled or oversedated. We therefore change position in only 20–30% of patients if 'stuck' at the splenic flexure for > 60 seconds or so, allowing several attempts at direct passage. The ability to perform such useful postural changes easily is an additional reason for reducing routine sedation (or avoiding it altogether when possible).

The 50-cm rule

The splenic flexure represents the 'half-time' point during a colonoscopy and is an excellent moment at which to ensure that the instrument is properly straightened to 50 cm from the anus and under control before tackling the proximal colon. The commonest reason for experiencing problems in the proximal colon is because the colonoscope has been inadequately straightened at the splenic flexure, persistence of loops making the rest of the procedure progressively more difficult or impossible. If the splenic flexure is passed with straight shaft configuration at 50 cm using the above rules, the rest of a total colonoscopy insertion should usually be finished within a minute or two.

Stiffening the colonoscope

If all else fails (about one case in 50 in our hands) use of an overtube or splinting-tube is almost guaranteed to hold the sigmoid colon straight and allow easy passage into the proximal colon. An overtube can only be inserted when the sigmoid colon has been completely straightened and the tip of the instrument is in the proximal descending colon or splenic flexure. Insertion may be impossible after

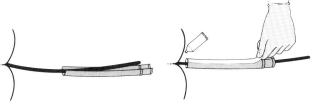

Fig. 9.63 (a) Insert the split-overtube onto the colonoscope shaft . . .

(b) . . . seal the slit with sticky tape, lubricate the shaft and tube . . .

(c) . . . insert gently holding the colonoscope shaft straight with the other hand.

hysterectomy, pelvis sepsis or in the presence of sigmoid colon diverticular disease with circular muscle hypertrophy.

The original extremely stiff wire-reinforced overtubes had disadvantages which have discouraged most endoscopists from using them routinely; the tube must be on the instrument before starting (or the scope completely withdrawn before it can be put on) and insertion can be traumatic and requires fluoroscopy. The principle of a soft-plastic split-overtube overcomes all of these disadvantages, especially new atraumatic prototypes made of frictionless and very flexible PTFE material (Gortex, Olympus). The split-overtube is softened in hot water, placed over the shaft of the colonoscope after this has been straightened to 50 cm at the splenic flexure. The overtube is sealed with adhesive tape and lubricated with jelly (Fig. 9.63a,b), then inserted (without fluoroscopy) as far into or through the shortened sigmoid colon as proves easy and comfortable for the patient (Fig. 9.63c). Resistance to insertion of the split-overtube means impaction against a fold, loop or flexure and discomfort means the same—both indications that further insertion or use of force could be dangerous (the same rules apply even when fluoroscopy is used). The tube is 45 cm long to accommodate long colons, but 'successful' insertion is usually only to around 30–40 cm, the handle of the overtube then being held by the assistant and the shaft of the colonoscope pushed in through it (Fig. 9.64). As soon as the colonoscope has been passed in satisfactorily (or at once if the overtube cannot be inserted successfully) it takes only a few seconds to remove the split-overtube again, strip off the tape and to return to normal handling of the instrument.

As well as its use for stiffening a looping sigmoid colon, the overtube can be invaluable for exchanging colonoscopes or removing multiple polypectomy specimens.

The 'reversed' splenic flexure

In about one patient in 20, if fluoroscopy is used, the instrument tip will be seen to be passing laterally rather than medially around the splenic flexure because the descending colon has moved centrally on a mesocolon (Fig. 9.65). This is of more than academic interest because, having passed laterally round the flexure and displaced the descending colon medially, the advancing instrument forces the transverse colon down into a deep loop. The instrument is then mechanically under stress and difficult to steer, and the hepatic

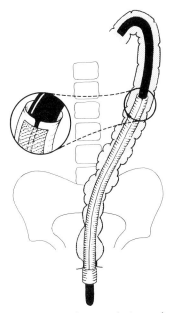

Fig. 9.64 A split-overtube inserted to 30–40 cm prevents looping of the sigmoid.

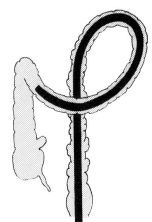

Fig. 9.65 A reversed splenic flexure due to a persistent descending mesocolon will result in a deep transverse loop.

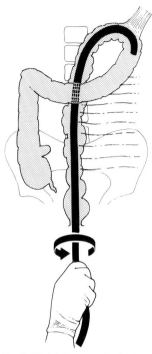

Fig. 9.66 (a) *Counter*-clockwise rotation . . .

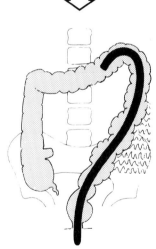

(b) . . . swings a mobile colon back to normal position.

flexure is approached from below at a very disadvantageous angle which makes it difficult to reach the caecum and impossible to pass the ileo-caecal valve. Even when the instrument tip can be hooked onto the hepatic flexure, the reversed loop configuration at the splenic flexure actively holds down the transverse loop and stops it being straightened and lifted up into the ideal 'question mark' shape.

If the reversed splenic flexure loop forms, an attempt should be made to convert it to the normal configuration. This can be done by twisting the shaft strongly *counter*-clockwise (rather than the usual clockwise twist). The tip should pivot around the phrenico-colic suspensory ligament (Fig. 9.66), then swing medially and, by maintaining counter-clockwise torque while pushing in, the instrument can be made to pass across the transverse in the usual configuration, forcing the descending colon back laterally against the abdominal wall (Fig. 9.66b). If there is difficulty in the proximal colon and a reversed splenic flexure is seen or thought to have formed, the situation cannot usually be converted back to normal without first withdrawing the tip to the splenic flexure, but the subsequent examination is so much quicker that the time spent is worth while. Although the counter-clockwise straightening manoeuvre is most easily performed under fluoroscopy, it is also quite feasible without fluoroscopy, using these guidelines and a little imagination whenever atypical looping is suspected in the proximal colon.

A reversed splenic flexure/mobile descending colon is the most frequent reason for an unexpectedly difficult adult or paediatric colonoscopy. It probably happens more commonly in children due to the relative elasticity of the attachments of the childhood colon. Sometimes the best solution, if the problem is suspected but fluoroscopy is not available and attempts at counter-clockwise de-rotation have failed, is simply to get a move on, push harder than usual (if necessary with extra sedation) and to stop as soon as a reasonable view of the right colon has been obtained. If a reversed splenic loop is present it is rare to be able to enter the ileo-caecal valve without successful de-rotation, because the looped and stressed instrument will not angulate sufficiently. If ileoscopy is essential, re-examination with fluoroscopy almost always allows de-rotation and successful insertion.

The transverse colon

Passing the transverse colon should present little problem if the sigmoid colon does not bow up into an 'N' loop, but in the mid-transverse colon there may be a surprisingly sharp bend where the colonoscope tip pushes downwards. Both at this bend and at the hepatic flexure a true 'face-on' view is obtained of haustral folds, which present a characteristic knife-edge appearance (Fig. 9.6); it is easy to confuse this bend with the hepatic flexure. The mid-transverse bend should be less voluminous, show no blue liver patch and may show aortic pulsation; it can also be distinguished by fluoroscopy, local palpation of the anterior abdominal wall or transillumination (if the room is darkened).

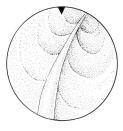 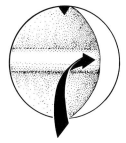

Fig. 9.67 In a redundant colon a longitudinal taenia coli shows the centre line.

Fig. 9.68 Follow the longitudinal fold (taenia coli) round an acute bend.

In a voluminous transverse colon the anti-mesenteric taenia coli may infold into the colon, acting as a highly useful pointer to the correct longitudinal axis to follow—rather like the white line down the centre of a road (Fig. 9.67). Appreciating this is particularly helpful at acute angulations, where a taenia can be followed blindly—to push round the bend and see the lumen beyond (Fig. 9.68).

Having passed the mid-point of the transverse, it can be slow and difficult to 'climb the hill' up the proximal limb of the looped transverse colon (Fig. 9.69a). The most important manoeuvre is to pull back repeatedly; the tip hooked around the transverse loop lifts it up, flattens it (Fig. 9.69b) and the tip often advances as the shaft is withdrawn ('paradoxical movements'). Very substantial and repeated in-and-out movements ('trombone playing') may be needed, the instrument advancing little by little towards the hepatic flexure. Hand pressure over the sigmoid colon during inward push or in the left hypochondrium to lift up the transverse loop, can be helpful. Deflation of the colon, clockwise or counter-clockwise torqueing movements and even change of position (usually to left lateral, sometimes to supine or prone) can all also help.

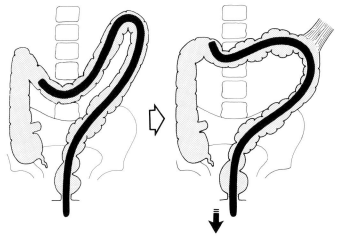

Fig. 9.69 (a) If passage up the proximal transverse is difficult . . .

(b) . . . pull back to lift and shorten it.

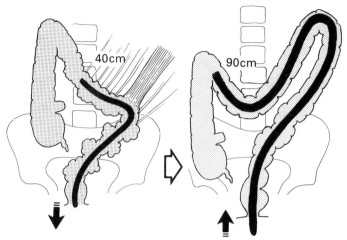

Fig. 9.70 (a) If the phrenico-colic ligament is lax withdrawal manoeuvres are ineffective . . .

(b) . .. and pushing in simply reforms the loop.

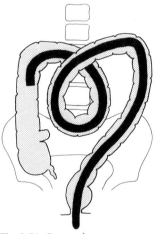

Fig. 9.71 Gamma loop.

During these 'lift' manoeuvres the fulcrum or cantilever effect (sometimes called 'balance beam effect') of the phrenico-colic ligament fixing the splenic flexure is crucial. In some patients this attachment is lax (Fig. 9.70a), and the colon is found to be hypermobile and unresponsive to any of the normally effective withdrawal or twisting movements (Fig. 9.70b). When this occurs the use of force is ineffectual but deflation, hand pressure, posturing and gentle perseverance will eventually win.

In occasional patients with a very redundant transverse colon, the formation of a spontaneous 'gamma' loop can be seen (Fig. 9.71); this is sometimes removed when the colonoscope is straightened out in the caecum, but often cannot be removed because the instrument falls back when withdrawn. It is usually impossible to enter the ileocaecal valve with a gamma loop in position, since friction makes the instrument tip less controllable.

Hand pressure

Since the major mechanical problem of colonoscopy is to stop the flexible shaft of the scope looping within the confines of the abdominal cavity, and to encourage it by any means to proceed straight on in an easy curve (the 'question mark' configuration), it is scarcely surprising that external hand pressure is valuable. The rationale for pressure in the lower left abdomen over the looping sigmoid colon has been described and illustrated (Fig. 9.11). The tendency of the sigmoid to re-loop at all stages of the examination has also been mentioned. Because of this tendency hand pressure over the sigmoid colon is a good bet to try whenever the instrument is looping—and its application has therefore been called 'nonspecific' hand pressure.

Other loops also cause problems which can be reduced by appropriate hand pressure, notably the drooping of the transverse colon into a deepening loop which results in the tendency for 'paradoxical movement' of the tip, which slips back more and more as the instrument shaft is pushed in. Pulling back when this occurs reverses the slippage so that the tip approaches the hepatic flexure again, aspiration collapses the colon and brings it nearer still, but changing the assistant's hand pressure to the left hypochondrial region will often pull the loop and the tip across the abdomen for the last few critical centimetres to reach the flexure. When such hand pressure fails to help, in the transverse or elsewhere, it is well worth the endoscopist optimizing both the view and the position of the instrument (by push, pull, rotation, deflation, angulation, etc.), then, whilst holding the instrument with one hand, palpating the patient's abdomen with the other to attempt to push the tip further in. This manoeuvre has been called 'specific' hand pressure. Pressure over the transverse is the most frequent and helpful example of 'specific' hand pressure, the left hypochondrial region being the most likely area to contribute, but pushing in the mid-abdomen or even the right hypochondrium can sometimes be dramatically helpful. Pushing over the central abdomen or the right iliac fossa can also help in reaching the caecal pole. At any time that a few extra centimetres of insertion are needed, but cannot be achieved, try abdominal hand pressure, first 'non-specific' (in the left lower abdomen) but, if this fails, 'specifically' according to the results of local palpation.

The hepatic flexure

One of the most frustrating problems for the colonoscopist is to have a clear view of the arc of the hepatic flexure but not be able to reach to it (Fig. 9.72a). If the flexure is only 2–3 cm away in spite of a reasonably straight colonoscope (around 70–80 cm), the sigmoid colon being held in control by hand pressure and clockwise torque, there is a sequence of actions which should ensure rapid passage around the hepatic flexure.

1 Assess from afar the correct direction around the flexure for after the tip reaches into it, it will angulate so close to the opposing mucosa that it is very difficult to steer, except by a predetermined plan (most commonly down and to the right). At all costs avoid impacting the tip against the opposing wall or it will catch in the haustral folds and there will be no view at all.

2 Aspirate air carefully from the inflated hepatic flexure, so as to collapse it towards, but not actually onto, the tip as it moves around (Fig. 9.72b).

3 Steer the tip in the predetermined direction around the arc of the flexure. Since the hepatic flexure is very acute, it takes some confidence to angulate nearly 180° around in the same direction without seeing well (Fig. 9.73). Use both angling control knobs simultaneously to achieve full angulation; adding clockwise twist may be helpful.

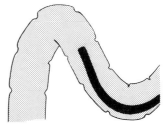

Fig. 9.72 (a) If the tip will not reach the hepatic flexure . . .

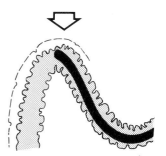

(b) . . . aspirate to collapse and shorten the flexure.

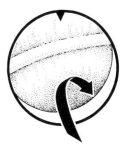

Fig. 9.73 Suck towards, then angle 180° around, the acute hepatic flexure.

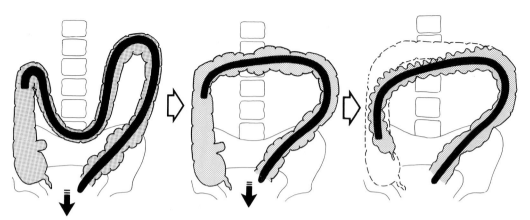

Fig. 9.74 (a) When around the hepatic flexure and viewing the ascending colon . . .

(b) . . . pull back to straighten . . .

Fig. 9.75 . . . and aspirate to deflate and fall down towards the caecum.

4 Withdraw the instrument gently for 30–50 cm (Fig. 9.74a) which lifts up the transverse colon and makes the colonoscope straighter and more manoeuvrable (Fig. 9.74b).

5 Once the ascending colon is seen, further aspiration again shortens the colon and drops the colonoscope down towards the caecum (Fig. 9.75).

In practice, a combination of these manoeuvres is used simultaneously, so that the hepatic flexure is sucked carefully towards the tip until the inner fold of the flexure is passed, the colonoscope is withdrawn (either by manipulation of the shaft or by leaning backwards whilst working the angling controls with both hands) whilst the tip is steered maximally around until it can be sucked down into the ascending colon. A parallel has already been drawn between the 'hook, withdraw and clockwise twist' situation in the transverse loop and hepatic flexure and the 'right twist–withdrawal' method of shortening the sigmoid 'N' loop at the sigmoid-descending colon angle; the same instrument manoeuvres apply to both, except that they must be exaggerated at the hepatic flexure because of its larger dimensions.

When things do not go according to plan, other tricks which help coax the colonoscope tip into and around the hepatic flexure include pressing in the left hypochondrium (to lift the transverse colon), getting the patient to inspire deeply and hold his breath (to lower the diaphragm and thus the hepatic flexure too), use of the split overtube to control the sigmoid colon, or change of position (to supine, prone or sometimes even right lateral) if the usual left lateral position has been ineffective. As in manipulating the transverse colon, applying brute force rarely pays off since sigmoid and transverse colon loops can take up most of the length of the colonoscope shaft. With the instrument really straightened at the hepatic flexure, only about 70 cm of shaft should remain in the patient; this is one of the situations where a distance check helps to ensure a straight colonoscope, and thus easy and painless insertion. The surface marking of the hepatic flexure by transillumination

(Fig. 9.31), if the tip becomes lost in this region, is posteriorly just above the right costal angle—not in the right hypochondrium as many people suppose. However, if no light can be seen be suspicious that the tip may still be in the splenic flexure; in a redundant colon it is possible to be over-optimistic and hopelessly lost.

The ascending colon and caecum

On seeing the ascending colon the temptation is to push in, but this usually results in the transverse loop re-forming and the tip sliding back. The secret here is to deflate; the resulting collapse of the capacious hepatic flexure and ascending colon will drop the tip downwards towards the caecum (Fig. 9.75); it also lowers the position of the hepatic flexure relative to the splenic flexure and with this mechanical advantage, pushing inwards should now be effective. Make short aspirations and steer carefully down the centre of the deflating lumen, then push the last few centimetres into the caecum. If it proves difficult to reach the last few centimetres to the caecal pole, change the patient's position to prone (even a small rotation may help) or supine. Once in the caecum the bowel can be re-inflated to get a view.

The caecum can be voluminous and its pronounced haustral infoldings and tendency to spasm may make it confusing to examine. In particular, it is possible to be mistaken about whether the pole has actually been reached. One should be very careful about assuming that true 'total colonoscopy' has been performed. The appendix orifice or ileo-caecal valve should be identified as landmarks, with or without fluoroscopy, or else iliac fossa transillumination or palpation should show the tip to be deep in the pelvis (Fig. 9.76) at the same time as the withdrawn colonoscope is at 70–80 cm. The caecal pole is often difficult to examine and not always completely clean, so a 'too good to be true' appearance may be the hepatic flexure and not the caecum; the lack of ileo-caecal valve and withdrawal distance of only 60–70 cm should warn of this possibility.

The ileo-caecal valve

To find the ileo-caecal valve pull back about 8–10 cm from the caecal pole and look for the first and most prominent circular fold at 5 cm from the pole. Scanning around this ileo-caecal fold, with the caecum moderately inflated, one part of the fold should be seen to be less perfectly concave than the rest. It may be simply flattened out, bulge in (especially on deflation, when it can make tell-tale bubbles), show a characteristic 'buttock-like' double bulge (Fig. 9.77) or, less commonly, have obvious protuberant lips or a 'volcano' appearance. It is rather uncommon to see the actual orifice or pouting lips of the valve from above, because they are normally situated on the upstream side of the ileo-caecal fold. With a modern colonoscope it is possible, if necessary, to retroflex the tip completely at the caecal pole and to identify the valve from below, sometimes only a slit-like orifice (Fig. 9.78).

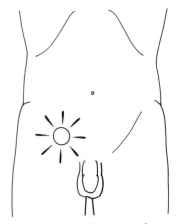

Fig. 9.76 Transillumination deep in the iliac fossa suggests the caecum.

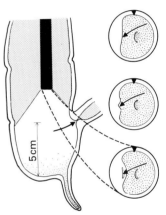

Fig. 9.77 The ileo-caecal valve, a bulge on the ileo-caecal fold: single bulge–double bulge or volcano.

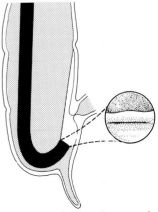

Fig. 9.78 A slit-like valve may only be visible in retroversion.

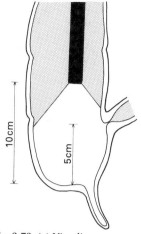

Fig. 9.79 (a) Visualize the ileocaecal valve and rehearse angulation . . .

Having located the bulge of the valve on the ileo-caecal fold, there is a sequence of actions to follow to angle in towards the valve and enter it (Fig. 9.79a–e):

(a) Rehearse at a distance the easiest combination of shaft twist and up/down angulation to point the tip towards the valve—pre-set and fix the lateral control if necessary.

(b) Pass the colonoscope tip down over the ileo-caecal valve fold in the region of the valvular bulge and angle in towards the valve, as predetermined in (a).

(c) Deflate the caecum partially, to make the valve supple.

(d) Withdraw the scope until the tip catches in the soft lips of the valve with a 'red-out' of transilluminated tissue.

(e) On seeing the 'red-out' stop withdrawal and insufflate air to open the lips—gently twisting or angling the scope a few millimetres if necessary—to find the dark lumen of the ileum at the orifice.

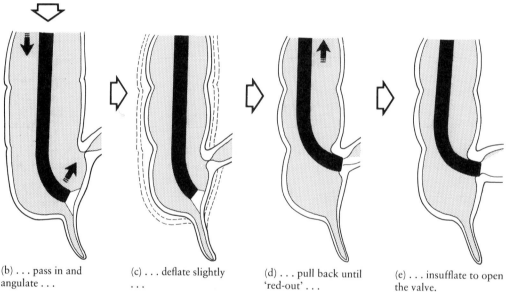

(b) . . . pass in and angulate . . .

(c) . . . deflate slightly . . .

(d) . . . pull back until 'red-out' . . .

(e) . . . insufflate to open the valve.

The mucosal surface changes from the pale, shiny vascular pattern of the colon of colonic mucosa, firstly to the red-out of the valve lips and finally to the slight granularity of the villous surface of the terminal ileum within the valve. Seeing this granularity may be the clue that the tip is poised for further minor adjustments to cause it to enter the lumen of the ileum itself.

Variable manoeuvres may be needed to enter the ileal lumen from the orifice of the valve; if considerable angulation has been used, the orifice may have been distorted upwards and *de*-angulation may straighten things out and let the tip slide in. If a distant or partial view can be obtained of the ileal opening, but the tip will not enter successfully, it may be possible to pass the biopsy forceps 4–5 cm into the opening either to obtain a blind biopsy or to act as an

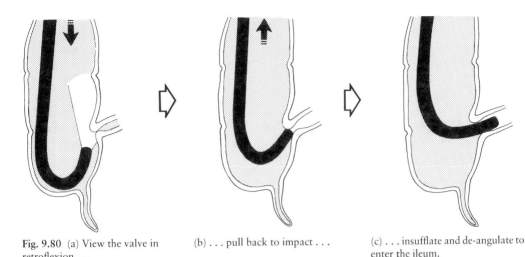

Fig. 9.80 (a) View the valve in retroflexion . . .   (b) . . . pull back to impact . . .   (c) . . . insufflate and de-angulate to enter the ileum.

'anchor' to fix the position of the tip relative to the valve and facilitate passage through it on the 'Seldinger' guidewire principle.

Multiple attempts may be needed for success in locating the valve and entering the ileum, if necessary rotating to slightly different parts of the ileo-caecal fold, hooking over it and pulling back to pass the area repeatedly. If the direct approach fails, it is possible to achieve success by retroflexion, with or without forceps in place as described above.

To enter the ileum in retroflexion (Fig. 9.80a), very acute angulation of the colonoscope tip is needed, with whichever combination of maximum up/down and lateral angulation or twist of the shaft achieves the best position. Fairly forceful inward push may be needed to impact low enough in the caecal pole to visualize the valve; with some video-endoscopes, the extra length of the bending section may preclude this. Once the valve is located, pull back to impact the tip within it (Fig. 9.80b), then insufflate to open the lips and de-angulate and pull back further to enter the ileum (Fig. 9.80c). The retroversion approach is particularly useful when the ileo-caecal valve is slit-like and invisible from above (Fig. 9.78). Those cases of inflammatory disease where the colonoscopist wants to see the terminal ileum are those where the valve is most likely to be narrowed and, although a limited view may be possible and biopsies taken, the valve may be impassable.

The terminal ileum

The terminal ileum surface characteristics are variable—matt in air, small finger-like villi waving under water, and often studded with raised lymphoid follicles resembling small polyps. Sometimes the ileum is surprisingly colon-like with a pale shiny surface and visible sub-mucosal vascular pattern. After colon resection the difference between colon and ileum may be imperceptible. Using 'dye-spray'

(1:4 dilution of washable blue ink, 0.2% indigo-carmine or 5% methylene blue) to highlight surface detail will rapidly discriminate between the granular or 'sand paper' appearance of ileal mucosa and the small circumferential grooves of the colonic surface, which gives a 'fingerprint' effect.

The ileum is soft, peristaltic and collapsible compared to the colon, and should be handled more like the duodenum. Greater distances can be travelled by gentle steering and deflation, so that the intestine collapses over the colonoscope, than will be achieved by force, which simply stretches it. At each acute bend it is best to deflate a little, hook round, pull back and then steer gently (and if necessary almost blindly) around and in before pulling back again to refind the view—the 'two steps forward and one step back' approach which applies throughout colonoscopy. Once the colonoscope tip is in the ileum it can often be passed up to 30–50 cm with care and patience, although this length of intestine may be folded onto only about 20 cm of instrument. Air distension in the small intestine should be kept to a minimum since it is particularly uncomfortable and slow to clear after examination.

Colonoscopic appearances

Better views are obtained during withdrawal than on insertion and the more painstaking examination is usually performed on the way out. However, in many areas, especially around bends, a different and sometimes better view is obtained on insertion. For this reason when a perfect view is obtained of a polyp during insertion (especially a small one) it is better to deal with it at once (snare, biopsy or photography) rather than have the humbling experience of not being able to find it again on the way out and to waste time. Another example of the difference between insertion and withdrawal is in the number of diverticular orifices seen in travelling around bends, compared with the few seen on coming out with the colon straightened.

The view is better on the way back because the colonoscope is in the centre of the lumen and is straight. However, the colon has been shortened during the insertion, and during withdrawal the most convoluted parts, such as the transverse and sigmoid colon, can spring off the tip at such speed that it is difficult to ensure a complete view. At sharp bends or marked haustrations there may therefore be blind spots during a single withdrawal; careful scanning and twisting movements should be used in an attempt to survey all parts of each haustral fold or bend, and some may need to be re-examined several times. At a flexure the outside of the bend may be seen on the first pass, but the colonoscope has to be re-inserted and hooked to get a selective view of the inside. The inside bends of the hepatic and splenic flexures and the sigmoid-descending colon junction are particular blind spots. As the straightened colonoscope emerges from the retroperitoneal tunnel of the descending colon it tends to spring free into the sigmoid colon; any inattention on the part of the colonoscopist means that 10 cm of sigmoid colon have been poorly seen and should be re-inspected.

Changes of position can also help to improve the accuracy of inspection. The splenic flexure and descending colon are rapidly filled with air and emptied of fluid by asking the patient to rotate towards the right lateral position. In any patient where accuracy is important, such as those with increased risk of polyps or possible bleeding points, it is our policy to rotate any fit patient to the right oblique position for inspection of the left colon, then back to the left lateral position again for a better view of the sigmoid colon and rectum.

The 'single-handed' technique (the endoscopist managing both controls and shaft) comes into its own during inspection on withdrawal. The endoscopist has precise control and the corkscrewing movements he makes by twisting the shaft are the quickest way of scanning a bend or haustral fold so that he can reflexly re-examine a problem area several times. With an assistant, difficulties of communication and co-ordination make it more difficult to be thorough and accurate.

As well as being obsessional the endoscopist must be honest, reporting not only what he sees but also when his view has been imperfect due to technical difficulty or bad bowel preparation. Even during an ideal examination the endoscopist probably misses 5% of the mucosal surface and in a problematic examination he may miss up to 20–30% (although he is unlikely to miss large protruberant lesions).

Normal appearances

The form and internal anatomy of the colon have been considered earlier in this chapter. The colonic mucosa normally shows a generalized fine, ramifying vascular pattern, which is most prominent in the rectum. The appearance depends on the transparency of the normal colonic epithelium, since the vessels seen are in the submucosa. If the epithelial capillaries are dilated (as may occur after bowel preparation) the vascular pattern may be partly obscured. If hyperaemia is marked (as in inflammatory bowel disease) there is no visible pattern. If the epithelial layer is thickened (as in the 'atrophy' of inactive chronic inflammatory disease) the mucosa appears pale and featureless even though biopsies may be essentially normal. The most convincing demonstration of how poorly the endoscopist normally sees the epithelial surface is to spray dye (25% dilution of washable blue ink or indigo-carmine 0.2%) onto the colonic mucosa. Small irregularities and lymphoid follicles stand out and there is a fine interconnecting pattern of 'innominate grooves' on the surface into which the dye sinks providing there is no excess of mucus on the surface.

There is a considerable size range of normal sub-mucosal vessels; even if they seem unusually prominent they should not be thought to be abnormal, and are not likely to be haemangiomatous unless the vessels are tortuous or serpentine. It is not surprising that there can be areas of mucosal trauma during insertion of the colonoscope, and red or even haemorrhagic patches may sometimes be seen on withdrawal especially in the sigmoid or where the looped sigmoid colon has impinged on the upper descending colon; it is wise to take biopsies to ensure that these appearances are not evidence of inflammatory change.

Abnormal appearances

It is not the purpose of this book to cover more than the most obvious points of endoscopic pathology. Fortunately for the endoscopist nearly all colonic abnormalities are either mucosal, with characteristic discoloration, or project into the lumen so that they are easy to see and excise or biopsy. Sub-mucosal lesions which may be very difficult to diagnose include secondary carcinomas, endometriosis, a few large-vessel haemangiomas and carcinoma underlying epithelial precancer in chronic ulcerative colitis.

Polyps

The normal mucosa is pale, so that sub-mucosal abnormalities projecting into the lumen such as hamartomatous polyps, lipomas or gas cysts may be pale. The very smallest polyps are also pale; those of 1–3 mm diameter may be transparent and invisible except on light reflex or by the dye-spray technique. From 4 to 6 mm there is no difference in appearance between a normal mucosal excrescence and a metaplastic, adenomatous or any other type of polyp. Adenomatous polyps over about 7–8 mm, being vascular, have a characteristic red colour which makes them easy to see. Even the smallest polyps are easy to pick out if the patient has been a purgative-taker, since the dusky appearance of melanosis coli (often most marked in the right colon) does not stain either polyps—which stand out like pale islands—or the ileo-caecal valve.

Flat, sessile, villous adenomas are also usually pale, soft and shiny, but these are rare above the rectum except in the caecum. Apart from lipomas or shiny, worm-like inflammatory polyps, which sometimes have a cap of white slough, all other polyps are best removed. Macroscopic differentiation is inaccurate and there is no sure way of anticipating which polyp will prove histologically to be neoplastic. A malignant polyp may be obviously irregular, may bleed easily from surface ulceration or be paler and is usually firmer than usual to palpation with the biopsy forceps. Such signs of possible malignancy warn to electrocoagulate the base thoroughly, to obtain a histological opinion on the stalk and to localize the polyp carefully in case subsequent surgery is indicated. Carcinomas are usually very obvious, larger and with a more extensive irregular base; carcinomatous ulcers are uncommon in the colon but look like malignant gastric ulcers. Conditions which can mimic malignancy are granulation tissue masses at an anastomosis, the larger granulation tissue polyps in chronic ulcerative colitis, and (rarely) the acute stage of an ischaemic process. Biopsy evidence should always be obtained, bearing in mind that the pathologist may only be able to report 'adenomatous tissue' since there may not be diagnostic evidence of invasive malignancy in the small pieces presented to him—which is why either a large forceps biopsy or snare-loop specimen should be taken whenever possible.

Inflammatory bowel disease

The degree of mucosal abnormality in different forms of inflammatory bowel disease can vary enormously. The mucosa can even appear *normal* with an intact vascular pattern or show the most minute haziness of vascular pattern, slight reddening or tendency to friability, and yet the pathologist can show very significant abnormality on the biopsies. The endoscopist is therefore wise not to rely too much on his eyes and must have an extremely low threshold for suspecting abnormality and taking biopsies, particularly if there is diarrhoea or any clinical suspicion of inflammatory disease.

Colonoscopic biopsies unfortunately rarely yield diagnostic granulomas in Crohn's disease, whereas the appearance of multiple small fat 'aphthoid' ulcers set in normal vascular pattern are characteristic. The differential diagnosis of the various specific and non-specific inflammatory disorders may not be easy; infective conditions, ulcerative, ischaemic, irradiation and even Crohn's colitis can look amazingly similar in the acute stage but biopsies will usually differentiate. Collagenous colitis, a rare cause of unexplained diarrhoea due to an extensive 'plate' of collagen deposition of unknown aetiology just under the epithelial surface, shows *normal* mucosa visually and the diagnosis can only be made histologically. The ulcer from a previous rectal biopsy or a 'solitary ulcer' of the rectum can look identical to a Crohn's ulcer, while tuberculous ulcers are similar but more heaped up and amoebic ulcers are more friable. Ulceration can also occur in chronic ulcerative colitis and ischaemic disease. The endoscopic appearances must be taken together with the clinical context and histological opinion. In the severe or chronic stage it is often impossible for either endoscopist or pathologist to help in differential diagnosis.

Unexplained rectal bleeding

This is a common reason for undertaking colonoscopy. Although colonoscopy gives an impressive yield of radiologically missed cancers and polyps, 50–60% of patients will show no obvious abnormality, which raises the spectre of whether anything has been missed. Haemorrhoids can be seen with the colonoscope (by retroversion in the rectum if necessary, but a proctoscope should be used for a proper view) and other rectal lesions may have been missed, so the colonoscopist should keep looking to the last. Haemangiomas are rare, but they can assume any appearance from massive and obvious sub-mucosal discoloration with huge serpentine vessels to telangiectases or minute solitary naevi, which could easily be missed in folds or bends. Angiodysplasias mainly occur in the caecum or ascending colon, but also in the small intestine or in the distal bowel;

they have variable appearances, always bright red, but they can be small vascular plaques, spidery telangiectases or even a 1–2-mm dot lesion; they may be solitary or numerous.

Special circumstances

Pain mapping

Functional bowel disturbance in the apparently normal colon can take many forms, and 'spastic colon' pain may present with equally variable referred-pain radiation patterns—to right or left loin, back or even into the thighs. An occasionally useful and very simple colonoscopic procedure is to map the pain experienced during distension at different sites in the colon produced by inflating a small balloon taped alongside the tip of the colonoscope (Fig. 9.81). A child's balloon, finger-cot or the cut-off finger of a rubber glove is bound with fine thread at the end of a small-bore flexible tube (include a short length of rigid tube inside the end, to stop it collapsing during binding). The bound neck of the balloon is taped to the junction of the shaft and bending section—placing the balloon at the tip can obscure the view—and two or three additional tapes secure it along the shaft. With a three-way tap and a 50-ml luer-lock syringe it is easy to inflate and deflate the balloon in representative sites during withdrawal of the colonoscope.

The balloon should not be inflated above 200 ml volume in the proximal colon and 100 ml distally, or mucosal stretch damage will occur. Because of variability in colon size, quantitation of volume inflated to pain experienced in different patients is unpredictable, but some patients with irritable bowel syndrome/spastic colon are notably hypersensitive to even 12–25 ml distension in the sigmoid colon. At each inflation site ask the patient about the quality and site of any pain experienced, and use this to map out referred-pain radiation sites and their correlation with the patient's 'usual' symptoms.

Colostomies and ileostomies

Providing that a finger can be inserted into the stoma, a colonoscope will also pass into the colostomy or ileostomy without trouble. The

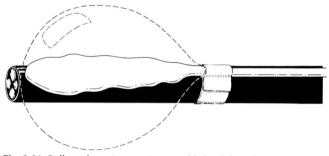

Fig. 9.81 Balloon for pain-mapping taped behind the colonoscope tip.

first few centimetres through the abdominal wall are sometimes difficult to negotiate and also to examine, partly because of the continual escape of insufflated air. It is quite normal for the stoma to change to an unhealthy-looking cyanotic colour and even for there to be a little local bleeding, but no harm ensues.

Through an ileostomy the distal 20 cm of ileum are easily examined but further insertion depends on whether adhesions have formed. As in the sigmoid colon, the secret of passage through the small intestine is to repeatedly pull the instrument back as each bend is reached, which convolutes the intestine onto the instrument and straightens out the next short segment; thus even though only 30–40 cm of instrument can be inserted, as much as 100 cm of intestine may be seen. Since the sigmoid colon will usually have been removed in a colostomy patient, examination of the proximal colon is usually very easy; if there is a loop colostomy both sides can be examined providing they have been suitably prepared.

Limited examination of an ileal conduit or continent (Kock's) ileostomy is also possible providing that an acutely angling endoscope is available; a paediatric gastroscope or colonoscope is ideal. Pelvic ileo-anal pouches are easy to examine with a standard instrument.

Paediatric colonoscopy

Neonatal examinations are best performed with a thinner (1 cm) and extra-flexible forward-viewing paediatric colonoscope, but from the age of 2 years upwards, adult colonoscopes can be used if necessary. The infant anus will accept an adult finger and so will take an endoscope of the same size, but the sphincters first require gentle dilatation over a minute or two, using any small smooth tube (such as a naso-gastric tube or a ballpoint pen cover). The main advantage of a purpose-built paediatric colonoscope is more the extra flexibility or 'softness' of its shaft than its small diameter, because it is easy with stiffer adult colonoscopes to overstretch the mobile and elastic loops of a child's colon. It is a mistake to use a paediatric gastroscope, which is thinner but much stiffer.

Bowel preparation in children is usually very effective. Pleasant-tasting oral solutions such as senna syrup or magnesium citrate are best tolerated. A saline or phosphate enema will cleanse most of the colon of a baby. Children of any age can be colonoscoped without general anaesthesia providing that generous pre-medication is used (except for neonates, who may sometimes be more safely examined with no sedation at all). A suitable oral sedative pre-medication (such as antihistamine) can be useful so that the child is relaxed before the procedure. A small intravenous catheter is inserted and followed by a small dose of i.v. benzodiazepine (Diazemuls 2–5 mg, or midazolam 1–3 mg) combined with a larger dose of pethidine (Demerol) 25–100 mg i.v., slowly titrated according to response. When the child is somnolent and tolerates digital examination easily, the rest of the colonoscopy can be certain to be equally well tolerated.

Per-operative colonoscopy

Per-operative colonoscopy is normally only justified if attempts at colonoscopy have failed in a patient with known polyps, where the small intestine is to be examined in a patient with continued blood loss, or where the colon proximal to a constricting neoplasm is to be inspected to exclude synchronous lesions.

For non-obstructed patients, oral lavage or full colonoscopy bowel preparation must have been used, as most standard pre-operative preparation regimes leave solid faecal residue. If the bowel has been completely obstructed, it is possible to perform on-table lavage through a temporary caecostomy tube. During per-operative colonoscopy, over-insufflation of air can fill the small intestine and leave the surgeon with an unmanageable tangle of distended loops. This can be avoided if the endoscopist uses carbon dioxide insufflation instead of air, or if the surgeon places a clamp on the terminal ileum and the endoscopist aspirates carefully on withdrawal.

To examine the small intestine at laparotomy (see Chapter 8) the long colonoscope can be used either per-orally by the usual route or through an intestinal incision; 70 cm of instrument are required to reach either the ligament of Treitz per-orally or the caecum per-anally. It helps for the surgeon either to mobilize or manually support the fixed part of the duodenum (see Fig. 8.3) if the colonoscope is passed orally. The small intestine must be very gently handled on the endoscope to avoid local trauma or postoperative problems. A very flexible single-channel endoscope is used to minimize stretching and it is also important to insufflate as little as possible. Clamps are sequentially placed on each segment of small intestine after it has been evacuated. The surgeon inspects the transilluminated intestine from outside (with the room lights turned off) whilst the endoscopist inspects the inside.

Hazards and complications

Colonoscopy (one perforation per 1700 examinations) is significantly more hazardous than barium studies (one perforation per 25 000 examinations)—one factor which needs to be borne in mind before advocating it too enthusiastically as a routine diagnostic procedure. Hypotensive episodes, and cardiac or respiratory arrest can be provoked by the combination of over-sedation and intense vagal stimulus from instrumentation. Hypoxia can occur in elderly patients who are over-sedated or suffer a vasovagal reaction during colonoscopy. Numerous perforations have been reported, usually due to inexperience and the use of excessive force when pushing in or pulling out. Either the tip of the instrument or a loop formed by its shaft can perforate. When surgery is performed soon after colonoscopy, small tears have been seen in the ante-mesenteric serosal aspect of the colon as well as haematomas in the mesentery. In several reported cases the spleen has been avulsed during over-aggressive straightening manoeuvres with the tip hooked around the splenic flexure.

Perforations have also occurred from air pressure including 'blow-out' of diverticula; unexplained pneumoperitoneum or ileo-caecal perforation has followed colonoscopy limited to the sigmoid colon. Instruments with single-button control of both air and water can produce dangerously high air pressures if the tip is impacted in a diverticulum or if insufflation is continued for excessively long periods, as for instance when trying to distend and pass a stricture. Great care and light finger pressure over the air button are indicated in the presence of diverticular disease. Diverticula are thin-walled and have also been perforated with biopsy forceps or by the instrument tip; it is surprisingly easy to confuse a large diverticular orifice with the bowel lumen.

The importance of using a prophylactic antibiotic combination in certain groups of patients has already been mentioned (for those with heart valve replacements, immunosuppressed or immunodepressed patients, especially babies, and with ascites or peritoneal dialysis fluid). Gram-negative septicaemia can result from instrumentation (especially in neonates or the elderly) and unexplained pyrexia or collapse should be investigated with blood cultures and managed appropriately.

Electrosurgery and snare polypectomy contribute additional specific hazards (see Chapter 10).

Safety during colonoscopy lies in being aware of possible complications and in avoiding pain (or over-sedation which masks the pain response, as well as contributing pharmacological side-effects). Before starting a colonoscopy it is impossible to know if there are adhesions, whether the bowel is easily distensible and whether its mesenteries are free-floating or fixed; pain is the only warning that the bowel or its attachments are being unreasonably strained and the endoscopist must respect any protest from the patient. A mild groan in a sedated patient may be equivalent to a scream of pain without sedation. Colonoscopy is *not* always technically possible; if there is a history of abdominal surgery or sepsis, or if the instrument feels fixed and the patient is in pain, the correct course is usually to stop. The experienced endoscopist learns to take his time, to be obsessional in steering correctly and to be prepared to withdraw from any difficult situation, and if necessary to try again. Too often the beginner has a relentless 'crash and dash' approach, and may be insensitive to the patient's pain because he causes it so often.

Despite these potential hazards, skilled colonoscopy is amazingly safe; it is certainly justified by its clinical yield and the high morbidity of colonic surgery (which would often be the alternative).

Instrument trouble-shooting

Colonoscopy can be difficult enough without adding problems in instrument performance. Ideally the functions of all instrument controls should have been checked before the examination, because they can be difficult to spot or tedious to remedy during it.

Vision

Check illumination and clarity of view beforehand. Is the light source functioning properly and the brightness control turned up? Is the view crisp or is there debris on the lens or light-bundle lenses which may need washing, polishing or even gentle scratching off? Colonic mucus and debris can be solidified by the protein-denaturing effects of strong antiseptics such as glutaraldehyde. Use a hand-lens to inspect the tip ocular closely and to help with local cleaning.

Air

If there is no insufflation from the tip, check the light source—is the air pump switched on, are the umbilical and water-bottle connections pushed in fully and the water bottle screwed on? Is the rubber 'O'-ring in place on the water-bottle connection? Is the air/water button in good condition and seated properly and the CO_2 button in position (where relevant) since it will otherwise allow air leakage?

As already mentioned, proper air insufflation is difficult to assess by bubbling under water, but very obvious when blowing up a rubber glove or balloon placed over the tip. Partial inflation can easily be missed during an examination, which becomes technically difficult and the colon apparently 'hypercontractile' because it collapses continually and inflates with difficulty. A great deal of wasted time can be avoided by noticing this defect before starting, or by withdrawing the scope at an early stage to check and rectify the problem.

Organic debris and mucus is the usual cause of poor insufflation, since this tends to reflux under the positive pressure within the colon back up the air channel when not in active use (and therefore at atmospheric pressure). A particular culprit is usually the small angled air (or air plus water) tube at the tip of the instrument. A single plug or an accretion of layers of proteinaceous material can solidify within this tube, especially after glutaraldehyde exposure. Paradoxically, the units with the greatest 'air-blockage' problems are often those with the highest cleaning standards, where full antisepsis is rigorously employed. The problem can be minimized by careful water-flushing of the air channel for at least 30–40 seconds immediately after each examination. Preferably, this should be achieved with a single-channel flushing device, since any adaptor which flushes both air and water channels simultaneously will simply by-pass an absolute or partial blockage in one channel without this being apparent. Using enzyme detergents is also very effective in the cleaning process, including domestic non-foaming versions for endoscope washing machines.

If a complete or partial blockage has occurred in the air channel, the quickest remedy is to try forcing first air, and if this fails water, by syringe down the CO_2 channel—remembering to press the CO_2 button at the same time. The CO_2 system connects directly with the air channel and so gives convenient access to it for flushing purposes. Water is preferable for forced perfusion since it is non-compressible and a smaller (5–10 ml) syringe gives greatest pressure. Some manufacturers have special 'flush buttons' which allow direct pressure syringing after replacing the usual air/water button. A messy alternative is to activate the regular air button, put a finger over the water-bottle port on the umbilical to avoid leakage and then to syringe through the air-input channel at the end of the umbilical using a suitable syringe attachment, such as a micro-pipette tip cut to size.

The angled air tube at the instrument tip is the logical place for a direct attack on a blockage problem. First try probing its slit-like opening, or even water-injecting this using a fine-gauge intravenous needle. If this proves ineffective it is possible, as a last resort, to remove the air pipe altogether. Although it may be more diplomatic to have this done by the manufacturer's service department, or at least by skilled technicians, removal, cleaning and re-insertion are actually an easy matter. A small jeweller's screwdriver is necessary and the covering layer of soft silicone sealant must be prized off, but under this will be found a simple slotted grub-screw which can be unscrewed for a turn or two, releasing the air pipe. The channel or the pipe are easily ram-rodded with a fine wire (such as the stilette of an ERCP cannula) or can be syringe perfused until all debris is removed, rapidly solving the problem.

If the air channel cannot be unblocked during the process of an examination, a simple dodge is to empty the water bottle, then to activate the water button to achieve air insufflation (use syringed water if lens washing is needed).

To check that the air pump is working properly (the lamp must be ignited in some light sources before the air pump operates), insert any syringe into the rubber air-output tube and the syringe plunger will rapidly blow out, demonstrating high pressure.

Water

Failure of the water system is relatively unusual, because mucus or debris do not reflux back up the filled water system as easily as up the empty air channel. None the less, particles of rubber 'O'-ring or other matter can become lodged in the water system. They should be quickly cleared by water-syringing with a micro-pipette tip into the small hose that normally lies underwater within the water bottle—remembering to press the water button simultaneously to obtain flow.

Suction

Particulate debris also easily blocks the suction channel. If in the shaft, this can be dislodged by water-syringing through the biopsy port. Removing the suction button and covering the opening on the control head with a finger is a quick way of improving suction pressure and can result in rapid clearance of the whole system (as when sucking polyp specimens). As a final resort the whole suction system can be cleared by retrograde syringing using a 50-ml bladder syringe to wash through tubing attached to the suction port on the umbilical. Push the suction button and also cover the biopsy port during this procedure to avoid unpleasant (refluxed) surprises.

Further reading

General reading

Hunt, R. H. and Waye, J. D. (1981) *Colonoscopy: Techniques, Clinical Practice and Colour Atlas.* Chapman and Hall, London.

Harned, R. K., Consigny, P. M., Cooper, N. B., Williams, S. M. and Woltzen, A. J. (1982) 'Barium enema examination following biopsy of the rectum or colon'. *Radiology*, **145**, 11–16.

Rankin, G. B. (1987) 'Indications, contraindications and complications of colonoscopy', in *Gastroenterologic Endoscopy* (ed. Sivak, M. V. Jr.), pp. 868–880. W. B. Saunders, Philadelphia.

McGill, D. B. (1985) 'The President and the power of the colonoscope'. *Mayo Clinic Proceedings*, **60**, 886–889.

Sakai, Y. (1981) *Practical Fiberoptic Colonoscopy*. Igaku-Shoin, Tokyo.

Sakai, Y. (1987) 'Technique of colonoscopy', in *Gastroenterologic Endoscopy* (ed. Sivak, M. V. Jr.), pp. 840–867. W. B. Saunders, Philadelphia.

Shinya, H. (1982) *Colonoscopy: Diagnosis and Treatment of Colonic Diseases*. Igaku-Shoin, Tokyo.

Bowel preparation

Davis, G. R. and Santa-Ana, C. A. (1979) 'Development of a lavage solution with minimal water and electrolyte absorption and secretion'. *Gastroenterology*, **78**, 991–995.

DiPalma, J. A., Brady, C. E. and Stewart, D. L. (1984) 'Comparison of colon cleansing methods in preparation for colonoscopy'. *Gastroenterology*, **86**, 856–860.

Thomas, G. (1982) 'Patient acceptance and effectiveness of a balanced lavage solution (Golytely) versus the standard preparation for colonoscopy'. *Gastroenterology*, **82**, 435–447.

Techniques

Arigbabu, A. O., Badejo, O. A. and Akinola, D. O. (1985) 'Colonoscopy in the emergency treatment of colonic volvulus in Nigeria'. *Diseases of the Colon and Rectum*, **28**, 795–798.

Berry, A. R., Campbell, W. B. and Kettlewell, M. G. W. (1988) 'Management of major colonic haemorrhage.' *British Journal of Surgery*, **75**, 637–640.

Bowden, T. A. Jr. (1989) 'Intraoperative endoscopy of the gastrointestinal tract: clinical necessity or lack of preoperative preparation?' *World Journal of Surgery*, **13**, 186–189.

Coole, P. K. W., Wheeler, J. and Rice, P. (1986) 'Carbon dioxide insufflated colonoscopy—an ignored superior technique'. *Gastrointestinal Endoscopy*, **32** (5), 330–333.

Danesh, B. J. Z., Spiliadis, C., Williams, C. B. and Zambartas, C. M. (1987) 'Angiodysplasia—an uncommon cause of colonic bleeding; colonoscopic evaluation of 1050 patients with rectal bleeding and anaemia'. *International Journal of Colorectal Disease*, **2**, 218–222.

Hussein, A. M. J., Bartram, C. I. and Williams, C. B. (1984) 'Carbon dioxide insufflation for more comfortable colonoscopy'. *Gastrointestinal Endoscopy*, **30**, 68–70.

Jensen, D. M. and Machicado, G. A. (1988) 'Diagnosis and treatment of severe hematochezia. The role of urgent colonoscopy after purge'. *Gastroenterology*, **95**, 1569–1574.

Kalvaria, I. Kottler, R. E. and Marks, I. N. (1988) 'The role of colonoscopy in the diagnosis of tuberculosis'. *Journal of Clinical Gastroenterology*, **10** (5), 516–523.

Kingham, J. G. C., Levison, D. A., Ball, J. A. and Dawson, A. M. (1982) 'Microscopic colitis—a cause of chronic watery diarrhoea'. *British Medical Journal*, **285**, 1601–1604.

Kozarek, R. A. (1986) 'Hydrostatic balloon dilation of gastrointestinal stenoses: a national survey'. *Gastrointestinal Endoscopy*, **32**, 15–19.

Rossini, F. P., Ferrari, A., Spandre, M. *et al.* (1989) 'Emergency colonoscopy'. *World Journal of Surgery*, **13**, 190–192.

Swarbrick, E. T., Bat, L., Hegarty, J. E., Dawson, A. M. and Williams, C. B. (1980) 'Site of pain from the irritable bowel'. *Lancet*, **443**, 446.

Waye, J. D. (1987) 'The differential diagnosis of inflammatory and infectious colitis', in *Gastroenterologic Endoscopy* (ed. Sivak, M. V. Jr.), pp. 881–899. W. B. Saunders, Philadelphia.

Hazards and complications

Bigard, M. A., Gaucher, P. and Lasalle, C. (1979) 'Fatal colonic explosion during colonoscopic polypectomy'. *Gastroenterology*, **77**, 1307–1310.

Bond, J. H. and Levitt, M. D. (1979) 'Colonic gas explosion: is a fire extinguisher necessary?' *Gastroenterology*, **77**, 1349–1350.

Botoman, V. A. and Surawicz, C. M. (1986) 'Bacteremia with gastrointestinal endoscopic procedures'. *Gastrointestinal Endoscopy*, **32**, 342–345.

Fleischer, D. (1989) 'Monitoring the patient receiving conscious sedation for gastrointestinal endoscopy: issues and guidelines'. *Gastrointestinal Endoscopy*, **35**, 262–265.

Habr-Gama, A. and Waye, J. D. (1989) 'Complications and hazards of gastrointestinal endoscopy'. *World Journal of Surgery*, **13**, 193–201.

Kozarek, R. A., Earnest, D. L., Silverstein, M. E. and Smith, R. G. (1980) 'Air-pressure induced colon injury during diagnostic colonoscopy'. *Gastroenterology*, **78**, 7–14.

Macrae, F. A., Tan, K. G. and Williams, C. B. (1981) 'Towards safer colonoscopy: a report on the complications of 5000 diagnostic or therapeutic colonoscopies'. *Gut*, **24**, 376–383.

10 Colonoscopic Polypectomy and Therapeutic Procedures

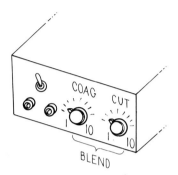

Fig. 10.1 Electrosurgical units should have cut, coag and blend circuitry.

Equipment

The equipment requirements for endoscopic polypectomy are few, and in many ways the fewer the better. It is preferable to be completely familiar with using one type of snare loop and one electrosurgical unit, since from this familiarity it becomes easy to recognize when polypectomy is going right and when it is not.

Any type of electrosurgical unit can be used for polypectomy. It will be used only at low power settings (15–50 W) and should have an automatic warning system in the circuitry in case a connection is faulty or the patient plate is not in contact. Most electrosurgical units have separate 'cut' and 'coagulate' circuits, which can usually be blended to choice (Fig. 10.1). As will be explained below, in electrosurgery the *type* of current is much less important than the *amount of power* produced. Since high dial settings (high power) of coagulating current have satisfactory cutting characteristics, and since in many units the 'cut' power output at any one setting is much greater than the 'coag' power output at the same setting, the difference in current type for polypectomy is often illusory. The chosen electrosurgical unit should be easily available, with good after-sales facilities and favoured by other local enthusiasts who can help with practical advice on its use.

Several makes of snare loop are available. For anyone doing a limited number of polypectomies it is advisable to have one snare type and best to use a commercial snare with handle (Fig. 10.2). The handle is convenient to manipulate; its position shows how far the snare loop has tightened which is *not* always obvious by eye or by feel, especially when snaring larger polyps.

Even with a commercial snare several points should be checked. The wire loop must open and close easily to give an accurate 'feel'. It should open wide enough to take a 2–3-cm polyp (and can be re-shaped by hand if necessary before polypectomy). The loop should close 15 mm into the snare tube (Fig. 10.3a) to squeeze a large stalk tightly even if the plastic snare sheath crumples slightly under pressure (see below); if it does not (Fig. 10.3b) the final cut relies entirely on high-power electrical cutting and may not coagulate the central stalk vessels enough. Conversely, if the wire closes too far into the tube (Fig. 10.3c) a stalk may be cut off by 'cheese-wiring'

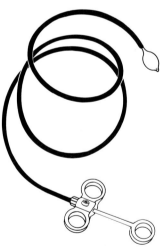

Fig. 10.2 Use one commercial snare type for familiarity.

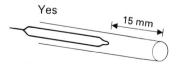

Fig. 10.3 (a) Snare closed—just right;

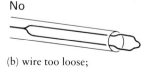

(b) wire too loose;

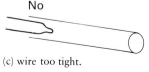

(c) wire too tight.

mechanically without adequate electrocoagulation. To avoid this make a mark on the snare handle to indicate the point when the loop is just fully closed (Fig. 10.4); check this before each polypectomy, especially if the particular combination of wire and handle may have been changed.

Snare wire thickness is also important. Most loops are made of relatively thick wire so that there is little risk of cheese-wiring unintentionally and a larger contact area which favours good local coagulation rather than electrocutting.

The endoscopist should therefore have a working snare, with a snare handle and several spare wires, and a purpose-built electrosurgical unit, and possibly a source of carbon dioxide (see p. 173). The chief characteristic of the working snare will be its longevity; it should last for hundreds of average polypectomies. 'Mini-snares' are available which may be more convenient for the majority of (smaller) polyps. Large polyps and difficult polypectomies can deform a snare before it is otherwise worn out. Misuse of a snare so that it sparks and over-heats at the tip will also shorten its life. Broken leads are potentially dangerous, especially if they make intermittent contact. A crude but effective test of the circuitry is to check for sparking between the *side* of the snare loop and the patient plate with dial setting at half power (Fig. 10.5) (sparking at the tip, already under stress, hastens breakage of the wire). For units not having automatic power-regulating circuitry a 40-W light bulb can be illuminated between snare loop and plate, which checks both the circuit and the power output of the unit.

Some other devices may be useful. An insulated 'hot biopsy forceps' is a good way of destroying small polyps up to 5-mm diameter and electrocoagulating telangiectases or angiodysplasia (see below). A polyp-retrieval forceps or grasping forceps is sometimes useful, but the snare loop itself is usually adequate for picking up the severed polyp and saves time in changing accessories. A sclerotherapy needle may be required and a washing or dye-spray cannula should be available.

Principles and practice of electrosurgery

The reason for using electrosurgical or 'diathermy' currents in polypectomy is to cause *heat*, with resultant coagulation of blood vessels. Coincidentally the cooked tissue becomes easier to transect with the snare wire, but this is of secondary importance.

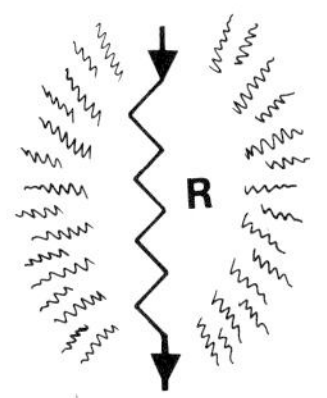

Heat is generated in tissue by the passage of any form of electricity (electrons) (Fig. 10.6). The use of a high-frequency or 'radio-frequency' current alternating in direction at up to a million times per second (10^6 c/s, 1000 kcs, 10 Hz) (Fig. 10.7) is only important because at such frequencies there is no time for muscle and nerve fibre depolarization before the current alternates again, therefore there is no shock due to massive muscle contraction. Electrosurgical current is thus not felt by the patient and there is equally no danger to cardiac muscle. Most modern cardiac pace makers are unaffected, providing that the current passage between

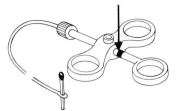

Fig. 10.4 Mark the handle when the loop is fully closed.

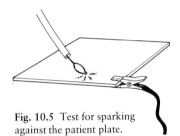

Fig. 10.5 Test for sparking against the patient plate.

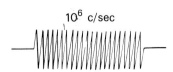

Fig. 10.6 Heat is generated by electricity (electrons) passing through a resistance—high-resistance wire or tissue.

10^6 c/sec

Fig. 10.7 Electrosurgical current alternates up to 1 000 000 times per second—heat but *no* shock.

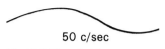

50 c/sec

Fig. 10.8 Household current alternates 50–60 times per second—heat and shock.

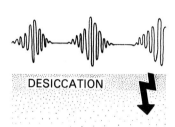

DESICCATION

Fig. 10.9 Coagulating current—intermittent high-voltage pulses pass desiccated tissue.

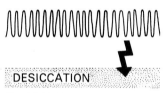

DESICCATION

Fig. 10.10 Cutting current—continuous (so high power) but too low a voltage to pass desiccation.

polypectomy site and patient plates (usually under the buttocks or on the thigh) is reasonably remote from the pacemaker; if in doubt consult a competent cardiologist. Because of deeply rooted fears about low-frequency household currents alternating 50–60 times per second (50 c/s) (Fig. 10.8) most people, patients, nurses and doctors, are unjustifiably nervous about electrosurgical currents which are inherently safe. At the lower power used in polypectomy, even the unlikely possibility of a direct burn to the skin of patient or operator is surprising but trivial, and actual burns are very rare because the heat resulting causes a strong protest long before actual damage occurs. The only danger from electrosurgical currents is that of the heat effects at the site of polypectomy.

It has already been mentioned that there is a theoretical difference between the pure 'coagulating' current, in which pulses of high-voltage electrosurgical current are used (the higher voltage causing the current to pass even desiccated tissue) (Fig. 10.9), and 'cutting' current with its continuous flow of lower voltage (which results in equal power, but because of low voltage will not pass the desiccated layer and thus does not heat too widely) (Fig. 10.10). 'Blended' current combines both wave-forms (Fig. 10.11). On most sources the 'cut' circuit is made to be more powerful than the 'coag' so that a dial setting of, say, 5 on 'cut' will naturally have more heating effect than 5 on 'coag'. The higher power and localized heating of 'cut' current vaporizes to steam these cells in contact with the wire, resulting in its localized cutting action.

Tissue heats because of its high electrical resistance (Fig. 10.6); but if the current is allowed to spread out and flow through a large area of tissue the overall resistance and heating effect falls (Fig. 10.12). To obtain effective electrocoagulation therefore, the flow of the current must be restricted through the smallest possible area of tissue—the critical principle of 'current density' (Fig. 10.13). This is basic to all forms of electrosurgery and explains why no noticeable heat is generated at the broad area of skin contact with the patient plate whereas intense heat occurs in

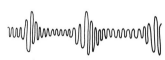

Fig. 10.11 Blended combines both characteristics.

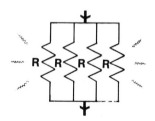

Fig. 10.12 Current flows more easily through larger areas of tissue resistance and so produces little heat.

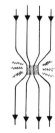

Fig. 10.13 'Current density' results from constricting tissue and greatly increases heating.

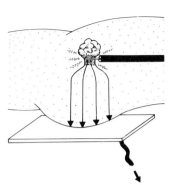

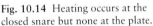

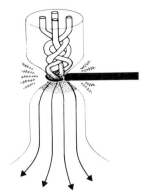

Fig. 10.14 Heating occurs at the closed snare but none at the plate.

Fig. 10.15 The whole plexus of stalk vessels must be electro-coagulated before section.

the closed snare loop (Fig. 10.14). Even a relatively small area of contact between buttock or thigh and patient plate is adequate, and extra moisture or electrode jelly is unnecessary at the power used for polypectomy.

The problem in polypectomy is to coagulate the plexus of arteries and veins at the core of the polyp stalk adequately before transection. Closing the snare loop both stops the blood flow and tends to concentrate current flow to this core (Fig. 10.15). The tightness of the loop is critical since the *area* through which current is concentrated (current density) decreases *as the square* of snare closure (πr^2). The heat increases as the square of current density, so heating increases overall *as the cube* of snare closure (i.e. slight increase of snare closure on a polyp stalk greatly increases the heat produced). Conversely, the fact that the closed snare loop is the narrowest part of the stalk means that the base of the stalk and the bowel wall should scarcely heat at all, which explains the rarity of bowel perforations during polypectomy.

Expressed graphically the heat produced in a polyp stalk increases directly with increased power settings on the unit dial (Fig. 10.16). It also increases directly as time passes (ignoring complicating features such as heat dissipation) (Fig. 10.17), but closure of the snare loop is much more important, resulting in a *cube* increase of heat as the snare closes (Fig. 10.18). If the snare is too loose it will hardly heat the tissue at all and if too tight will heat it too fast. In the snaring of a large polyp this rapid increase of heating can have the unfortunate effect that, as the snare starts to close down through the stalk, the heat produced increases dramatically and results in electrocutting of the central core, which is the part that needs slow and controlled coagulation. The soft stalk of a small polyp should coagulate rapidly; a larger stalk requires a slightly higher power setting and more time before visible coagulation occurs. Visually it is difficult to be absolutely sure of the diameter and consistency of the stalk; the 'feel' of the

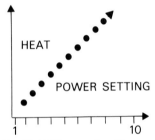

Fig. 10.16 Heat produced is directly proportional to power . . .

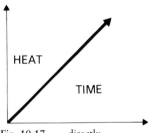

Fig. 10.17 . . . directly proportional to time . . .

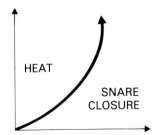

Fig. 10.18 . . . but increases as the cube of *snare closure*.

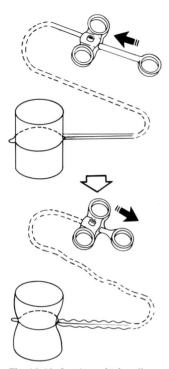

Fig. 10.19 Snaring a thick stalk . . . the snare sheath may crumple before closure is adequate.

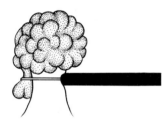

Fig. 10.20 Polyp tissue can be trapped in the snare reducing its efficiency.

stalk may also be inaccurate, especially with snares having a thin and compressible Teflon tube (Fig. 10.19), so that the snare handle appears 'closed' when the stalk is not adequately narrowed. It is safest to start at the low power setting (corresponding to only 15–25 W) and to increase the power in steps if no visible coagulation has occurred.

Since the essential principle of polypectomy is to electrocoagulate or cook the stalk tissue before section, there must be visible whitening as the protein denatures and swelling or steam as the tissue boils. However, if all water boils off electrons will no longer flow through the desiccated tissue, and the wire has to be pulled through mechanically. Inevitably it takes a little time at the safer lower current settings to boil the tissue but if this takes more than 15–20 seconds the risk of heat dissipation and damage to the bowel wall increases and it may be more realistic to increase the power setting so as to speed things up. It should, however, be unusual to need a power setting equivalent to more than 35–50 W.

The risk of inadequate central coagulation increases with a stalk > 1-cm diameter, particularly if it is firm and relatively non-compressible. The vessels in such a thick stalk may be large and thick-walled; in addition high power is needed to start the electro-coagulation peripherally and too sudden cutting can eventually occur. Additional factors such as current leakage may contribute and are discussed later. When no coagulation is occurring in a large polyp stalk despite a power setting of 35–50 W and bursts of current amounting to 20 seconds in total, all possible variables must be checked.

1 Check that the circuitry and connections are correct and also that the snare has been properly assembled and closes adequately (in some makes, the snare wire can be too loose at the handle and must be tightened).

2 Check the polyp stalk.
  (a) Has the stalk been correctly snared or is the head of the polyp trapped out of sight (Fig. 10.20)?
  (b) Would a change of patient position improve the view of the stalk (Fig. 10.21)?

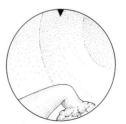

Fig. 10.21 Bad view of a polyp?
. . .
. . . change the patient's position.

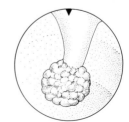

Fig. 10.22 Bad position for snare placement? . . .
. . . rotate the instrument.

(c) Would rotation of the colonoscope shaft put the forceps or snare in a better position, so that the view is not lost during polypectomy (Fig. 10.22)?

(d) Can the snare loop be re-opened and positioned higher up the stalk where it is narrower?

(e) Is it a thick stalk where sclerotherapy injection should be made before further snaring (or be available in case of immediate haemorrhage) (Fig. 10.23a)?

If there is any fear of complications or the operator is inexperienced this may also be the moment to disengage the snare and leave the procedure to someone else.

Starting polypectomy

It can be difficult even for an expert to snare some polyps and easy for a beginner to miss them or to get inadequate views; it is unwise to do polypectomies during the first 50 colonoscopies. Before starting, it is sensible to practise with the equipment under controlled conditions, with meat or a piece of resected bowel. Short strips of steak, cut to the diameter of a pencil, make good 'stalk substitutes'. The narrower end of the strip is held in the snare loop with the broader end wetted to make good contact and rested on the patient plate. Alternatively, a small portion of fresh colon resection specimen can be placed on the patient plate; a pseudo-polyp of mucosa is lifted up with forceps and the snare loop closed onto it.

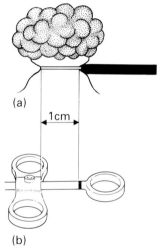

(a)

(b)

Fig. 10.23 (a) Thick stalks risk haemorrhage—think of sclerotherapy. (b) The distance to the closure mark indicates stalk size.

An over-enthusiastic but inexperienced assistant can 'cheese-wire' through the polyp stalk before adequate electrocoagulation by closing the snare handle completely and too forcibly; this is particularly likely to occur if the snare wire is thin or the polyp stalk is small. Most snare wires are made of reasonably thick braided wire and only thicker highly-vascular stalks present a real risk in this respect. To avoid it, make a mark on the snare handle to indicate where it should have reached when the loop is snugged tight by snaring a small object such as a match and use an indelible marker to register this position (Fig. 10.23b). If in doubt the endoscopist himself should be responsible for snare closure, especially for small polyps. When first using an electrosurgical unit, start with the lowest dial setting and work up with bursts of 2–3 seconds at each setting. Discover the lowest dial setting which will cause visible electrocoagulation in the smallest 'stalk' of meat, and compare this with the ferocious effect of using a very high setting—the resected part can become fused by the heat back onto its stalk, making it difficult to see when severance has occurred. Note also the possibility of causing desiccation and the resulting mechanical difficulty of achieving section.

Develop a standard routine or drill for each polypectomy and thereafter stick to it, checking each connection, the plate position and the unit dial setting before starting. Before polypectomy, try to assess whether the stalk is thin and soft—when low power should suffice—or whether the stalk is thicker when it may prove necess-

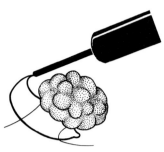

Fig. 10.24 Backward snaring is sometimes useful.

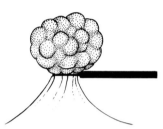

Fig. 10.25 Usually snare at the narrowest part of the stalk.

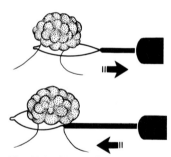

Fig. 10.26 To avoid the loop pulling off during snare closure push the loop against the stalk *before* closing.

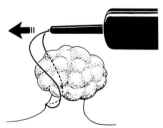

Fig. 10.27 To disengage a trapped snare, push it upstream over the polyp head.

ary to use higher power for a longer time. Visual assessment of stalk size can be difficult due to the distorting effect of the wide-angle endoscope lens; comparing stalk size to the 2-mm width of the protruded plastic snare sheath and pushing it around to assess its length and mobility can be helpful.

For single-handed snaring, open the snare loop within the instrument channel, so that on protruding the snare the loop opens spontaneously without needing to use the handle. Rotatable snares usually prove to be a disappointment in practice, since they are only fully torque-stable when the instrument is straight, whereas problem polypectomies usually occur when the tip is angled and the loop will not respond predictably.

Lassoing a polyp head efficiently takes practice. It is usually best to have the plastic sheath of the snare protruding a few millimetres into the field of view, then to open the loop fully, and after this to manoeuvre only with the instrument controls or shaft so that the snare loop is placed over the polyp head almost entirely by manipulation of the endoscope. It may help to open the snare in the colon beyond the polyp, and then to pull the colonoscope slowly back until the polyp head comes into the field of view and into the open loop. Alternatively, the loop can be pushed backwards over a difficult polyp head (Fig. 10.24), or even rotated laterally over it by appropriate movements of the instrument.

Ideally, the snare loop should be closed near the top of the stalk at its narrowest part, providing a short segment of normal tissue to help in pathological interpretation (Fig. 10.25). With longer stalks—especially if there is any suspicion of malignancy—it may be possible and desirable to snare lower down. Before closing the loop, make sure that the sheath of the snare is pushed against the stalk (push technique), which ensures that the loop will tighten exactly at that point; if the sheath is not pushed, the action of closing the loop may simply pull the wire off the polyp head (Fig. 10.26) unless the sheath is simultaneously advanced (pull technique). If there is any doubt that the snare is properly over the polyp head, try shaking the snare or opening and closing the loop repeatedly so as to help it to slip down around the stalk, angling the colonoscope tip in the relevant direction even if this means losing a proper view. Initial snare closure should be gentle; it may be in the wrong place and once the wire has cut into polyp tissue it may be difficult to release and reposition. If a snare loop does get stuck in the wrong position or if it becomes apparent that the polyp cannot be safely transected, releasing the snare loop is made easier if it is lifted up over the polyp head and pushed upstream—with the whole colonoscope if necessary (Fig. 10.27). Alternatively, if the loop is completely trapped, a second small-diameter instrument (gastroscope or paediatric colonoscope) can be inserted alongside the first scope and the biopsy forceps used to coax the trapped wire free. Remember that it is possible (depending on type) either to dismantle the snare or to sacrifice it by cutting it with wire cutters, withdrawing the colonoscope and leaving the loop *in situ*. Either the polyp head will fall off or another attempt can be made with a new snare or, if necessary, a different endoscopist.

Problem polyps

Large polyps

Having appreciated the principles of current density in electro-coagulation it should be obvious why removal of large sessile polyps (Fig. 10.28a) or broad-stalked polyps presents problems to the endoscopist. Fortunately, many so-called 'sessile' polyps are simply semi-pedunculated and can be pulled up by the snare onto an adequate and compressible pseudo-stalk. Other larger lesions can be removed in small pieces, whilst the technique of adrenaline injection or sclerotherapy of the stalk removes much of the risk of transecting thick stalks (see below).

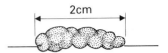

Fig. 10.28 (a) Sessile polyps can be risky to snare in one portion . . .

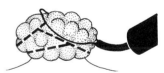

Having snared a polyp, the closed snare should always be moved to and fro; if the mucosa moves, but not the bowel wall, there is no danger that the full thickness of the wall has been 'tented' (Fig. 10.28b); whereas, if the colon moves too, the snare should be repositioned to take only a smaller part. If a polyp base is > 1.5 cm in diameter, without a stalk, the safe course is to take the head 'piecemeal' in a number of bits (Fig. 10.29), each of which will cut through with no risk of full-thickness burn and little risk of bleeding since the vessels of the head are much smaller than those in the stalk. Sometimes a sessile polyp is better removed by surgery, but this must be a matter of opinion and clinical judgement; sessile polyps up to 5-cm diameter can be removed, providing that the hazards and the trauma involved are appreciated by all concerned and that the endoscopist is very experienced. It is better to make repeated piecemeal attempts at different sessions to lessen the chance of full-thickness heat damage to the bowel wall, to give time for histological assessment (surgery will be indicated if any piece contains malignancy) and to allow the site to be checked for recurrent polyp tissue. The endoscopic approach is the obvious one in a patient who is a bad operative risk and prepared to accept repeated endoscopy. In a younger patient, or if there are technical difficulties, it may be better sometimes to admit that the risks of surgery are not excessive compared to the trials of aggressive endoscopy, which may not remove all neoplastic tissue, or laser which destroys the evidence.

(b) . . . because 'tenting' results.

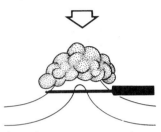

Fig. 10.29 Piecemeal removal is safer (although less satisfactory for the pathologist).

During snaring of a large-stalked polyp, the head will flop about, inevitably touching the bowel wall in several places. 'Leak' currents flow at each point of contact which results in inefficient heating of the stalk (Fig. 10.30) and the possibility of a 'contra-lateral burn'—often out of the field of view. The burn hazard is more theoretical than real but the possibility can be reduced by moving the whole polyp around during coagulation so that no one point gets all the heat, or by making sure that the area of point contact is larger than that of the stalk. During a difficult poly-pectomy of a large polyp, try to keep a view of the snared stalk and

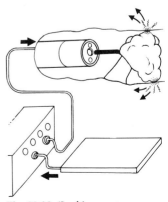

Fig. 10.30 'Leak' current can result in contralateral burns.

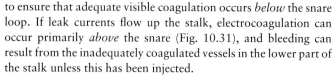

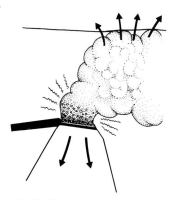

Fig. 10.31 A large area of contact reduces risk of contralateral burn, but also reduces current flow and heat coagulation in the lower stalk.

to ensure that adequate visible coagulation occurs *below* the snare loop. If leak currents flow up the stalk, electrocoagulation can occur primarily *above* the snare (Fig. 10.31), and bleeding can result from the inadequately coagulated vessels in the lower part of the stalk unless this has been injected.

It is wise to keep asking the patient if there is any pain, since full-thickness heating of the bowel wall causes slight immediate peritoneal pain, as a warning symptom before there is any serious risk of damage. If pain occurs and deflation does not remove it (it is easy to over-insufflate during a problematic examination) the procedure should be abandoned until another session at least 3 weeks later—when healing should have occurred and the area can be properly assessed. Large sessile polyps in the rectum within 12 cm of the anal verge are better and more safely removed by local proctological techniques under anaesthesia, so as to allow anal dilatation and a two-handed approach, including ligature and suture if necessary. Partial electrocoagulation of such rectal polyps by the endoscopist forms scar tissue which greatly complicates the method of sub-mucosal adrenaline injection and scissor excision used by skilled proctologists.

Stalk injection

Pre-injection or sclerotherapy of thick stalks, before snaring and snare transection, has revolutionized the endoscopist's approach to large polyps and effectively removes the risk of causing uncontrollable immediate or delayed haemorrhage. The technique is exceedingly easy and requires only judgement as to whether adrenaline alone should be used, or adrenaline + sclerotherapy solution. Adrenaline (1–10 ml 1:10 000 dilution in 0.9–1.8%) used alone is entirely safe but short-lived in effects and is employed for short broad stalks (Fig. 10.32), some sessile polyps and for any bleeding point. For long-stalked polyps, adding sclerosant solution (ethanolamine, sodium tetradecyl sulphate or ethoxysclerol) in equal volume to adrenaline 1:10 000 dilution but employing only 1 ml injection causes aggressive local vascular coagulation and

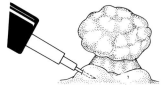

Fig. 10.32 (a) Inject broad-stalked polyps with adrenaline before snaring to avoid bleeding.

oedema in the stalk, with longer term effects which should remove the risk of delayed haemorrhage. Using sclerosant in addition to adrenaline, however, introduces the possible risk of bowel wall damage, peritonism or perforation; sclerosant *is only indicated for long stalks, 1 cm or more in diameter*, where the risks of haemorrhage would otherwise be significant. Using adrenaline alone, the solution is injected at one or more sites into the base of the polyp and causes visible blanching from vessel contraction within a minute or so; employing isotonic or slightly hypertonic saline slows dissipation from the site. Because some leakage frequently occurs, it is helpful to add a drop of methylene blue to the injection solution so that any efflux is obvious and the needle can be re-inserted elsewhere. The actual injection should be slow, the assistant feeling tissue resistance during successful infiltration—compared to no resistance during leakage. The endoscopist sees a blue stain

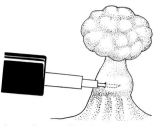

(b) For long-stalk polyps with a risk of bleeding inject sclerosant and adrenaline.

(if methylene blue is used), then blanching and swelling of the stalk and finally mauve coloration of the ischaemic head. Transection can then be made through the upper part of the stalk or above the injected area in the certain knowledge that there will be no bleeding at all; a relatively high-power current is therefore appropriate and perfectly safe. The injection sclerotherapy technique is useful in any patient where polypectomy must be undertaken in the presence of coagulopathy or anti-coagulation.

Recovery of very large polyps

Polyps of ⩾3 cm in diameter can be difficult to extract through the anus and may become fragmented if excessive traction is needed on the snare or retrieval forceps. Getting the patient to bear down 'as if to pass wind' at the same time as traction is applied may help relaxation of the sphincters (cover the perineal area to avoid explosive surprises!). Having the patient squat on the floor is more natural and physiological if withdrawal fails in the left lateral recumbent position; the minor embarrassment of this manoeuvre is well worth while for the rapid delivery that invariably results. Alternatively, a split-overtube can be inserted into the rectum over the colonoscope, the polyp pulled into the end of the tube and the whole assembly removed together. If for some reason the polyp is dropped in the rectum, the alternative is to use a large rigid proctoscope and tissue-grasping/sponge-holding forceps to grab the polyp and pull it and the instrument out together (for removal of piecemeal fragments see p. 235).

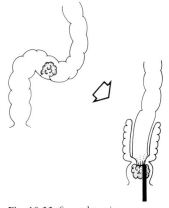

Fig. 10.33 Snare-loop intus-susception can be used for very large polyps in the distal sigmoid.

Pull-down technique

The largest broad-stalked polyps are found in the sigmoid colon; before attempting or abandoning a hazardous polypectomy, the technique of pull-down or snare-loop intussusception deserves consideration. Polyps situated in the mid-sigmoid colon at 30–35 cm from the anus occasionally present spontaneously to the anus and can be snared and pulled down by snare-loop intus-susception (Fig. 10.33) for local removal by a colorectal surgeon under general anaesthesia, providing that there are no peri-colic adhesions (diverticular disease, pelvic surgery, etc). The home-made snare (Fig. 10.34) is ideal for this purpose, since the braided wire is thick and unlikely to cut through the polyp stalk and there is no handle; if only a commercial snare is available wire cutters will be needed to cut the wire and outer below the handle with operation and fixation using haemostat forceps. After snaring the stalk, the colonoscope is pulled back, guiding the polyp head around any tight bends to the recto-sigmoid junction. At this point the colonoscope is withdrawn leaving the snare *in situ* and held closed with an artery forceps. Providing the polyp head can be just felt by a palpating finger, the technique will be successful, the extra pelvic relaxation of general anaesthesia allowing it to be delivered to the anus. The patient is anaesthetized with muscle relaxants;

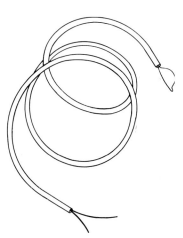

Fig. 10.34 Home-made (handleless) snare.

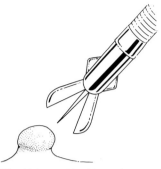

Fig. 10.35 (a) Hot-biopsy forceps grasp the small polyp and pull up . . .

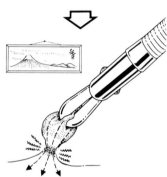

(b) . . . coagulate until 'snow on Mount Fuji' . . .

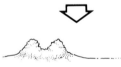

(c) . . . then pull off the biopsy leaving the base coagulated.

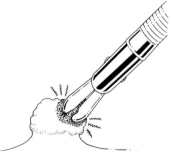

Fig. 10.36 Local burning at the forceps means the base is too large for hot biopsy.

gentle traction brings the polyp down to the dilated anus where it is grasped, locally excised and sutured.

Small polyps—'hot biopsy'

During colonoscopy, often in patients with larger polyps to be snared, it is common to see one or more tiny polyps (2–5 mm diameter) which are below the normal resolution of the radiologist. Tiny polyps are just as awkward to snare as larger ones, and can be difficult to retrieve, even using the filtered polyp suction trap. There has therefore been a tendency for some endoscopists to ignore small polyps or to describe them as 'metaplastic/hyperplastic', wrongly inferring that small polyps have no neoplastic potential. On biopsy, 70% of such small polyps prove to be adenomas, and only around 10% of those in the colon (as opposed to the rectum) are hyperplastic/metaplastic. Small polyps in the colon should therefore be destroyed or removed on sight. The best method is to use 'hot-biopsy' forceps (Fig. 10.35a). These are biopsy forceps with an electrically insulated plastic sheath, connected to the electrosurgical unit. The patient is placed on the return plate and connections made as for polypectomy, a similar coagulation power setting being used as for snaring of a medium-sized polyp (15–25 W equivalent). The polyp or part of its head is grasped in the jaws of the forceps, and the colonoscope is then angled or withdrawn slightly to pull up the grasped polyp onto a 'pseudo-pedicle' like a small mountain (Fig. 10.35b). Ensure that the black insulating plastic of the forceps is visible, so that the metal parts of the jaws do not contact the endoscope. Next apply the coagulating current for around 2–3 seconds; since the pseudo-pedicle is the narrowest part, it will heat and coagulate (Fig. 10.35b). The extent of this coagulation is easily seen as whitening, which should only spread just over half-way down the mountain—like snow on Mount Fuji—enough to destroy the narrow neck of tissue under the polyp but not involving the bowel wall significantly. Pull off the biopsy at this point in the knowledge that, even if some of the head is left uncoagulated, basal tissue and blood vessels will have been destroyed (10.35c).

Providing that a high enough power setting is used to finish coagulation in around 2–3 seconds, the heat produced in the basal tissues will not conduct back to the metal parts of the forceps and the biopsy specimen protected within the jaws is therefore unharmed with successful histology being achieved in at least 95% of cases. Polyps > 5–7 mm in diameter are not suitable for this technique using standard forceps, since the base will be broader than the area of contact of the forceps; only a small burn will therefore result at the surface of the polyp (Fig. 10.36) and there will be inadequate damage of the base. Alternatively, especially if little appears to be happening during hot biopsy, the current fanning out from the point of contact of the hot-biopsy forceps with a too-large polyp will heat tissue at a distance—invisibly and dangerously

(Fig. 10.37). Coagulating for too long or attempting to destroy too-large polyps with the hot-biopsy technique risks full thickness heating or perforation (especially in the proximal colon or small intestine) and increases the possibility of delayed haemorrhage by damaging larger sub-mucosal vessels. If a polyp proves to be too large for rapid and localized hot-biopsy electrocoagulation *stop*, take the biopsy, and remove the rest of the tissue by conventional snare polypectomy. Only polyps 2–5-mm diameter which 'neck' easily are suitable for the hot-biopsy technique and all polyps larger than this should be snared.

The complications of hot biopsy should be few if the principles described above are applied with common sense. A few perforations have occurred, presumably due to over-coagulation. On the other hand, inadequate coagulation heats and vasodilates the area locally and bleeding can result—immediate or delayed. Apart from a few delayed haemorrhages at 24–72 hours, we have had no complications from use of the hot-biopsy technique on over 3000 patients. By restricting hot biopsy *only* to small polyps which pull up to a satisfactory narrow neck and then coagulate locally and rapidly, changing back to snare polypectomy for all others, we have had no recent bleeds.

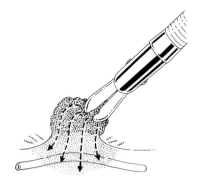

Fig. 10.37 Current fanning out from the point of contact will heat (invisibly) at a distance—risking delayed bleeding or perforation in polyps too large for hot biopsy.

Multiple polyps

Fortunately 90% of polyp patients have only one or two polyps; it is very uncommon to find more than five polyps unless the patient has polyposis coli (in which case prophylactic surgery is needed). Some multiple polyps (metaplastic/hyperplastic, Peutz–Jeghers, juvenile, lymphoid, lipomatous, or inflammatory) are not neoplastic, so that it may sometimes be preferable to await results of standard biopsies before undertaking heroics.

In the rare circumstance that a patient has six or more polyps, it is essential to examine the whole colon before snaring to be certain that other smaller polyps are not present. Very careful inspection is necessary; the most accurate method is to use a fine spray of surface dye (such as washable blue fountain-pen ink 20% or indigo-carmine 0.2%) (p. 46) which will emphasize any small polyps as white islands on a blue background and facilitate accurate biopsy. If histology shows adenomas, an unexpected diagnosis of polyposis can be made. The dye-spray technique is also invaluable in excluding polyposis coli in members of a known polyposis family.

Snaring and retrieving multiple polyps is tedious since it means passing the colonoscope several times, but this is preferable to surgery and can be facilitated using a split-overtube (see above). Ideally, the polyps are snared and removed from above distally, keeping a careful map of the location of each one. Smaller polyps can be hot biopsied or snared and aspirated through the suction line into a mucus trap (Fig. 10.38) or the newer filtered polyp suction trap (Fig. 10.39) which, by rotating to the appropriate position, ensures that each polyp is trapped in a separate small

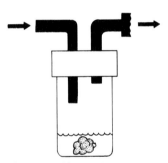

Fig. 10.38 Obstetric/bronchoscopic sputum trap.

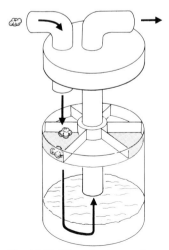

Fig. 10.39 Filtered polyp suction trap.

chamber whilst removing all excess fluid. When an overtube has been used or if a split-overtube is inserted, the colonoscope can be withdrawn with one or more polyps and re-inserted easily. In the absence of an overtube and if colonoscopy has been too difficult to justify repeated withdrawal and re-insertion of the instrument, an unsatisfactory compromise is to retrieve the larger or more sinister-looking polyps, having destroyed or snared the others. With all the removed polyps withdrawn to the descending colon or below, the colonoscope is passed back proximal to the splenic flexure and 500–1500 ml of warm tap water syringe-injected through the instrument channel so as to wash them distally. The proximal colon is then gently air-insufflated until the patient feels minor distension, the colonoscope is withdrawn from the anus and a disposable or phosphate enema administered on the endoscopy table so that the patient should pass most of the polyps or polyp fragments into a commode within a few minutes.

Malignant polyps

It is sometimes not obvious at the time of snaring that a polyp is malignant. Malignancy may be suspected if a polyp is irregular, ulcerated, firm or has a particularly thick stalk; firmness to palpation is probably the best single discriminant. If malignancy is possible, it is important to be certain that transection has been made low down the stalk (to give the pathologist a proper assessment) and that all visible polyp tissue has been removed, but without risking perforation. The endoscopist should report whether or not the polyp has been completely removed. If necessary, an early repeat examination can be taken, preferably within 2 weeks since at a longer interval there may be no visible ulcer to indicate the polypectomy site.

Because of the possibility of malignancy, each polyp must be retrieved and identified separately on an anatomical polyp map. It is inadequate to say that a polyp was removed at '70 cm from the anus' since this might represent mid-sigmoid colon or caecum. 'Tattooing', using India ink injected intramucosally at the time of polypectomy, is an excellent way to mark the site of a suspicious or partially removed polyp. Sterile black ink (either a sterile carbon particle suspension or autoclaved 20% dilution of commercial drawing ink) is injected using a long sclerotherapy needle inserted flat just under the mucosal surface (Fig. 10.40). Since some leakage often occurs, resulting in near 'black out', polypectomy and retrieval of specimens should be complete before tattooing. A permanent blue–grey stain is left, which makes follow-up inspection very easy.

When a stalked polyp is reported as malignant by the pathologist, the clinician or the endoscopist is faced with a dilemma. If the cancer is of 'low' or 'moderate' grade of malignancy, or 'well' or 'averagely well' differentiated and confined to the head or upper part of the stalk with a margin of at least 3 mm above the electrocoagulated tissue at the transection line, most experts would

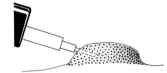

Fig. 10.40 A 1-ml India ink tattoo marks a polypectomy site permanently.

not recommend surgery, providing that endoscopic removal also appeared complete. The likelihood of resectable metastases under these circumstances is extremely small, whereas the mortality of surgery is significant. However, if the polyp was sessile or if invasion extends histologically to the resection line, involves lymphatic vessels or is poorly differentiated (anaplastic), most would favour operation unless the patient is a poor surgical risk. Judgement is involved, balancing risks and clinical factors. It may be difficult not to operate in a young patient, mainly for emotional reasons. In older patients the decision is not so obvious; very few patients have been found at operation to have locally involved lymph nodes but some with no residual cancer have died as a result of unnecessary surgery.

Complications of polypectomy

The most frequent complication is bleeding, which is usually visible immediately after section. Bleeding should occur in < 1–2% of polypectomies, the previous problems with haemorrhage from large polyp stalks having been largely removed by the technique of injection sclerotherapy. Secondary haemorrhage may occur 1–14 days after polypectomy, particularly after removal of large-stalked polyps or use of hot biopsy on too-large polyps. Patients who have had polypectomy should know of the possibility of delayed bleeding and the unlikely possibility of needing to report to an emergency department for observation. Delayed haemorrhage normally stops spontaneously but transfusion may occasionally be required.

Immediate haemorrhage is usually a slow ooze but can be an arterial spurt of frightening proportions as viewed endoscopically. Every possible attempt should be made to stop an arterial bleed *immediately*—either by quickly re-snaring the remaining stalk or by immediate injection, using a sclerotherapy needle, of up to 5–10 ml of 1:10 000 adrenaline solution sub-mucosally or into any residual stalk. If the stalk has been re-snared, simple strangulation alone with taping of the snare handle for 10–15 min is usually sufficient, without further electrocoagulation. If bleeding recurs on releasing the snare, attempts to stop it can be made with further electrocoagulation or by injection, if necessary using a second instrument (paediatric colonoscope or gastroscope) passed up alongside the first. In the unlikely event that arterial bleeding persists in spite of all efforts, the most elegant solution is to perform selective arterial catheterization and embolization or infusion of pitressin (success has been reported using pitressin or somatostatin by intravenous infusion alone). A surgical team must be alerted and adequate supplies of blood ensured. If venous oozing has occurred and the source is not immediately obvious, the most effective action is to infuse large volumes of ice-water containing adrenaline (5 ml 1:10 000 adrenaline per 50 ml water) in the region of the bleeding. This helps to prevent formation of clots, which are impossible to aspirate and, with posturing to the right side if necessary to visualize the distal colon, should allow location of the polypectomy site. Persistent or secondary haemorrhage in the left colon will be indicated by repeated calls to stool and the passage of fresh clots, whereas in the right colon the rate of bleeding is more difficult to assess because of the long delay before volumes of altered blood are expelled.

Frank perforation with an electrosurgical snare is fortunately a rare occurrence. Full thickness heat damage to the bowel wall, also called 'post-polypectomy syndrome' or 'closed perforation', is an occasional sequel to a difficult polypectomy such as piecemeal removal of a sessile polyp. The patient experiences localized abdominal pain and fever for 12–24 hours following polypectomy, without free gas on X-ray or sign of generalized peritonitis. This is due to inflammatory reaction of the peritoneum and is followed by adherence to omentum or small bowel; it is therefore self-limiting. Conservative management with bed-rest and systemic antibiotics is indicated, but surgical advice is wise, especially if the symptoms and signs do not abate rapidly.

Safety

It cannot be over-emphasized that polypectomy is potentially hazardous and that rigorous adherence to all possible safety factors is essential. Assuming that the correct equipment has been acquired it must be carefully handled and maintained. Never bend or coil the connecting leads tightly or they will fracture; if a lead looks or feels partially fractured, replace it or have it mended at once. If polypectomy is not proceeding according to plan, check the connections, patient plate and circuitry before anything else.

As already explained the greatest single safety factor lies in a strict routine regularly repeated for each polypectomy, because human error is much more likely than failure of the equipment. A military-type approach has much to commend it: any request from the endoscopist being repeated out loud by the assistant so that each knows what the other is doing. The assistant and the endoscopist must check on each other to watch that all is in order during the procedure, having checked the equipment (including marking the snare handle at the point of closure) beforehand.

The endoscopist must see that the bowel preparation of the patient is adequate to give a good view and a dry field in which to work. If bowel preparation is poor (most likely during flexible sigmoidoscopy), either use carbon dioxide instead of air (because of the important possibility of methane/hydrogen explosive mixtures) or take great care to insufflate and then aspirate repeatedly to dilute any gas present. In a well-prepared bowel (other than with mannitol) there is no explosion hazard and air can be safely used (see caveat on mannitol bowel preparation, p. 165).

Ideally, patient medication with aspirin, non-steroidal anti-inflammatory agents and other medications affecting platelet adhesion will be withdrawn 5 days before, and for 14 days after, the procedure to minimize the risk of delayed haemorrhage. Only a very experienced operator should undertake polypectomy in a patient on anticoagulants, the patient being warned of the need for immediate repeat endoscopy should bleeding occur.

Current leakage through the endoscope (to the patient or operator) can be avoided by attaching a bypass lead or 'safety cord' between the patient plate and a metal part of the endoscope (normally close to its insertion into the light source). Such leakage currents present an insignificant hazard at the power levels used in polypectomy, and any endoscope can be used for electrosurgery without bypass. Wearing rubber gloves (removing the large contact area of the bare hands on the endoscope) theoretically risks a minute burn on the eyebrow if the endoscopist activates the unit and pulls the snare wire into contact with the metal tip of a non-bypassed instrument, but there is no danger.

Polypectomy outside the colon

Although the principles and techniques described refer primarily to polypectomy in the colon, they are essentially the same as for gastric polypectomy or polypectomy in the small intestine and the same rules can be followed. There may be a higher risk of bleeding when snaring polyps in the stomach and duodenum. Where feasible pre-injection of adrenaline before snaring is a wise routine and we give H_2-antagonists for 1 week afterwards. Snare-loop biopsy (Ménétrièr's disease, etc.) is particularly useful in the stomach but some caution is needed since it is easy to take a much bigger bite than intended when using a wide-angled instrument in a large viscus.

Gastric polyps are easily lost after snaring so that antispasmodics and a quick eye and hand are desirable. Small gastric polyps are not so easy to destroy using 'hot-biopsy' forceps, apparently because the thickness of the gastric mucosa stops it 'tenting up' into the necessary narrow pseudo-pedicle. The wall of the duodenum and small intestine is thin and there is a corresponding need for caution in snaring and electrosurgery.

Other therapeutic procedures

Balloon dilatation

Balloon dilatation of short colonic strictures, particularly anastomotic narrowings due to sepsis or inflammatory change, has been made easy by 'through the scope' (TTS) balloons made of non-distensible polyethylene (as used in the upper GI tract). Balloons of at least 18 mm diameter should be used whenever possible and those 5-cm long are easiest to 'dumb-bell' in a stricture, whereas 3-cm balloons slip out of the narrowing on inflation. Because of the length of colonoscopes and their looping tendency, it is particularly important that any TTS balloon has been completely deflated and silicone-lubricated before insertion, and the instrument shaft should be straightened as much as possible to enable the balloon to be pushed through without force. Balloons should always be fluid-distended, using either water or dilute contrast material. Remember that small syringes (5–10 ml) exert the greatest pressure, whereas large syringes (50 ml) evacuate the balloon most efficiently.

Colonic strictures are frequently found at an angulation, which may make passage of a balloon difficult. There can therefore be a place for initial passage of a flexible guidewire followed by a suitable balloon. In the left colon, endoscopic insertion of a guidewire can be followed either by a balloon or bougie. Dilators can be used under fluoroscopic control (or if a balloon is being used), with the instrument also inserted for visual control.

Tube placement

Colonoscopic placement of drainage tubes or recording devices is possible as far as the ileo-caecal region, ideally with an internal removable stiffening wire to stop early tube displacement. The technique is particularly important in prolonged post-operative ileus or episodic 'pseudo-obstruction' of the colon (Ogilvie's syndrome), where endoscopic deflation avoids the need for surgery. The easiest technique is the 'piggy back' method in which a loop attached to the leading end of the tube is grasped by forceps (Fig. 10.41). A variation which allows better suction during the procedure (the colon may be unprepared and foul) is to use a thin loop of cotton thread at the end of the tube, held by a loop of strong monofilament nylon passed through the suction channel; once in the proximal colon a sharp tug on the nylon breaks the cotton loop and the tube is free.

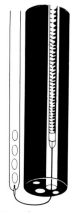

Fig. 10.41 Deflation tube carried up alongside colonoscope.

De-rotation of volvulus

If passage of a rectal tube will not deflate a sigmoid volvulus and allow it to de-rotate, the colonoscope can be passed as a steerable flatus tube. Large-channel 'therapeutic' colonoscopes allow a deflation tube (with a stiffening guidewire) to be inserted through the instrumentation channel. After the tube or endoscope tip is passed gently into or through the twisted segment, deflation alone is usually sufficient for the torsion to reverse spontaneously; actual endoscopic manipulation is usually unnecessary. However, if the segment appears blue–black and gangrenous, surgery is indicated because of the high risk of perforation.

Use of the colonoscope to reduce intussusception in the proximal colon is generally unrewarding, because not enough inward push can be transmitted around the looped colon. Should reduction by X-ray contrast fail, it might be possible to combine an inflated balloon around the instrument tip with pressure-injection of diluted water-soluble contrast medium down the instrument channel.

Obliteration of angiodysplasia

The electrocoagulation of angiodysplasia has been mentioned previously. Since these occur mainly in the thin-walled proximal colon, great care should be taken with whichever modality is used—electrocoagulation (mono- or bi-polar), heater probe and especially laser. The object of the exercise is to damage the superficial part of the lesion, which extends also into the sub-mucosa, in such a way as both to coagulate the vessels nearest the surface (and most liable with trauma to result in superficial damage) and to cause re-epithelialization by normal mucosa. It is preferable to cause a ring of local heating points around the periphery of larger lesions, followed by one or more applications near the centre, rather than to apply excessive heat in one area alone (Fig. 10.42). Err on the side of too little heat; even minor whitening and oedema will progress to produce remarkable local ulceration within 24 hours. It is easy enough to repeat the examination a few weeks later to check results, but difficult to justify perforation from over-aggression during the first procedure. The careful use of hot-biopsy forceps is particularly effective with smaller lesions, which can be grasped, the mucosa tented up and selectively heated. It is unnecessary to take a biopsy, the jaws being simply re-opened after minimal visible coagulation. Larger lesions should be tackled last because mechanical trauma can cause them to bleed and obscure other lesions which may be present, and for the same reason the most dependent lesions are treated first. Protruberant cavernous haemangiomas (blue-rubber bleb naevus syndrome) are better managed by sclerotherapy.

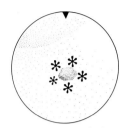

Fig. 10.42 Point coagulations around an angiodysplasia before heating the centre.

Tumour destruction

Use of laser photocoagulation to vaporize inoperable or obstructing tumour tissue in the recto-sigmoid is described in Chapter 5. A similar effect can be achieved, more laboriously but very cheaply, by multiple injections of 100% ethanol using a sclerotherapy needle, the procedure being repeated every day or two until the desired clearance is achieved. The use of a wire resectoscope loop, similar to that employed during transurethral prostatectomy, has also been described, under water or in air.

Further reading

Barlow, D. E. (1982) 'Endoscopic applications of electrosurgery: a review of basic principles'. *Gastrointestinal Endoscopy*, **28**, 73–76.

Cranley, J. P., Petras, R. E., Carey, W. D., Paradis, K. and Sivak, M. V. (1986) 'When is endoscopic polypectomy adequate therapy for colonic polyps containing invasive carcinoma?' *Gastroenterology*, **91**, 419–427.

Giardiello, F. M., Welsh, S. B., Hamilton, S. R. *et al.* (1987) 'Peutz-Jeghers syndrome: perhaps not so benign'. *New England Journal of Medicine*, **316**, 1511–1514.

Haggitt, R. C., Glotzbach, R. E., Soffer, E. E. and Wruble, L. D. (1985)

'Prognostic factors in colorectal carcinomas arising in adenomas: implications for lesions removed by endoscopic polypectomy'. *Gastroenterology,* **89**, 328–336.

Hoff, G. (1987) 'Colorectal polyps. Clinical implications: screening and cancer prevention'. *Scandinavian Journal of Gastroenterology,* **22**, 769–775.

Jass, J. R. (1989) 'Do all colorectal carcinomas arise in pre-existing adenomas?' *World Journal of Surgery,* **13**, 45–51.

Mathus-Vliegen, E. M. H. and Tytgat, G. N. J. (1986) 'Laser ablation and palliation in colorectal malignancy'. *Gastrointestinal Endoscopy,* **32**, 393–396.

Nivatvongs, S. (1986) 'Complications in colonoscopic polypectomy. An experience with 1555 polypectomies'. *Disease of the Colon and Rectum,* **29**, 825–830.

Wadas, D. D. and Sanowski, R. A. (1987) 'Complications of the hot biopsy forceps technique'. *Gastrointestinal Endoscopy,* **33**, 32–37.

Waye, J. D. (1987) 'Techniques of polypectomy—hot biopsy forceps and snare polypectomy'. *American Journal of Gastroenterology,* **82**, 615–618.

Waye, J., Geenen, J. and Fleischer, D. (1987) *Techniques in Therapeutic Endoscopy.* W.B. Saunders, Philadelphia.

Williams, C. B. and Price, A. B. (1987) 'Colon polyps and carcinoma', in *Gastroenterologic Endoscopy* (ed. Sivak, M. V. Jr), Chapter 45, pp. 921–945. W. B. Saunders, Philadelphia.

The Endoscopy Nurse/Assistant

11

Although a doctor has overall charge of an endoscopy unit, its success and safety is largely dependent on the main endoscopy assistant, usually a senior (head) nurse. She is there most, or all, of the time, and patients, relatives and other staff have more contact with her than anyone else. Her precise duties will depend on the number of nurses in the unit, on the volume of work and the presence of other support staff such as secretaries, technicians, radiographers, domestic staff and orderlies. In small units, an endoscopy nurse may find herself filling many roles. To cover holidays and illness any unit must have at least three nurses trained to take charge, with arrangements made for adequate replacement. It is essential to have two nurses in each endoscopy room (one 'technical', one 'patient') when complex and therapeutic procedures are being performed. Other nurses supervise reception and recovery of patients, and cleaning of the instruments. Large units with many rooms in action can function efficiently with some staffing economies because of the ability to overlap activities and adapt schedules to the staff available. The total staffing required is best assessed by using some form of relative value scale (Chapter 3), which reflects the complexity of procedures, rather than simply the total number.

Patient care

The primary role of an endoscopy nurse is to safeguard the patient before, during and after the procedure, as well as ensuring the highest technical and hygienic standards throughout. Modern endoscopy should be quick and atraumatic, but most patients are anxious and the nurse has a crucial role in explanation and reassurance. An endoscopy nurse should interview all patients prior to the procedure, both to reassure and to see that the preparation and other preliminaries are understood. For out-patients a personal explanation is more effective and supplements the written instructions (Chapter 13). Explanations should be reinforced when the patient arrives in the unit—where first impressions are particularly important. One of the nurse's main contributions is to ensure that the atmosphere is friendly and humane, and that the patient's valuables (including teeth and spectacles) and accompanying relatives are looked after. But there are very specific tasks concerning patient safety. The pre-procedure assessment includes checking:

(a) that preparatory instructions have been carried out;
(b) that appropriate medical records (and X-rays) are available;
(c) the list of current medications (especially anticoagulants and antidepressants);
(d) any history of allergy to medication (and iodine for ERCP);

243

(e) toleration of any previous endoscopy, and sedation;

(f) cardiac history which might warrant antibiotic prophylaxis against endocarditis;

(g) that informed consent has been obtained and documented;

(h) that there are appropriate transport arrangements.

The patient should not be allowed to enter the endoscopy room until everything is prepared, with instruments and accessories preferably concealed from view. The nurses supervise the checking and administration of medication. Doctors in a hurry may tend to give sedative drugs too quickly, with sudden and profound reactions.

During the procedure, the doctor is usually preoccupied with the endoscopic view. The nurse caring for the patient should keep a check on the patient's vital functions, particularly respiration (since respiratory depression is the first sign of over-sedation). Pulse oximeter monitoring has become standard and provides objective assessment.

Throughout the examination, the 'patient nurse' maintains a reassuring presence, aspirates secretions when relevant and must also be prepared for emergencies. Happily these are very rare, but many patients are frail and ill, especially those undergoing emergency procedures. For all complex procedures, the 'patient nurse' is complemented by a 'technical nurse' who manages all of the equipment and assists with biopsies, photographs and therapeutic devices.

After the examination, the patient (and belongings) must be delivered safely back to the recovery area and, if sedated, to the accompanying relative or friend—with relevant instructions for that day and any subsequent appointments. With in-patients, the nurse should ensure that ward staff are given details of the procedure, medication and appropriate after-care.

Nursing documentation

The patient nurse must keep some record of her safety activities. The extent of this documentation will vary in different units according to customs in the institution, and the wishes of the head nurse and endoscopy director. An example of a nursing record sheet is shown (Fig. 11.1). This 'flow sheet' is designed to cover the activities from the initial endoscopy request through preparation, procedure, recovery, and up to discharge from the unit. It becomes part of the patient's permanent record—just like an anaesthetic record.

Care of equipment

Endoscopy nurses are responsible for the care of much delicate and expensive equipment. Satisfactory cleaning and disinfectant procedures are of paramount importance, and are detailed in Chapter 12. Nurses also need to maintain a comprehensive register of all unit equipment, with details of repairs and replacements; repair bills are minimized by good maintenance. The chief nurse will

THE BEST HOSPITAL ENDOSCOPY UNIT

Name:

History number:

GI endoscopy flow chart

Birth date:

Doctor:

Appointment:

Request by: Date:

Phone number (H):
                              (W):

Procedure:

Procedure to be done by:

Clinic/Ward:

Problem:

Patient/Floor informed: Yes/No

Request approved by:

Prep given:

Previous GI procedures/Surgery (dates):

Risks

Allergies :   Iodine/Demerol/Antibiotics/Local anaesthetics

Other:

Cardiac: Surgery/Valves/Endocarditis: Needs antibiotics: Yes/No   Given: Yes/No

Chest/Renal/Diabetes/Infection/Glaucoma/Pregnant ?

Details

Medications: Anticoagulants/Antidepressants/Sedatives/Aspirin

Current:

Taken today:

Pre-procedure interview/Phone call: Date:

Comments: Signature/Title:

Weight: BP: Pulse: Resp:

Reviewed educational material:

Prep for procedure: Prep results:

Dentures/Loose teeth/Caps: PT: Hgb:

Travel arrangements: APTT: Hct:

Abd assessment: Consent signed: Yes/No

Comments: Special equipment anticipated:

                                     Signature/Title:

Fig. 11.1 A nursing record sheet (pre-procedure) (continued overleaf).

GI endoscopy nurse report

Patient name:

Procedure: Date:

Performed by: Scope number:

Time   Start: End:

i.v. started by unit/   Site: With: Fluids:

Assessment/Consent completed: Yes/No   Monitor attached: Yes/No

TIME	BP	PULSE	RESP	O_2S_{AT}	LOC	MEDICATIONS (dose in mg) Local anaesthetic spray	COMMENTS Yes/No

Biopsies taken: Yes/No   Number of containers: Cytology: Yes/No

Diathermy used: Yes/No   Ground plate location: Settings:

Photos: Yes/No   35 mm/Polaroid/Videotape

Comments:

Signature/Title:

POST-PROCEDURE

TIME	BP	PULSE	RESP	LOC	COMMENTS

LOC = Level of consciousness

6 = Fully awake
5 = Easily aroused
4 = Arousable, may be
    confused

3 = Aroused only by vigorous
    stimuli, cannot communicate
2 = Responds only to pain
1 = Unresponsive

Discharged to: Time: With:

Discharge instruction sheet given:

Comments:

Signature/Title:

Fig. 11.1 (*continued*) A nursing record sheet (procedure and post-procedure).

often provide the main interface with equipment manufacturers and suppliers.

Organization and standards

The head nurse is the main organizer of the unit and co-ordinator of its activities. Along with the secretarial and medical staff she will organize bookings and arrangements with other relevant departments (radiology, pathology, etc.). If there is no secretary in the unit, she will also have responsibility for records, photographs and videotape recordings.

The head nurse will play a major role in setting the routines and standards of the unit, and in insisting (tactfully) that they are maintained. This applies particularly in units which have trainees— who are often reluctant to display their ignorance. There are many examples of ways in which an alert nurse can protect the patient (and doctor).

1 Standards can slip in the checking and administration of drugs; when several different syringes are drawn up ready for use, the doctor may pick up the wrong one. Labels are helpful.

2 Allergies and drug interactions are hazardous, but the doctor can easily overlook a particular patient's current medication.

3 It is easy for doctors, between efforts to complete an examination, report on it and prepare for the next patient, to make errors in labelling specimens or report forms.

4 Inexperienced doctors may mishandle the equipment, insufflate too much air, or use force to pass unlubricated forceps down an acutely angled instrument; an experienced nurse can gently insist on correct technique.

5 Even an experienced endoscopist can fail to check electrical connections and settings during electrosurgery; the nurse should understand the procedure and notice the error.

6 The need for proper standards of hygiene is obvious, and applies to staff as well as to the instruments. The fact that sepsis is rare can lead to a sense of false security which the nurse must help combat (see Chapter 12).

There are many potential stresses and problems in an endoscopy unit; it can be just as busy and dramatic as an operating room, and often has far fewer staff. Sessions may start early or finish late, and busy periods may be interspersed with slack ones. Different doctors with varying personalities and habits will use the unit, and patients of all types will pass through it. Unit nurses have to accommodate all these changes of technique, tempo and temperament. Endoscopy nurses who combine all these virtues with good humour greatly enhance the efficiency and safety of the unit and complement the best efforts of the endoscopist.

Professional activities and training

Endoscopy nurses are a relatively new breed whose responsible position and technical expertise are underestimated in many institutions, as compared to the high standing of operating room staff. Both morale and skills can be maintained and developed by contacts with others in the field by visiting different units or participating in teaching meetings. Many countries welcome endoscopy nurses and assistants as associate members of the endoscopy society or group; others have professional associations specifically for endoscopy nurses and assistants. These associations are interesting for the individual, provide a forum for teaching, and help to set guidelines and standards for endoscopy practice. Endoscopists are well advised to enable and encourage their nursing staff to participate in such activities.

Further reading

Drossman, D. A. (1987) *Manual of Gastroenterology Procedures* (2nd edn). Raven Press, New York.

Revenscroft, M. M. and Swan, C. H. J. (1984) *Gastrointestinal Endoscopy and Related Procedures*. Chapman and Hall, London.

Cleaning and Disinfection   12

Whereas in the early years of flexible endoscopy there was some laxity of standards, there can be few endoscopists who are now unaware of the need for proper cleaning and disinfection of endoscopes and accessories—and all endoscopy units worthy of the name have adopted rigorous standards. The need to face up to laborious and time-consuming cleaning routines was forced by a combination of AIDS awareness, individual case reports of *Salmonella* transmission and the realization that catastrophic, sometimes fatal, septic cholangitis is a frequent complication of ERCP unless the highest standards are applied. Even if the endoscope itself has been properly disinfected, catastrophe can originate from bacterial colonization of the water bottle or inside the spiral wire of the biopsy forceps; even when instruments and accessories have been scrupulously managed the results are useless if a washing-machine water reservoir or the mains water supply itself proves to be contaminated with *Pseudomonas*.

Clearly, there is room for a little common sense. Use of sterile water, a fresh water bottle per patient and even disposable accessories may be of fundamental importance during ERCP, but may be overkill for a routine flexible sigmoidoscopy list. On the other hand, sick patients (especially if very young or very old) can be immunodepressed and at comparably increased risk to occult AIDS patients; others may be on immunosuppressive therapy after transplant, etc. Whereas certain procedures and certain patients are obviously at high risk, in a busy endoscopy practice the correct attitude is 'one standard for all', since it is impossible to identify either carriers of pathogenic bacteria or viruses or those who may be at an increased susceptibility to them. This is the principle behind the policy of 'universal precautions', in which high standards throughout are the routine so that everyone, staff and patients alike, knows that they are protected. We have always insisted on high standards of personal and professional hygiene, for aesthetic as well as purely medical reasons, especially now that others must be taught what is essential in modern endoscopy. What follows is a synthesis of the recommendations of UK and USA professional associations and represents a reasonable 1990 viewpoint. We realize that changes of materials, disinfectants and working practices may outdate these current views. For more detailed accounts the reader should consult other source material, in consultation with manufacturers' representatives and/or infection control experts who should regularly visit the unit.

Disinfection or sterilization?

Higher standards are needed in endoscopy than in a bar or restaurant because of the selective concentration in a clinical environment of risky organisms and at-risk patients. However, true 'sterilization', in the surgical sense of guaranteed destruction of all microbial life, including spores, is unachievable for flexible endoscopes and also unnecessary for examinations of the GI tract—in contrast to those that are intravascular or within closed body cavities, or for specific procedures such as biopsy or injection sclerotherapy where the mucosa is breached (with potential or actual access to the bloodstream). With equipment not suitable for autoclaving the aim is for 'high-level disinfection', sufficient to inactivate bacteria and viruses, which is much more easily achievable. Disinfectants are assessed on their 'log kill' capability on the basis that, for a given concentration, perhaps 99.9% of test organisms may be rapidly inactivated by the disinfectant whereas the remaining few may be more resistant. As a generalization, much of the effect of a disinfectant is in the first few seconds, with full clinical efficacy by a minute or two of exposure. 'Exposure' presumes chemical contact, which may be achieved in the test system but not in working practice if mucus, blood and other organic matter acts as a physical barrier, reacts chemically to neutralize the disinfectant or, as is often the case, a combination of both. Glutaraldehyde, for instance, reacts with organic matter, denaturing it into a hard impenetrable layer which protects underlying infective agents—hence the need for excellent preliminary mechanical and detergent cleaning.

'Infectivity' is an important parallel concept. For most infections such as hepatitis B or salmonellosis a substantial dose (probably many thousands) of the infective agent is needed to penetrate body defences and cause clinical illness. On the other hand introducing a single *Pseudomonas* organism into the perfect culture medium of a stagnant biliary system could theoretically achieve colonization and cholangitis. Infectivity is also the experimental gold standard for assessing the success or failure of a disinfection regime; since this requires a suitable animal model (for viruses, often chimpanzees) it is not surprising that literature data are extremely thin and the disinfectant concentrations or exposure times employed may be significantly different from those in normal medical use. The 'recommendations' for disinfectant exposure are therefore based on a body of expert clinical, bacteriological and virological experience, with an extra 'safety factor' deliberately built in. Concentrations (up to 2% in the case of glutaraldehyde) and time of exposure (4–5 min for glutaraldehyde) are such as to give a high probability that even partially-inactivated disinfectant reaching some areas with difficulty will still be effective. Most infective agents, with the notable exception of mycobacterial spores, are rather easily inactivated; reassuringly, the AIDS virus is extremely sensitive to disinfectants and even hepatitis B virus (contrary to early reports) no more resistant than representative bacteria.

The choice of disinfectant is inevitably constrained by the materials used in endoscope construction, particularly the delicate silicone rubber covering of the bending section, the bonding agents used in lens mounting and elsewhere, and the waterproofing rubber seals in the control head. Even in this respect there is some latitude; for instance short (3–4 min) repeated exposure of the bending section to 70% ethyl alcohol is reported to have no damaging effect during thousands of test immersions, whereas long continued exposure is damaging. As various alternative cleaning or disinfecting agents become available there is a need for manufacturers to assess them and validate their use. However, since slightly different materials may be used it can be difficult to get general agreement from all manufacturers.

Accessories

Disinfection of accessories is essential, with particular attention to those which are used parenterally and especially if their design makes access for cleaning and disinfectant solutions difficult. For metal and heat-resistant plastic or Teflon accessories there is a clear advantage in using standard steam autoclave procedures for sterilization. In high-risk situations in which this full sterilization is essential (such as variceal sclerotherapy or interventional biliary therapy), and whenever equipment can be relatively cheaply manufactured, disposable products are increasingly employed so as to avoid the significant time, tedium, staff risks and uncertainty involved in cleaning re-usable accessories.

Mechanical cleaning

Thorough cleaning to remove all blood, mucus, other body secretions or organic debris is the first and main essential in the disinfection process so that the chemical agent(s) subsequently employed can penetrate for effective bacterial or viral inactivation. Detergents of any kind, but especially enzyme detergents, are useful in removing organic matter and blood, both in areas which can be reached for brushing, swabbing or other methods of physical cleaning and for perfusing the inaccessible parts such as the air and water channels of an endoscope. Non-foaming domestic enzyme detergents can be used in endoscope washing machines. Accessories, which include the air/water and suction buttons, tooth guard, water bottles and the cleaning brushes, themselves must all be similarly scrupulously cleaned. Fuller details are given below.

Water supply

Excellence of the water supply should not be assumed. Surprisingly large particles can be passed, with potential to contribute to endoscope channel blockage or to clog the filters of a washing machine; various in-line water filters are available, from those that

remove only larger foreign bodies to true bacterial filters producing a sterile water supply. This can be of critical importance, for
the water supply or its pipework can become the source of
Pseudomonas contamination, rendering useless during the final
rinse of an instrument all the careful disinfection which has gone
before.

Disinfectants

Glutaraldehyde

Glutaraldehyde (2% alkaline solution) or related products consti-
tute the only disinfectant which can currently be globally recommended for endoscopic use. It destroys all viruses and bacteria
within 4 min, is non-corrosive and has a low surface tension which
helps penetration. Glutaraldehyde is however related chemically to
formaldehyde and has similar toxic qualities on human skin
and mucous membranes, with the capability of causing severe
dermatitis, sinusitis or asthma. Unless closed-system washing
machines and excellent ventilation/extraction systems are used,
there is a serious risk of sensitization of nursing staff, the risk
increasing with increasing levels and time of exposure. Heavy
domestic-grade rubber gloves should be worn when using glutaraldehyde since normal thin medical glove material is permeable to
it, and goggles and/or a face mask can protect against splashes.

Second-line disinfectants

The British Society of Gastroenterology recommendations recognize that, mainly in those units where poor past practice or
individual idiosyncrasy has led to glutaraldehyde sensitization,
there may need to be an alternative 'second-line' dinsinfection
regime. No alternative single disinfectant can be recommended as
being bactericidal, viricidal and compatible with endoscopic
instrumentation, but a bactericidal detergent for 2 min, followed
by a 70% ethyl alcohol soak for 4 min (ethyl alcohol is more
viricidal than isopropyl) is accepted as an effective alternative
regime.

The drying properties of alcohol are also made use of in the
suggestion that, as well as the outside of a previously disinfected
endoscope being wiped with an alcohol swab, the air, water and
suction channels should be perfused with 70% alcohol before
storage (then air-dried again). This removes any residual water,
which otherwise leads to a risk of bacterial re-growth when the
endoscope is stored overnight. Hang instruments upright in a
well-ventilated cupboard; in no circumstances should the trans-
portation suitcase be used for storage between examinations,
because its absorbent lining cannot be disinfected and the closed,
potentially moist, atmosphere inside can encourage growth of
micro-organisms.

Although alcohol perfusion before storage and re-use of the

scope 'from the cupboard' has not been sanctioned in the UK as an alternative to repeating the full disinfection regime before an endoscopy list, this simplified practice has been validated in respected units over many years without laboratory evidence of bacterial re-growth (viruses cannot multiply in isolation). We consider it safe to re-use a gastroscope or colonoscope after disinfection and overnight storage, but disinfect again after weekend storage. ERCP scopes are disinfected before every use.

Staff protection

The need to avoid splashes of disinfectant, and also of blood or body fluids, is obvious. Opinions differ on the need for protective clothing between those who change completely and endoscope in mask, goggles, protective apron and gloves, to others who take inadequate precautions. We prefer to change clothes and to wear gloves, but then rely on common sense to avoid contamination. If using a fibrescope to inject varices it makes sense to cover the face and eyes; if using a video-endoscope, so that the operator stands more remotely, it is unnecessary. Frequent hand washing, rigorous use of paper towels or gauzes when handling soiled accessories, putting soiled items directly in a sink or designated area (not on clean surfaces), covering sores or skin wounds with a waterproof dressing and general maintenance of good hygienic practice throughout the unit is more logical and safe than dressing up as for outer space and then being unthinkingly messy. Needle-stab injuries are a particular worry during endoscopy; a rigid attitude towards immediate disposal of sharps, avoiding re-sheathing of needles, taking extreme care if a needle is used in handling specimens and avoiding use of spiked biopsy forceps, all contribute to safety. The literature suggests that, even when a needle stick has occurred, HIV seroconversion is fortunately almost unknown. Hepatitis B is a greater risk; immunization should be a routine for all endoscopy staff, with their antibody status checked.

Facilities

A purpose-built cleaning area is essential for safe and efficient practice. In a one-room facility this may be within the room itself, but for two or more rooms a dedicated cleaning room is needed, preferably centrally. It should have clearly defined 'clean' and 'dirty' areas, a double sink and separate hand-wash basin, endoscope washing machine(s), an ultrasound cleaner, and ample storage. Good ventilation/extraction facilities are essential.

Washing machines

A variety of endoscope 'washing machines', manual, semi-automatic and automatic, are available. Most take only a single scope, some take two or more at a time. Some require special three-phase electricity supply and high-pressure water input; others are mobile with tanks that must be filled or emptied by hand before and after the session. Some include the control head of the instrument and its accessories in the wash/rinse/disinfect/rinse/dry cycles; others do not. In deciding which machine to purchase an on-site trial is strongly advised, to ensure that staff concerned are satisfied, that all routine scopes can be handled by it, and that the machine is suitable for the space available.

Remember that a washing machine does *not* remove the need for scrupulous mechanical cleaning. What it *does* do is to reduce exposure to glutaraldehyde, ensure properly timed perfusion cycles and release staff for other more productive activities during the disinfection period. Care is needed for periodic disinfection of the washing machine itself, especially any reservoirs, and attention must be paid to the tendency for gradual dilution of the disinfectant re-used in it. Advice may be needed from the manufacturer's representative as to how often to renew the disinfectant (usually at least weekly), or the concentration can be assayed directly with test strips.

A suggested routine for endoscope cleaning

All endoscopes marketed now are fully immersible and have been designed to facilitate cleaning and disinfection. Their major advantage over earlier equipment lies not just in their immersibility, but in the ability to irrigate all channels with positive pressure. Most endoscopes have three channels: suction/biopsy, air and water. Side-viewers fitted with a bridge/elevator have a fourth smaller channel which carries the bridge elevator cable and others may have a separate injection channel. All channels must be included in the cleaning and disinfection process, as all are potential reservoirs for transmissible infection.

Cleaning

1 External cleaning

Totally immerse the instrument in warm water and neutral detergent. Wash the outside of the instrument thoroughly with gauze swabs. Brush the distal end with a soft toothbrush, paying particular attention to the air/water outlet nozzle and bridge/elevator where fitted. All valves are removed (air/water, suction, biopsy), and on colonoscopes the CO_2 valve and distal hood are also removed. Clean and disinfect these as described above. Have additional valves and hoods available for busy lists. Clean the biopsy channel opening and suction port using a cotton bud.

2 Brushing through the suction biopsy channel

Use a cleaning brush suitable for the instrument and channel size, and brush through the suction channel several times until clean, as described below, and clean the cleaning brush itself in detergent with a soft toothbrush each time it emerges.

(a) Introduce the cleaning brush via the *biopsy* port, through the shaft, until it emerges from the distal end at least three times.

(b) Pass the cleaning brush through the *suction* port (having removed the suction button) and down the shaft until it emerges from the distal end at least three times.

(c) Pass the cleaning brush from the suction port in the other direction, through the *umbilical*, until it emerges from the suction connector at least three times.

After the channel has been thoroughly brushed, either put the endoscope into a washing machine to complete cleaning and disinfection, or alternatively follow the manual method described below.

3 Flushing of internal channels

Flush each internal channel with detergent fluid. This should be done independently for each separate channel. Alternatively, an all-channel irrigator device may be used, but if so ensure that detergent is seen to emerge through the air/water nozzle at the distal end of the insertion tube and out of the water and suction (and on colonoscopes, CO_2) connectors on the light guide. It is essential to confirm that all air is expelled from the channels.

On scopes with a bridge/elevator, attach the bridge channel adaptor and flush this additional channel using a 2-ml syringe. Some endoscopes also incorporate an auxiliary washing channel which should be similarly flushed.

4 Rinsing

Flush all channels as above using clean water followed by air to expel as much water as possible prior to disinfection. In some areas the water supply may contain small particles which can lead to blockage. Under these circumstances, sterile water should be used (filtered or bottled).

5 Disinfection

If a closed system is not available, this should be carried out under a fume canopy wearing gloves, and avoiding splashing. Totally immerse the instrument in 2% glutaraldehyde. Fill each internal channel with disinfectant and leave the instrument for the recommended contact time. Before and after the list this is 20 min, and between cases 4 min. A clock timer should be used for accuracy.

6 Rinsing

Following disinfection, rinse the instruments internally and externally to remove all traces of disinfectant.

7 Drying

Dry the endoscope externally paying particular attention to the light guide connector and eye-piece. Flush air through each channel. Reconnect the endoscope to the light source and fit disinfected valves and distal hoods. Switch on the light source and expel fluid from the air/water channel by simultaneously occluding the water bottle connector on the endoscope and depressing the air/water valve. Connect the instrument to suction and dry the suction channel by depressing the suction valve several times.

Between patients

Immediately the scope is removed from the patient, flush the air/water channel for 10–15 seconds to eject any refluxed blood or mucus (a special cleaning air/water channel adaptor is available for some endoscopes to flush these channels automatically). Aspirate detergent through the biopsy/suction channel for about 10–15 seconds to remove gross debris. Disconnect the instrument from the light source and carry out the cleaning and disinfection procedure as above (disinfect for 4 min).

End of list

Clean and disinfect as indicated above, but leave in disinfectant for 20 min to reduce the risk of overnight colonization. Following the disinfection period, rinse thoroughly and dry. After the instrument has been rinsed and dried, the outside can be swabbed, and the channels perfused with 70% ethyl alcohol and air-dried again before the instrument is hung up for storage.

Check the angulation of the instrument and inspect the condition of the fibre bundle before storage hanging in a well-ventilated security cupboard.

At the end of each list, or alternatively before starting in the morning, the instruments should be leak-tested, inflating the shaft under pressure to expose any possible puncture in the rubber of the bending section which avoids subsequent inward leakage of fluid resulting in damage and expensive repair bills.

Documentation and validation

Some form of documentary record should be made after an endoscope is cleaned and disinfected, at the simplest a tag left on it with the date and time, but better still with a completed and initialled proforma (which may then be kept for medico-legal purposes). Routine bacteriological test cultures are not thought necessary once a disinfection routine has been established and initially validated, but are wise whenever there is any change of routine and may be undertaken on an occasional basis, especially for ERCP instruments. A bile culture taken during ERCP, looking for

Pseudomonas, is probably the most critical test as well as the most clinically relevant.

Each instrument should additionally have its own log-book page for repairs and overhauls.

Cleaning/disinfection/sterilization of endoscopic accessories

All ancillary equipment used during endoscopic procedures can transmit infection. In particular, those accessory items which are designed to breach the mucosa provide a potential portal of entry to the systemic circulation for any organisms present. Except where disposable accessories are used, it is necessary between patients to clean and disinfect/sterilize accessories (including cleaning brushes and cleaning attachments) using the following procedures.

1 *Wash* immediately after use in fresh detergent solution.

2 *Dismantle* as far as possible: remove handles and withdraw inner parts where these exist—for example, remove snare wires from sheaths and inner tubes from injection needles.

3 *Brush* away adherent debris with cleaning brush or toothbrush.

4 *Flush* detergent solution through lumens of all hollow components using syringe attachments where these are available.

5 *Ultrasonic clean* (with any lumen filled with fluid). It is almost impossible to thoroughly clean items with a spiral metal structure, such as biopsy forceps and Eder–Puestow dilatation flexible tips, without this facility.

6 *Rinse* thoroughly, flushing lumens of hollow items well.
Then either:

7 *Disinfect*. Immerse equipment in the disinfectant(s) of choice with lumens filled for the required length of time.

8 *Rinse* thoroughly, flushing all disinfectant out of the lumens.

9 *Dry*.

10 *Lubricate* all moving parts.

11 *Store* equipment, then re-disinfect, immediately before use.
Alternatively, and preferably:

12 *Sterilize* after following procedures **1–6**, accessories being stored in sterile packs which avoid the need for re-disinfection. Methods available for sterilizing accessories include:

  (a) Steam autoclaving (where recommended by the manufacturer, since some plastics melt) (see list below).

  (b) Ethylene oxide gas.

  (c) Low-temperature steam and formaldehyde.

Use of sterilization is desirable for biopsy forceps, and sterilization or use of disposable products is strongly recommended for injection needles. A portable electric autoclave on site is practical and inexpensive. Water bottles should be disinfected or autoclaved before and after the list.

Current accessory recommendations

Makers recommendations

Olympus

All Olympus autoclave accessories can be recognized by the letter (S) which supersedes their product codes in the Olympus/Keymed flexible accessories catalogue or by a light green identification marking on the accessory body, e.g. water bottles. If in doubt consult the inspection manual.

Pentax

Pentax accessories with pink handles are autoclavable and their catalogue numbers have the letter (S) after the product code.

Fujinon

All Fujinon accessories with purple handles are autoclavable. ERCP cannulae are autoclavable.

Hobbs

The majority of accessories are not autoclavable but can be sterilized by ethylene oxide gas.

Endovations

All the Endovations range are designed for single use only.

Wilson–Cook

All new biopsy and grasping forceps are autoclavable.

Other suitable accessories currently in production will, in future, be manufactured using autoclavable components as new fittings become available. Equipment which is intrinsically intolerant of autoclave sterilization may be sterilized by ethylene oxide gas. Certain products are designed for single use only.

Logistic consequences of disinfection

Following the above recommendations means that proper cleaning of an endoscope and its accessories, whether manually or by machine, cannot be achieved in less than 12–15 min unless hazardous short-cuts are taken. It follows that at least two endoscopes are required for a busy list (as well as others for back-up purposes in case of breakage), and that a nurse or assistant will be kept busy full time in managing the cleaning routines. Disassembly, cleaning, disinfection and re-assembly of accessories, and their packing and transmission for sterilization, is both time-consuming and requires appropriate numbers of extra accessories. These are conveniently stored in see-through sealed bags for immediate use when required.

Antibiotic prophylaxis for GI procedures

Bacteraemia occurs after many GI procedures. There is a risk of sepsis during biliary intervention, for which prophylactic antibiotics are recommended (see regime below). There has been much discussion and writing recently concerning the possible risk of inducing endocarditis after GI procedures. Literature data are not sufficiently precise to provide any absolute guidelines but the suggestions below conform to current opinion. There is, however, no substitute for the informed judgement of the physician; where the clinical situation appears not to be covered by these guidelines, or where there are conflicting opinions among several physicians, the endoscopist, whilst considering the wishes of the referring physician, will make the final decision.

Guidelines

Patients with prosthetic heart valves undergoing any invasive GI procedure (optional in proctoscopy, barium enema, percutaneous liver biopsy and laparoscopy): ampicillin 1–2 g i.m. or i.v. and gentamicin 1.5 mg/kg i.m. or i.v. at 1–2 hours prior to the procedure (substitute vancomycin 1 g i.v. over 1 hour for allergy to ampicillin).

Other specific cardiac conditions (congenital malformations, rheumatic or acquired valve disease, previous endocarditis) when undergoing oesophageal dilatation or variceal sclerotherapy: amoxycillin 3 g at 1 hour prior to the procedure (optional 1.5 g repeat dose 6 hours later). (Substitute vancomycin and gentamicin, as above, when penicillin allergy is present.)

Biliary sepsis prophylaxis. All patients having ERCP (or PTC) in whom biliary tract obstruction is present or suspected, or in whom a therapeutic intervention is planned (sphincterotomy, dilation, stent placement, stone extraction, etc.): ampicillin (or vancomycin) and gentamicin as above.

Further reading

Axon, A. T. R. (1988) 'Infection and disinfection: special review', in *Annual of Gastrointestinal Endoscopy* (ed. Cotton, P. B., Tytgat, G. N. J. and Williams, C. B.), pp. 181–193. Gower Academic Journals, London.

Axon, A. T. R. and Cotton, P. B. (1983) 'Endoscopy and infection'. *Gut*, **24**, 1064–1066.

Babb, J. R., Bradley, C. R., Deverill, C. E. A., Ayliffe, G. A. J. and Melikian, V. (1981) 'Recent advances in the cleaning and disinfection of fibrescopes'. *Journal of Hospital Infection*, **2**, 329–340.

Hanson, P. J. V., Clarke, J. R., Nicholson, G. *et al.* (1989) 'Contamination of endoscopes used in AIDS patients'. *Lancet*, July 8, 86–88.

Shorvon, P. J., Eykyn, S. J. and Cotton, P. B. (1983) 'Gastrointestinal instrumentation, bacteremia and endocarditis'. *Gut*, **24**, 1078–1093.

Weller, I. V. D. (1988) 'Cleaning and disinfection of equipment for gastrointestinal flexible endoscopy: interim recommendations of a Working Party of the British Society of Gastroenterology'. *Gut*, **29**, 1134–1151.

'Cleaning and disinfection of equipment for gastrointestinal flexible endoscopy: interim recommendations of a Working Party of the British Society of Gastroenterology'. *Gut*, **29**, 1134–1151, 1988.

Documentation, Teaching and Certification 13

Documentation

Reporting and recording are essential parts of any service. The documents and system should be designed around local needs and limitations, and it is wise to look at a number of ideas from established units, and to incorporate those which fit. The advent of affordable microcomputers—especially easy-to-use systems for endoscopy—transforms the management and record-keeping systems of the past. Some of the factors to be considered are outlined here and in Chapter 3, and examples are given.

Requests and registration

In many units, endoscopies are performed on a 'service' basis with no opportunity to assess the patient until he arrives for the procedure. A request form (Fig. 13.1) will simplify booking arrangements, indicate the degree of urgency for the procedure and any special transport or medical problems (e.g. an 85-year-old living at a distance may need admission).

It is also necessary to have a booking register (which can be simply a large desk diary) and checklists for X-rays received/returned, biopsies sent off, reports received, etc.

Fig. 13.1 Endoscopy request form.

Lab use	THE BEST HOSPITAL GASTROINTESTINAL UNIT		GI
In-patients Walk/chair/stretcher	Request tick Endoscopy (upper GI) Colonoscopy	No.	
Out-patients Transport required yes/no Transport arranged	ERCP Jejunal biopsy Pancreatic function Gastric function	Surname Mr First names Mrs Miss D of B	
Patient's address and tel. no.	Other	Ward/Dept.	
	Clinical problem (include X-ray details and potential contra-indications)	Consultant date	
		Referring doctor (PRINT)	
		Urgent/Non-urgent	
Appointment Patient informed Ward informed			
Form No. 9561	use ball-point pen		

THE BEST HOSPITAL ENDOSCOPY UNIT

Upper GI endoscopy (OGD)

Upper GI endoscopy—or oesophagogastroduodenoscopy (OGD)—is a visual examination of the lining of your oesophagus, stomach and the first part of your intestine. This is performed by passing a small, long flexible telescope through your mouth, under sedation. The doctor will be able to look for any abnormalities which may be present. If necessary, small tissue samples (biopsies) can be taken during the examination (painlessly) for detailed laboratory analysis.

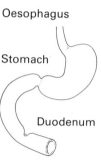

    Some treatments can also be done through the endoscope. These include stretching (dilating) narrowed areas of the oesophagus, stomach or duodenum, removing polyps and swallowed objects, and treatment of bleeding vessels and ulcers by internal injection, or application of heat (using electrical diathermy, laser or heat probes).

Preparation

Your stomach must be empty, so do not eat or drink anything after midnight. If you must take prescription medication, use only small sips of water. Do not take antacids.

What will happen

The doctor and/or nurse will explain the procedure and answer your questions. Please tell them if you have had any other endoscopic examinations, or any allergies or bad reactions to medications. You will be asked to sign a consent form, giving your permission for the examination. You will need to put on a hospital gown, and to remove your eyeglasses, contact lenses and dentures.

    A local anaesthetic will be sprayed onto your throat, to make it numb. You may be given medication by injection through a vein to make you sleepy and relaxed. While in a comfortable position on your left side, the doctor will pass the endoscope through your mouth, and down your throat. A guard will be placed to protect your teeth. The instrument will not interfere with your breathing, nor cause any pain. The examination takes 10–30 minutes.

Afterwards

You will remain in the clinic area for up to 1 hour, until the main effects of any medication wear off. Your throat may feel numb and slightly sore. You should not attempt to eat or drink until your swallowing reflex is normal (at least 1 hour). After this you may return to your regular diet unless otherwise instructed. You may feel slightly bloated, due to the air which has been injected through the endoscope; this will quickly pass.

    If you have had a sedative injection, a companion *must* be available to drive you home. For the remainder of the day you should not drive a car, operate machinery, or make important decisions, as the sedation impairs your reflexes and judgement.

Risks?

Endoscopy can result in complications such as reactions to medication, perforation of the intestine, and bleeding. These complications are very rare (less than one in 1000 examinations), but may require urgent treatment, and even an operation. The possibility of complication is greater when the endoscope is used to apply treatment. Be sure to inform us if you have any pain, black tarry stools, or troublesome vomiting in the hours or days after endoscopy.

Questions or problems?

Contact the nurse in charge, Endoscopy Unit (Tel: . . . . .) 8 a.m. to 4.30 p.m. Monday to Friday. At other times, in case of emergency, call the Hospital Operator to contact the gastroenterologist on duty.

Fig. 13.2 Upper GI endoscopy explanation sheet.

THE BEST HOSPITAL ENDOSCOPY UNIT

Colonoscopy

Colon

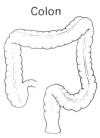

Colonoscopy is a visual examination of the lining of your colon (large intestine). A long flexible tube (colonoscope) is passed through the rectum, and around the colon. Through this telescope the doctor will be able to look for any abnormalities that may be present. If necessary, small tissue samples (biopsies) can be taken during the examination (painlessly) for laboratory analysis. Polyps (abnormal growths of tissue) can also be removed, using an electric snare wire.

Preparation

To allow a clear view, the colon must be completely free of waste material. You will be given a laxative solution to drink the day before examination, and instructions to remain on clear fluids. Do not eat or drink anything after midnight. If you must take prescription medication, use only small sips of water. Avoid taking aspirin products or any iron preparations for 2 days before the examination.

What will happen

The doctor and/or nurse will explain the procedure and answer your questions. Please tell them if you have had any other endoscopy examination, or any allergies or bad reactions to medications. You will be asked to sign a consent form, giving your permission to have the procedure performed. You will be asked to put on a hospital gown, and to remove your eyeglasses, contact lenses and dentures.

You will be placed in a comfortable positon on your left side, and may be given medication by injection through a vein to make you sleepy and relaxed. The doctor will pass the colonoscope through the anus and into the rectum, and advance it through the colon. You may experience some abdominal cramping and pressure from the air which is introduced into your colon. This is normal, and will pass quickly. You may be asked to change your position during the examination, and will be assisted by a nurse. The examination takes 15–60 minutes.

Afterwards

You will remain in the clinic area for up to 1 hour, until the effects of any medication wear off. A companion *must* be able to drive you home as the sedation impairs your reflexes and judgement. For the remainder of the day you should not drive a car, operate machinery, or make important decisions. We suggest that you rest quietly.

Risks?

Colonoscopy can result in complications, such as reactions to medication, perforation of the intestine, and bleeding. These complications are very rare (less than one in 1000 examinations), but may require urgent treatment, and even an operation. The risks are slightly higher when the colonoscope is used to apply treatment, such as removal of polyps. Be sure to inform us if you have any severe pain, black tarry stools or persistent bleeding in the hours or days after colonoscopy.

Questions or problems?

Contact the nurse in charge, Endoscopy Unit (Tel: . . . . .) 8 a.m. to 4.30 p.m. Monday to Friday. At other times, in case of emergency, call the Hospital Operator to contact the gastroenterologist on duty.

Fig. 13.3 Colonoscopy explanation sheet.

Appointments and information sheets

Patients need to know when and where to come and also what to expect. It will be some years before the public understands that endoscopy is a simple procedure. An informative and reassuring written explanation saves much unnecessary worry (Figs 7.8, 13.2 and 13.3). For certain techniques (e.g. colonoscopy), the instructions about diet must be precise and can include such welcome information as the inclusion of alcoholic drinks in a 'clear fluid' regime.

Name: History no: Date of birth:

THE BEST HOSPITAL ENDOSCOPY UNIT

Consent for endoscopy

I, ... and/or ....

authorize the performance upon ....

of the following procedure/s (mark through those not applicable):

1 Upper gastrointestinal endoscopy   2 Colonoscopy   3 Flexible sigmoidoscopy   4 Endoscopic retrograde cholangiopancreatography (ERCP)

with: ....

and other procedures as deemed necessary or advisable during the endoscopy procedure. I understand that the responsible physician will be

Dr ....
　　　　　(Name or initials)　　　　　　　　　　　　　　　　　(Last name)

I consent to the administration of such medications as may be considered necessary or advisable to provide relaxation.

The nature and purpose of the procedure, alternative methods of treatment, and the risks involved have been explained to me. I have had the opportunity to study the specially prepared procedure information sheet(s). No guarantee has been given as to the results that may be obtained.

I agree that any tissues and body fluids removed, and any X-ray or photographic records taken, during the course of the endoscopy procedure described above may be examined, preserved and/or disposed of in whatever way may be considered proper for purposes of diagnosis and treatment.

Witness: ....   Signed: ....
　　　　　　　　　　　　　　　　　　　　　(Patient or person authorized to consent for patient
　　　　　　　　　　　　　　　　　　　　　and relationship)

Date: ....   Time: ....

Notes or comments: ....

....

....

Fig. 13.4 Consent form for endoscopy.

Patients in hospital should be visited before the procedure by a doctor or nurse of the endoscopy team. Other nursing staff often have little knowledge about endoscopy, and their explanations can provoke further anxiety; the chief endoscopy nurse should ensure that in-patient floors have up-to-date information and instructions about endoscopy procedures.

Consent forms

Some units do not ask patients to sign consent forms, but in many countries detailed informed consent is mandatory. An example is shown in Fig. 13.4.

Reports and records

When patients are recovered outside the unit, a transit form should accompany them, giving details of medication and other instructions (Figs 13.5 and 13.6). If sedation is used, it is sensible to give the

---

THE BEST HOSPITAL GASTROINTESTINAL UNIT

telephone extension:

To Nurse in charge of Mr/Mrs/Miss ....

Dr.. has performed ....

completed at: .... date: ....

drugs given:
Diazepam   mg
Midazolam   mg
Atropine   mg
Buscopan   mg   Local anaesthetic to throat
Pethidine   mg   yes/no
Glucagon   mg
Secretin
Other

Nursing instructions   nil by mouth until: ....

....

Please report pain, distension or fever.

Special observations required: ....

....

Fig. 13.5 Form giving details of medication.

THE BEST HOSPITAL ENDOSCOPY UNIT

Patient discharge instructions after GI endoscopy

You have undergone a procedure called: Upper GI endoscopy (OGD)/Colonoscopy/ERCP/ Sigmoidoscopy/with: ....

This procedure has been performed by Dr ....

1　It is essential that someone accompany you home if you received sedation, and if so you should not: drive a car, operate machinery, or drink any alcohol. The effects of the test and medications should wear off by the next day and you will be able to resume normal activities.

2　Diet: You may resume your normal diet unless otherwise instructed by your doctor.

3　You may resume your normal prescription medicines.

4　There may be some slight soreness where the instruments have been, but this will wear off in a day or so.

5　Some bloating may be experienced if air has remained in your gastrointestinal tract (stomach and/ or bowel) and will resolve within a few hours.

6　Things to report to your doctor:
　　— severe pain or vomiting
　　— passage or vomiting of blood
　　— temperature greater than 101°
　　— redness, tenderness and swelling at site of IV that persists greater than 48 hours.

7　Further advice about your condition and treatment will be given at your next clinic appointment.

8　If specimens have been taken for analysis, the results may take several days.

9　If you have any questions or concerns, call the Endoscopy Unit (Tel: ....) 8 a.m. to 4.30 p.m. Monday to Friday, or at other times call the Hospital Operator and ask for the gastro-enterologist on call.

Fig. 13.6 Patient discharge instructions after GI endoscopy.

patient a written outline conclusion of the endoscopy findings since he is likely to forget anything he is told soon afterwards; a computerized system makes an additional printout appropriate to the patient very easy to produce.

The main variables affecting design of records are the volume of work and data, and whether or not a typist is always immediately available. Any system must provide immediately available facts on in-patients and urgent cases, allow for copies to all referring doctors, and permit reliable subsequent recall of data.

A handwritten report is quick, but often illegible and fails to provide copies or recall. Stamped organ outlines (Figs 13.7–13.9) can be used to indicate the site of lesions and biopsy specimens. Tubular structures such as the oesophagus, duodenum and colon are easy to represent in two dimensions, but the stomach is more difficult.

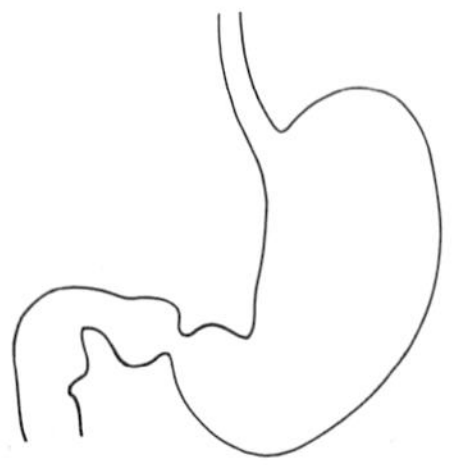

Fig. 13.7 Upper GI.

Fig. 13.8 ERCP.

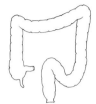

Fig. 13.9 Colonoscopy.

Writing or typing the report on 'chemical carbon' paper can provide two top copies (gummed if necessary) and a card for filing (Fig. 13.10). Alternatively, a dictated report can be typed onto pre-printed stationery, a word-processed form or a computer database so as to produce a full report (Fig. 13.11) which is photocopied.

Amongst other details, any report must indicate the type of medication and the instrument used, the extent of examination, the name of the endoscopist and whether or not the examination was technically satisfactory. A report of a 'difficult' endoscopy by an inexperienced doctor should obviously carry less weight than a report by an expert indicating a 'good view of all areas'. A 'yes/no' format is convenient for a positive record of whether specimens, etc. have been taken or not.

THE BEST HOSPITAL GASTROENTEROLOGY DEPT.	If label used fix duplicate to 2 copies	
	Surname	Forename
Reason for referral: X-ray date: result:	Age/D.O.B.	C.R. No.
	Doctor	IP/OP
Endoscopist(s) Medication Instrument Biopsy ☐ Cytology ☐ Photo ☐ Video ☐		
CONCLUSION:		
ENDOSCOPY: GASTRODUODENOSCOPY Date:		

Fig. 13.10 Record card for filing.

THE BEST HOSPITAL ENDOSCOPY UNIT

NAME: ....   Series number:

ADDRESS: ....   REFERRED BY: ....

COPIES TO: ....

Indication/History/X-ray ....

....

REPORT ON: ....   Date: ....

Medication: ....   Instrument: ....

FINDINGS:

Histology/Cytology

Signed: ....

Fig. 13.11 Report sheet.

Permanent records—computerization

The patient's permanent record should contain data useful to the endoscopist and the endoscopy unit in addition to that contained in the actual clinical report. To standardize input and facilitate the management of complex information from thousands of records, a computer database system cannot be bettered, providing it is well thought out and appropriate to the needs of the particular endoscopy unit.

A few units co-operate successfully with hospital computer departments, but whereas mainframe computers require a professional intermediary to retrieve data, the newer microcomputers cost less than an endoscope and can be programmed to be managed entirely by untrained personnel. Two limitations of microcomputers have been removed with the production of hard-disc memory storage capable of holding many millions of characters, and the development of 'user-friendly' programs for data entry and analysis. Whether the data are entered by secretarial staff alone or also by nursing and medical staff (either onto paper or directly on the keyboard) depends on local wishes and circumstances. In our units, the patient details and administrative data are entered by the secretary/receptionist and doctors then enter the medical data, produce and sign the printouts for the case record and referring doctor. With a little practice and a suitable program, data entry takes surprisingly little time. Having all staff involved with the computer as a central part of the patient's management and using it as the only documentation ensures that the records are accurate for medico-legal or research purposes.

There are many advantages of directly-operated microcomputers over other forms of record keeping. The record structure can be carefully defined, with safeguards so that key questions must be answered before the program will proceed or the report record is complete; only sensible replies are accepted by the computer and irrelevant keys are made non-operative. It is easy to produce and modify automatically word-processed forms, listings and reports from the data entered and there can be substantial free-text sections so that the computer format is not restrictive. The computer can also deal with large amounts of data for analysis but individualize so that relevant points (drug sensitivities, previous technical problems, sedational requirements, etc.) for a particular patient are automatically presented for any follow-up visit. Multi-user operation or a network system means that several screens can work simultaneously and the patient data are instantly available (or can be entered) in different places (e.g. reception/secretary/endoscopy room) without the problems of physical transfer. Computer management is virtually indispensable for any unit offering proper follow-up/surveillance services, not only because of the need to spot non-attenders and follow correct schedules, but because the sheer volume of correspondence becomes overwhelming without the ability to print off batches of letters automatically, correctly addressed and dated.

Computers also impose constraints however. Care has to be taken in planning the record structure so that useful data are asked for in an amount acceptable to the user but feasible in data-entry terms, also that the program is foolproof and able to cope with multiple repeat visits and also human frailties (such as misspelling of surnames). Hardware is no longer a limiting factor and an easy facility for regular 'back-up' is of critical importance. In a clinical environment it is also essential that the equipment used is of high quality with rapid service facilities available.

Image documentation

For clinical purposes the ideal is to have a colour print of any lesion to attach to the report sent to the referring clinician and this is now attainable, either by off-screen or endoscopic Polaroid photography, ideally with a 'slave' monitor incorporating a memory so that endoscopy is not delayed. The best results are obtained by special units which receive and show, in sequence on-screen, the actual red/blue/green components from which the normal televised colour image is created, with a long exposure time to allow for the slow response of present 'instant' film emulsions.

Video-printers perform a similar function with the advantage of being able to incorporate multiple endoscopic images on a single sheet, with as many copies as required. Representative images of even a normal endoscopy can be issued with the report, thus removing one of the major criticisms of endoscopy compared to the permanent images available after an X-ray examination. With the advent of cheap mass-storage media capable of handling the vast amount of information needed to create a higher resolution colour graphic image, it is becoming realistic to consider permanent storage of visual information accessible from the patient database. This will, to a large extent, remove the inadequacies and difficulties of present routines for film storage, labelling and retrieval.

Lecture slides

Colour transparencies (35- or 60-mm film) give good results for meetings, but the delay in processing and the inconvenience of handling transparencies limits their clinical impact.

Films should be returned from processing in strip form; having the pictures ready mounted takes too much storage space. The results should be viewed as soon as possible, when the clinical details are still fresh in the mind. The outstanding pictures are selected and mounted, the failures thrown out and the rest stored. Most endoscopists take a relatively large number of photographs because it is not always possible to predict which lesions will be clinically important. There is no purpose in keeping poor photographs, because even if they show rare lesions, no one will wish to look at them. The easiest storage system is to keep strips for individual patients in separate envelopes or a loose leaf or similar negative file, each strip being marked with the patient's name, diagnosis and a comment on the quality of the photographs. This makes it relatively easy to find good pictures of a particular condition or those of a particular patient.

Video-recording and endoscopic television

The miniaturized 'chip CCD' (charge-coupled device) television cameras and video-endoscopes now available make endoscopic television easy for anyone with access to the necessary funds, and transforms endoscopic procedures for patients, nursing staff and medical colleagues as well as allowing video-taping for a permanent record. Clinical video-tapes of abnormalities for discussion or review with colleagues should be highly selective, preferably not lasting more than a minute or two and with a clear running commentary. Televised teaching demonstration meetings, combining the internal endoscopic appearances, an external camera view and X-ray fluoroscopic images where appropriate, have tremendous impact in allowing larger groups to see, discuss and compare endoscopic techniques. Many hospitals now have access to suitable video equipment including video projectors and the necessary switching or mixing gear. It remains very expensive to mix several pictures on a single screen, but having one projector for the overall view and several monitors for the endoscopic or fluoroscopic images works well (Fig. 13.12).

Teaching and learning endoscopy

Flexible endoscopy is a manual technique like driving a car or playing a musical instrument; some people learn more quickly than others and some may never become particularly adept. Practice is the only certain way of learning, but it helps if correct habits are instilled at any early stage. Because patients are involved some form of apprenticeship is essential, with an experienced endoscopist overseeing the early examinations during which patient and instrument are at risk. How long the apprenticeship continues varies according to circumstances, but as well as performing at least 50 endoscopies under supervision, a trainee should make use of available written, slide or film material, practise under supervision on teaching models, attend teaching courses and see several different endoscopy centres. All of these methods have their advantages.

Apprenticeship

Watching an expert is useful, providing that the expert actively explains what he is doing and seeing. In countries where endoscopy is a well-established speciality with numerous staff, the trainee may watch through the 'teaching attachment' or on the video-monitor for months before he is allowed to handle the instrument. In other countries where endoscopy is newer and existing endoscopists are mainly self-taught, the approach is more relaxed and the beginner may be 'thrown in at the deep end'. He finds himself being asked to use an expensive instrument he does not understand in an organ with unfamiliar anatomy and gets a poor view of appearances he cannot interpret. One answer is to 'phase' trainee introduction to a set period (e.g. 5–10 min) or a defined part of the examination (e.g. insertion to the cardia or the proximal sigmoid colon), the extent of examination and responsibility being gradually lengthened. The trainee can be entrusted with some of the routine duties in the endoscopy room, helping the nurse and learning correct techniques in handling and cleaning the endoscopes. An old or broken instrument available in partly stripped-down form can help to demonstrate the complexity of the equipment and the need to treat it with respect.

The teacher needs considerable patience and the ability to adapt to the different physical and personality traits of different pupils. Some need calming down, to learn to be more cerebral and more humane in their actions; others need speeding up to become gradually more positive and fluent. Generally speaking, a slow, thoughtful endoscopist with integrity can learn to excel, whereas those that start erratic usually remain so.

Endoscopic technique builds up by learning to combine visual interpretation with the correct mechanical response. Attention to

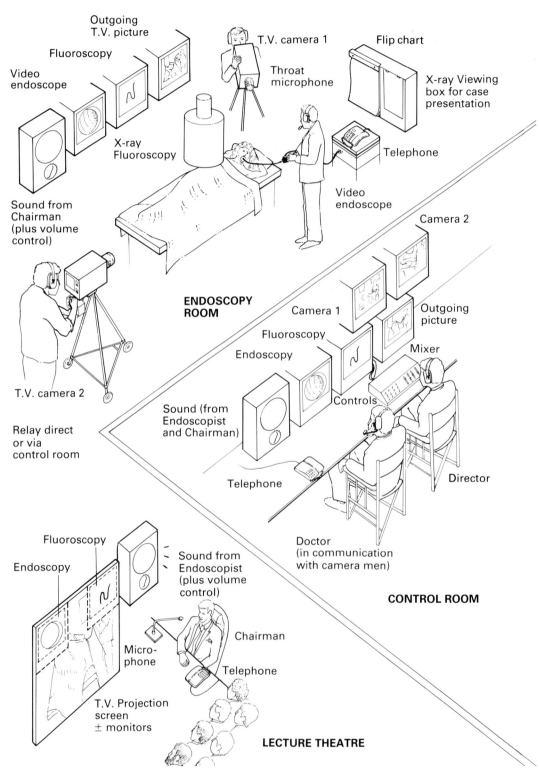

Fig. 13.12 Diagrammatic layout for endoscopic television teaching between endoscopy room and lecture theatre.

the detail of finger movements, shaft twist and even body position are all important. The teacher may need, for instance, to hold his own hand over that of the trainee on the shaft of the instrument to demonstrate the requisite amounts of to-and-fro or twisting movements, or to check that when the pupil intends to angle either up or down he is actually moving the control knob in the correct direction first time. Regrettably, there are too few experienced endoscopists combining the necessary skills themselves with the amount of time and interest required to teach successfully.

There is a range of teaching material which can be useful between endoscopic sessions. A collection of books, atlases and selected reprints can be assembled with little effort. Teaching video-tapes and education slide tapes liven up the topic and help to show that there are different approaches to endoscopy. Home-made slide-tape sequences are also not difficult to produce and help the teacher to avoid tedious repetition. National endoscopic societies have an important role in ensuring availability of teaching material (viz. American Society for Gastrointestinal Endoscopy Teaching Library).

Models and simulators

No model can simulate exactly the varying and variable anatomy of the human GI tract, especially its combination of elasticity and contractility. None the less, half an hour spent practising on a stomach or colon model under expert guidance, followed by another half an hour alone, is very helpful in understanding spatial relationships and in co-ordinating the view down the endoscope with the correct movements of the controls. It is easy to see, explain and practise on a model how to perform retroversion at the cardia, why the pylorus must be correctly positioned with a side-viewer, why upwards angling approximates to the papilla, or why clockwise rotation undoes an alpha loop. Once seen and understood, these things are never forgotten and with the opportunity to practise them repeatedly without involving a patient, the trainee develops self-confidence and better understanding of correct instrument handling. Supervision is important (the teaching attachment is useful for this) not least because instruments can be damaged on models as well as in patients.

A newer approach, not yet either fully developed or evaluated, may be the use of electronic endoscopy simulators. The severe constraints of the limited budgets available for medical teaching mean that the sophisticated but enormously expensive simulators available to train pilots in aviation are regrettably not applicable to endoscopy. The prototypes available currently for endoscopy teaching make use either of video-disc technology to show actual endoscopic images or computer-graphic techniques to produce a cruder image simulated mathematically in real time. The trainee handles a dummy endoscope, the steering controls, shaft movements and air/water/suction buttons which are converted by transducers and switches into electrical output so as to modify the image display according to the handling of the instrument. The microcomputer incorporated in the system, in addition to control-ling the image, will produce screen prompts and a 'score' to give interactive teaching without the presence of an expert teacher, and can also evaluate the progress of the trainee in different simulated circumstances on an objective basis without patient trauma or danger of instrument damage.

Certification of competence

Professional organizations in many countries have struggled with the need to certify when endoscopists are competent. This is an issue with complex ramifications, and it is pertinent sometimes to re-member that most specialities (including surgery) do not certify competence specifically by procedure. In addition, certification is only meaningful if there is any disadvantage in not being certified.

Both the UK and American national organizations with which we are familiar have discussed these issues again recently. The perspec-tives are different. In the UK, the relative lack of medical staff means that most trainees gain a lot of experience, but often with relatively little supervision. The British Society of Gastroenterology is setting up a mechanism for certifying trainees in four different groups of techniques: diagnostic upper GI endoscopy, therapeutic upper GI endoscopy, colonoscopy and ERCP. Certification will be done by accredited trainers, who have to prove their own competence and the adequacy of their facilities. In the USA, fellows may do less procedures, but the much shorter period of training and both medico-legal and financial concerns mean that they are fully super-vised. They keep a log book of all endoscopies, and expect to be certified as competent at the end of the training period (whether this be 2 or 3 years). However, for the individual trainee, the crucial question is whether the hospitals to which attachment is sought (for private practice) will award 'privileges' for performing these procedures. The issues here become even more complex, since they involve not only the question of competence, but also the perceived needs of the community and also of the established specialists. Heads of gastroenterology and endoscopy departments have actually been held partly responsible for complications of procedures performed by people they have certified to be competent.

It must be recognized that not all trainees can expect to become competent in all of the GI procedures. Furthermore, at least in the USA, the number of specialists within a single community may be such as to dilute the work load for any individual below the threshold for continuing competence. It is therefore logical to consider different levels of endoscopic training. Most clinical gastroenterologists will be trained in upper endoscopy and colonos-copy with their standard therapeutic applications (polypectomy, sclerotherapy, and endoscopic haemostasis). This level can be called standard training. Some family practitioners may wish to be trained only in flexible sigmoidoscopy; some surgeons and research gastro-enterologists may need only to perform diagnostic upper GI endos-copy and flexible sigmoidoscopy. A small proportion of trainees will go on after standard to advanced training in more specialized (rarer and more dangerous) procedures, including ERCP and its therapeutic applications, laser therapy, laparoscopy, etc. Restricting advanced techniques to a selected group of trainees is not universally popular, since many wish to keep their options open. However, such selection is inevitable if quality is to be maintained, and if we are to produce experienced trainers for the next generation. Another emphasis is that (with rare exceptions at the basic level) no one should be taught diagnostic procedures without learning the therapeutic applications. It is illogical to do a colonoscopy without being able to perform polypectomy, and equally so (as well as potentially hazardous) to undertake ERCP in a patient with jaundice without the skills to provide drainage. It follows that these endoscopic trainees will spend additional time in attaining competence—whilst their colleagues may obtain specialized training in other directions, such as laboratory research.

Both in the UK and USA, much responsibility is placed on the shoulders of the trainer (in the USA the 'endoscopy program training director') whose job it is to organize training, ensure that facilities and trainers are adequate, and to certify competence at an appropriate time.

There has been much discussion about the number of procedures which trainees should perform. Speed of achievement of competence will vary enormously between individuals, and also in different institutions. Previous attempts to set guideline numbers have largely been misinterpreted to mean that a trainee is competent once a particular number is reached. It is helpful to look at numbers only as guidelines, and we prefer the term 'thresholds for competence'. When a trainee has achieved this number in his log book, he must formally ask his training director to assess his skills and certify competence, or guide him towards more appropriate further experience.

Further reading

Sivak, M. V. Jr (1989) 'Endoscopic documentation: overview', in *Annual of Gastrointestinal Endoscopy* (ed. Cotton, P. B., Tytgat, G. N. J. and Williams, C. B.), pp. 149–159. Current Science, London.

14 Postscript—Problems and Horizons

Forecasting is always difficult; predicting trends in endoscopy is especially difficult. It is really only possible to analyse current trends and attempt to extrapolate from them. Our attempts to forecast in the second edition of this book less than a decade ago have met with mixed success. We did predict the immersible endoscope, and speculated about the impact of 'intra-cavity television'—by which we surely meant video-endoscopy. We predicted (correctly) that a few new procedures would be described, and that some would prove to be worth while. However, most of our thoughts were targeted at the professional strains which the success of endoscopy has engendered—the turf issues between gastroenterologists, surgeons (and radiologists), and the difficulties involved in meeting the increasing demand for endoscopy procedures: 'Toys have turned into tools, and the excitements of conception have fathered a service obligation.' These concerns continue to dominate, and have come into somewhat closer focus.

Inevitably, the concerns of endoscopic communities vary in different countries. The authors now have very different congregations and perspectives. Money has a major influence. Hospital budgets in the UK are fixed on an annual basis, and rarely increase in real terms. In general, one sub-speciality can expand only at the expense of another. It is a truly UK paradox that a specialist with a reputation sufficient to draw patients from all over the nation will be unpopular within his institution simply because these activities consume an increasingly large proportion of a fixed budget. In the UK there are still relatively few trained endoscopists, facing a rapidly increasing demand for diagnostic and therapeutic procedures. Examinations are often done with obsolete equipment and inadequate facilities, with insufficient trained assistance. Despite this, there is some very innovative research, and some careful evaluation studies—many of which are performed in the hope of refining (i.e. reducing) the indications for endoscopy.

The pressures are reversed in private health care systems or those where insurance rewards on a fee-for-service basis; doctors and institutions alike then have a vested interest in maximizing endoscopic activity. There is appropriate heavy investment in facilities, equipment and staff, whether the profits are to be used to fund research or recreation. Inevitably there may be less scrutiny of indications for procedures, and more opportunity for abuse. The free-market system also means that there are far more gastroenterologists (maybe too many), and no shortage of trainees. The training period in the USA is short by comparison with the long apprenticeship in the UK, but this has one major advantage—it forces both trainers and trainees to structure the programme appropriately, and to evaluate its results. These concerns come to a focus over 'certification of competence', discussed in Chapter 13.

The role of surgeons in gastrointestinal endoscopy continues to be debated; both academic and financial pressures impinge. With a few notable exceptions, surgeons failed to recognize the potential of flexible endoscopy when diagnostic techniques were first introduced. Indeed, many surgeons (and some academic gastroenterologists) were frankly dismissive. The increasing interest now shown by surgeons is not surprising, since so many endoscopic procedures are replacing orthodox operations. Bile duct stones provide a good example. Whereas endoscopists used to deal only with those crumbs which fell from the surgeon's table, they now increasingly have the first bite, leaving to the surgeon their occasional failures and rare disasters. Most polyps in the colon are now firmly in the province of the endoscopist; even large, sessile or malignant lesions are being managed endoscopically. These changes have important implications for the training of surgeons—and have made gastroenterologists more conscious of complications and medico-legal problems. Unfortunately some endoscopists think of surgeons only as additional ancillaries to be used when problems occur, but many of these risky procedures can be undertaken only with the wholehearted backing of surgical colleagues. The best interests of the patient can nowadays only be protected by a team approach.

Whether endoscopes and endoscopic techniques 'belong' to surgeons or gastroenterologists is a sterile issue. It is more productive to think of therapeutic endoscopy as simply a new form of surgery, and to attempt to break down the artificial barriers which interfere with its best use. Professional associations (and training programmes) should serve the future of medicine and the well-being of patients, and should be changed when they become too rigid to accommodate healthy developments. This difficult area has recently been reviewed by a prominent surgeon in the field, Ted Schrock. Some internists and family practitioners in the USA have embraced flexible sigmoidoscopy, particularly as a screening tool. In other countries, endoscopy is practised by some gastrointestinal radiologists. All of these specialists have groups or associations which champion their causes, and it is not productive for gastroenterologists to pretend that they have control. The best we can do is to lead by providing an excellent example of training, clinical service, and research. It is a piquant point that some research-orientated departments of gastroenterology (in the USA) are now forced to embrace endoscopy since their income depends increasingly upon it.

Many gastroenterologists (certainly trainees) think of endoscopy in terms of individual procedures and patients, and are primarily concerned with indications, techniques and results. For many of us there is the wider and much more complex problem of managing endoscopy departments. When this book was conceived about 10 years ago there were few institutions with more than one procedure room, or more than one or two GI nurse/assistants. Now there are many centres with five or even ten endoscopy rooms, with dozens of endoscopists and a small army of supporting staff, including nurses, technicians and secretaries. Many will have radiographic staff, data analysts, messengers (porters) and cleaners. In earlier days our main interface outside the endoscopy room was with a few professional colleagues and the distributors of endoscopic equipment. Now we have to communicate effectively with many other specialists and service departments, and have complex logistic and financial problems. Equipment for a modern, multi-procedure area will be very costly, especially if radiographic equipment is included, and the annual turnover of a major American endoscopy centre may well exceed one million dollars. Few gastroenterologists are trained in management skills; some learn well, others do not. Within an individual unit, the head endoscopy nurse and the medical director usually form the administrative team, with appropriate technical and secretarial back-up. The importance of functional design and fully-trained staff have already been emphasized. We have also made reference to the importance of documentation, but this issue is much wider than the endoscopy report itself. In order to plan and evaluate, it is essential to have accurate records of the work load of the department, and how it is changing. Currently, 'medical audit' and 'quality assurance' are the words in regular use, which simply reflect the logic of knowing how well a job is being done. This demands attention to detail in the keeping of patient, administrative and financial records, and a commitment to excellence by all concerned in the organization. The complexity of these records demands computerization. The morale of a team depends almost entirely on its leaders, who can make the practice of endoscopy a joy—or a pain.

The use of endoscopes as research tools is still sadly neglected. Endoscopic ultrasound is moving from the experimental to the clinical phase, but there has been relatively little study of the gut wall, or its intricate secretions in health or disease. Now that more research-orientated departments of gastroenterology are building up their endoscopy divisions (both to be able to pay for their research activities and teach their fellows), we can hope for better future collaboration between the basic scientists and their clinical colleagues. This could also encourage more endoscopists to use scientific discipline in the evaluation of their own work.

And as for the future—who knows? By the time you read this, we should all be wiser.

Further reading

Schrock, T. R. (1987) 'Endoscopic surgery: healing the wound'. *Gastrointestinal Endoscopy*, 33, 345–347.

Index